EATING AGENDAS

SOCIAL PROBLEMS AND SOCIAL ISSUES

An Aldine de Gruyter Series of Texts and Monographs

SERIES EDITOR

Joel Best

Southern Illinois University at Carbondale

EATING AGENDAS

Food and Nutrition as Social Problems

Donna Maurer and Jeffery Sobal

EDITORS

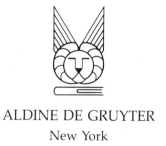

ALDINE DE GRUYTER
New York

About the Editors

Donna Maurer is a doctoral candidate, Department of Sociology, Southern Illinois University at Carbondale. Her research centers on the cultural aspects of the vegetarian movement, microlevel processes of dietary change, and food consumption and sharing as forms of communication.

Jeffery Sobal is an Associate Professor, Division of Nutritional Sciences, Cornell University, where he teaches undergraduate and graduate courses that apply social science perspectives to food, eating, and nutrition.

ALDINE DE GRUYTER
A division of Walter de Gruyter, Inc.
200 Saw Mill River Road
Hawthorne, New York 10532

This publication is printed on acid free paper ∞

Library of Congress Cataloging-in-Publication Data

Eating agendas : food and nutrition as social problems / Donna Maurer
    and Jeffery Sobal, editors.
        p.   cm. — (Social problems and social issues)
    Includes bibliographical references and index.
    ISBN 0-202-30507-4 (cloth : acid-free paper). — ISBN
0-202-30508-2 (paper : acid-free paper)
    1. Nutrition policy.   2. Food—Social aspects.   3. Nutrition—
Social aspects.   I. Maurer, Donna, 1961–   .   II. Sobal, Jeffery,
1950–   .   III. Series.
TX359.E38   1995
363.8—dc20   94–49387
                                                                                      CIP

Manufactured in the United States of America

10 9 8 7 6 5 4 3 2 1

Contents

Preface

People must eat to survive, which makes food an important commodity in everyone's life. Food, however, takes on far more than a biological reality. We may associate eating with great pleasure as well as with disease and death. When usual food, eating, and nutrition practices go awry, people may define them as social problems.

People's concerns about food often incorporate both cultural and structural elements. For example, cultural food practices possess symbolic meanings that people may use to express themselves and communicate, which suggests that some foods may be more culturally significant than others; these foods may be more prone to a problematic status. Structural patterns of food production, distribution, and consumption emerge as social institutions and food industries. When people designate food conditions as problematic, they may blame these social institutions and industries as sources of the problems.

Sociologists pay attention to food as a social problem when people go hungry (Sorokin 1922), but food and nutrition traditionally have been only a marginal sociological concern. Notable early exceptions include Thorstein Veblen's (1899) consideration of the significance of food as a status marker and George Simmel's (1910) examination of the sociology of a meal. More recently sociological research, teaching, and practice have given increased attention to food, eating, and nutrition in research, teaching, and practice (Mennell et al. 1992; Sobal 1992; Sobal et al. 1993; Whit 1994). Sociologists have addressed the gendered nature of food preparation and distribution (Charles and Kerr 1988; DeVault 1991) and the public's concerns about food safety (Beardsworth 1990; Hoban et al. 1992).

Until recently, the major public concern has been whether enough food is available. As food systems developed capacities to provide increasingly stable supplies of adequate food, people could focus more on food's qualitative aspects. Questions of quantity became replaced with concerns about ensuring the best possible food supply for health, leading to questions such as: Are pesticides and additives dangerous? What foods promote longevity? Does biotechnology create a healthier or more dangerous food supply?

People have many choices in contemporary industrialized food systems. They can choose to eat large quantities of a range of foods or restrict their diets to alter their body weight. Matters of taste and ethics also come into play, and people may choose to take on an ideological food identity such as "gourmet" or "vegetarian." When people have more choices and increasing opportunities to make their grievances known, they are also more likely to view the quality of their food as problematic.

Theoretical Approaches to Examining Food and Social Problems

Social problems analysis typically takes one of two major orientations: objectivist and constructionist (Holstein and Miller 1993). Objectivist analyses of food, eating, and nutrition problems are the most common, and fit within positivist social facts paradigms (Ritzer 1983). The number of constructionist analyses is increasing, however, in line with growing application of social definition paradigms in many disciplines (Ritzer 1983).

The Objectivist Orientation

An objectivist approach to social problems takes a positivistic stance, seeking to describe the reality of some social problem in the world (Spector and Kitsuse 1977). Objectivists assume that when specific negative conditions reach an intolerable point, they self-evidently become recognized as social problems. This type of analysis usually focuses on the prevalence, patterns, and severity of a particular problem. Objectivists see hunger, for example, as a condition where insufficient food exists to supply the physiological needs of some individuals. They define hunger as a social problem to the extent that hungry people exist.

An objectivist analyst of hunger may document epidemiological patterns of hunger, determine their causes, and propose solutions that may include engineering social institutions. Sociological examples of objectivist analysis include the comparison of competing reasons for people's use of meal programs (Sosin 1992) and the examination of soup kitchen participants (Rauschenbach et al. 1990). Nutrition scientists characteristically take an objectivist approach, generating descriptions of food and nutrition problems and developing interventions to minimize or eliminate such problems. For example, the entire rapidly expanding field of nutritional epidemiology is designed to understand the etiology, prevalence, and consequences of nutritional risks for the population (Margetts and Nelson 1991; Willett 1990).

The Constructionist Orientation

Most people would recognize the condition of massive hunger as a social problem. The difficulty is evaluating the point at which a particular condition should be addressed as problematic. There are always people without enough to eat, but how is this determined to be a problem at a local, national, or international level? Also, many food-related conditions are not so universally recognized as problems. For example, in the food "scare" about Alar in apples in 1989, some groups of people—particularly industry representatives—claimed that the concern about eating apples was completely unwarranted. Others, especially parents with small children, demanded that grocery stores indicate the potential dangers and many stopped eating apples altogether. Endless potentially problematic conditions exist, but only a limited number can come to the forefront of public attention (Hilgartner and Bosk 1988).

While an objectivist might designate certain categories of conditions as problems, a constructionist examines the processes by which people come to identify certain phenomena as problematic (Schneider 1985; Spector and Kitsuse 1977). Constructionists focus on process rather than "facts," viewing social problems as collective definitions. Consequently, constructionists set aside rigid social problems categories, and instead consider the *claims* that people make regarding these conditions. From a constructionist standpoint, a *social problem* has no independent ontological status; it is *dependent* on public definition. As social constructions, problems have life cycles that may or may not correspond with the objective prevalence or severity of the condition (Best 1989:139–140; Downs 1972).

Why is it useful to study social problems as processes as opposed to (or in addition to) the study of social problems as objective "facts"? Objectivist studies of social conditions tend to reify empirical data and position the sociologist as the moral arbiter of "good" and "bad." The study of social problems as a *process*, on the other hand, enables the development of a sociological theory of how issues become recognized as problematic and how this definitional process is associated with other structural and cultural conditions.

Varieties of Social Constructionism

While all constructionists recognize the negotiated, intersubjective nature of knowledge (including scientific knowledge) (Aronson 1982; Kitsuse and Cicourel 1963), they disagree on constructionism's direction and potential applications. Strict constructionists maintain that only the process itself should be described (Ibarra and Kitsuse 1993; Spector and Kitsuse 1977). Any recourse to "facts" results in "ontological gerrymandering," which grants privileged status to certain information that the sociologist regards as "true" (Woolgar and Pawluch 1985). Strict constructionists view the use of such facts as a return to objectivism—which they see as detracting from a "pure" social constructionist theory (Troyer 1992).

Although strict constructionists have called for research that makes no recourse to "facts" and therefore makes no claims of its own, such pure constructionism remains elusive. Some theorists argue that strict constructionism is vacuous because it can explain only the broadest generalities of social processes (Best 1993; Rafter 1992). In their recent prologue to a collection of constructionist research, strict constructionist advocates Sarbin and Kitsuse (1994:14) admit that "None of the chapters in this volume is an exemplar of strict constructionism. . . . It is questionable whether researchers can sustain any method that would be consistent with [its] requirements." Since any form of analysis requires leaving the claimsmakers' narratives, even the aspiring strict constructionist creates a set of sociological claims that can itself be analyzed sociologically.

A more moderate contextual constructionist stance maintains that claims need to be addressed in their cultural and structural contexts, even though it may require the use of some objectified "facts" (Best 1993). Contextual constructionists do not necessarily "debunk" popularly assumed objectivist explanations (a practice that incurs the strongest accusations of ontological gerrymandering). Instead, they suggest that a constructionist perspective enables the explanation of the rise and fall of a variety of social problems with reference to interest groups, government, science, the media, historical conditions, and cultural values. Contextual constructionism also permits the differentiation between sets of claims—as some sets may be more worthy of study than others. Strict constructionists have difficulty with this approach, as they view *all* claims as equally valid and sociologically interesting.

Jeffery Sobal
Donna Maurer

References

Aronson, N. 1982. "Nutrition as a Social Problem: A Case Study of the Entrepreneurial Strategy in Science." *Social Problems* 29:474–487.

Beardsworth, A. 1990. "Trans-science and Moral Panics: Understanding Food Scares." *British Food Journal* 92(5):11–16.

Best, J. (ed.). 1989. *Images of Issues: Typifying Contemporary Social Problems.* Hawthorne, NY: Aldine de Gruyter.

———. 1993. "But Seriously Folks: The Limitations of a Strict Constructionist Interpretation of Social Problems." Pp. 109–127 in *Constructionist Controversies: Issues in Social Problems Theory,* edited by G. Miller and J. A. Holstein. Hawthorne, NY: Aldine de Gruyter.

Charles, N., and M. Kerr. 1988. *Women, Food, and Families.* Manchester: University Press.

DeVault, M. 1991. *Feeding the Family: The Social Organization of Caring as Gendered Work.* Chicago: University of Chicago Press.

Downs, A. 1972. "Up and Down with Ecology: The Issue-Attention Cycle." *The Public Interest* 28:38–50.

Hoban, T. J., E. Woodrum, and R. Czaja. 1992. "Public Opposition to Genetic Engineering." *Rural Sociology* 57(4):476–493.

Holstein, J., and G. Miller (eds.). 1993. *Reconsidering Social Constructionism: Debates in Social Problems Theory.* Hawthorne, NY: Aldine de Gruyther.

Ibarra, P. R., and J. I. Kitsuse. 1993. "Vernacular Constituents of Moral Discourse: An Interactionist Proposal for the Study of Social Problems." Pp. 21–54 in *Constructionist Controversies: Issues in Social Problems Theory,* edited by G. Miller and J. A. Holstein. Hawthorne, NY: Aldine de Gruyter.

Kitsuse, J. I., and A. V. Cicourel. 1963. "A Note on the Uses of Official Statistics." *Social Problems* 11(2):131–139.

Margetts, B. M., and M. Nelson. 1991. *Design Concepts in Nutritional Epidemiology.* New York: Oxford Medical Publications.

Mennell, S., A. Murcott, and A. H. Van Otterloo. 1992. *The Sociology of Food and Eating.* Newbury Park, CA: Sage.

Rafter, N. 1992. "Some Consequences of Strict Constructionism." *Social Problems* 39(1):38–39.

Rauschenbach, B. S., E. A. Frongillo, Jr., F. E. Thompson, E. J. Andersen, and D. A. Spicer. 1990. "Dependency on Group Kitchens in Urban Areas of New York State." *American Journal of Public Health* 80:57–60.

Ritzer, G. 1983. *Contemporary Sociological Theory,* 2nd ed. New York: Alfred A. Knopf.

Sarbin, T. R., and J. I. Kitsuse (eds.). 1994. "A Prologue to *Constructing the Social.*" Pp. 1–18 in *Constructing the Social.* London: Sage.

Schneider, J. W. 1985. "Social Problems Theory: The Constructionist View." *Annual Review of Sociology* 11:209–229.

Simmel, G. 1910. "Soziologie der Mahlzeit." *Der Zeitgeist.* Supplement to *Berliner Tageblatt.* Translated by Michael Symons. Pp. 328–334 in *Eating into Thinking: Explorations in the Sociology of Cuisine.* Unpublished Ph.D. thesis, Flinders University of South Australia.

Sobal, J. 1992. "The Practice of Nutritional Sociology." *Sociological Practice Review* 3(1):23–31.

Sobal, J., W. A. McIntosh, and W. Whit. 1993. "Teaching the Sociology of Food and Nutrition." *Teaching Sociology* 21(1):50–59.

Sorokin, P. A. 1922, 1975. *Hunger as a Factor in Human Affairs*. Gainsville: University Press of Florida.

Sosin, M. R. 1992. "Homeless and Vulnerable Meal Program Users: A Comparison Study." *Social Problems* 39(2):170–188.

Spector, M., and J. I. Kitsuse. 1977. *Constructing Social Problems*. Menlo Park, CA: Cummings.

Troyer, R. 1992. "Some Consequences of Contextual Constructionism." *Social Problems* 39(1):35–37.

Veblen, T. 1899, 1953. *Theory of the Leisure Class*. New York: Mentor.

Whit, W. 1994. *Food and Society: A Sociological Approach*. Flint, MI: General Hall.

Willett, W. 1990. *Nutritional Epidemiology*. New York: Oxford University Press.

Woolgar, S., and D. Pawluch. 1985. "Ontological Gerrymandering: The Anatomy of Social Problems Explanations." *Social Problems* 32(3):214–237.

I

Introduction

1

Food, Eating, and Nutrition as Social Problems

JEFFERY SOBAL and DONNA MAURER

Different aspects of food, eating, and nutrition have attracted the attention of sociologists and other social scientists. Various food and nutrition issues can be constructed as social problems. Quantity of food is problematic in cases of hunger and famine, and excess food consumption is an issue in obesity and eating disorders. Quality of food is problematic because of biological qualities related to food safety and environmental impact, and because of social qualities related to the meanings of food. Major interest groups involved with food and nutrition problems include consumers, industry, government policy makers, program workers, the media, and scientists. Past social problems work on food and nutrition topics has dealt with some of these areas, and the chapters in this book expand this body of work.

The authors in this book all address food and nutrition issues from a social constructionist perspective. They use the perspective in different ways, however. Some use social constructionism to shed light on previously unexamined issues, while others attempt to make original contributions to constructionist theory. Some chapters address old topics in new ways, such as Karen Way's portrayal of anorexia nervosa as both a "normalized" and stigmatized condition that results in comparatively little attention paid to anorexia nervosa as a social issue. Other authors, such as Thomas J. Hoban, show how other sociological approaches (in this case, theories of risk perception) can be integrated with social constructionism to provide additional insight. Still others, such as Wm.

Alex McIntosh and David Miller and Jacquie Reilly, provide critiques of the social constructionist approach and consider potential drawbacks of its applications. In the following sections, we provide a general thematic overview of the chapters in this book.

Quantity of Food

The most fundamental problem is getting enough food, and the lack of adequate food has the potential to become an important social issue. Although there is a large and growing literature on hunger (which recently has been reframed as food insecurity [Dodds et al. 1992]), little attention has been given to how lack of food emerges as a social problem. Janet Poppendieck extends her earlier work (1986) and provides a historical portrait of how three major "discoveries" of hunger in the United States shaped definitions of hunger as a social problem by typifying hunger in different ways. Wm. Alex McIntosh considers how hunger is defined as a social problem from objectivist and constructionist perspectives, and suggests that a third perspective, derived from people's experiences of hunger, is also important in understanding hunger as a social problem.

Contemporary society offers more than ample food to most people, and many gain weight. Researchers in the past have addressed the problem of weight loss with both individual and collective explanations. For example, group dieting rituals serve to solve both the individual's excess weight as a manifest problem and the need for social support as a latent problem (Allon 1974, 1975) and entrepreneurs may capitalize on people's desires to lose weight by offering programs in organizational settings (Laslett and Warren 1975). The consumption of too much food comes under the responsibility of medical institutions as a problem in the process of medicalization (Conrad 1992; Conrad and Schneider 1992). Jeffery Sobal examines the medicalization of obesity, which as a deviant condition has shifted from being under moral social control as badness to medical social control as sickness and most recently under political social control as discrimination. Karen Way addresses the various claims about the severity and prevalence of eating disorders that claimsmakers use in constructing anorexia nervosa as a social problem.

Quality of Food

The potential risks of eating include severe negative consequences such as poisoning and infection, and problems in the safety of the food supply easily become regarded as social problems. Food scares may evolve into moral panics when they are amplified by the media and other social institutions (Beardsworth 1990). Ideological shifts in society may give rise to new food concerns and subsequent reactions of the food industry (Belasco 1993). For example, increasing concern about children is associated with the development and spread of folklore about poisoned Halloween food treats (Best 1990; Best and Horiuchi 1985). In this collection, Alan Beardsworth considers three types of food ambivalence and how people deal with them in contemporary culture. These food ambiguities underpin many current issues regarding food safety and ethics.

Another basic food issue relates to the meanings that people attach to various foods. Industrial organizations and other groups may attempt to utilize or manipulate the cultural meanings associated with particular foods, such as butter and coffee, to forward their particular agendas. For example, Ball and Lilly (1982) examine how interest groups supporting butter suppressed margarine production until the 1950s, when other interest groups reversed the situation and redefined margarine as a more desirable product. In a similar vein, Troyer and Markle (1984) address the continuing emergence of claims about coffee drinking as a social problem; while the deleterious effects of coffee may receive considerable press attention, people are unlikely to consider coffee as a social problem because of its innocuous connotation as a "moral" beverage. In this volume, Donna Maurer examines how claims-makers manipulate symbol systems in the vegetarian literature to construct meat as a social problem.

The Food Industry

In developed societies, the food industry manages the safety of food production and processing, with distrustful consumers often believing that industrial decisions are out of their control. Social problems analysis of food industry activities has focused on the controversy over the marketing of infant formula to new mothers, which led to an international boycott of Nestle products in the 1970s (Ermann and Clements 1984; Gerber 1991; Gerber and Short 1986). In this volume, Clifton Anderson discusses the emergence of an information war between consumers and the food industry, with both sides making claims about problems in the food system by strategically employing scientific information, and Thomas J. Hoban examines consumer distrust of industry's use of biotechnology, considering how people's risk perceptions operate to define and defuse claims about biotechnological issues.

Government Food Programs and Policies

Governments also deal with food and nutrition issues by offering social programs to citizens, often provoking a great deal of criticism. For example, DeVault and Pitts (1984) examine the emergence of the Food Stamp program, as hunger became defined as a national social issue in the 1960s in response to social movements and civil rights legislation. In this volume, Kim D. Travers discusses how professional nutritional science discourse structures how food program staff view program participants in Canada. Mark R. Rank and Thomas A. Hirschl examine the social forces that influence participation in the U. S. Food Stamp program, and the claims about food as a social problem generated by food stamp recipients, policy analysts, and the public.

Government plays a major role in the development and resolution of food and nutrition problems. In this volume, Unni Kjærnes describes how the Norwegian government proactively framed food and nutrition as social problems, first attracting public awareness and then gaining consensus and support for dealing with the food and nutrition problems they had defined. David Miller and Jacquie Reilly examine the government's slow response to food scares in the United Kingdom, which led to the emergence of the scares as social problems beyond the control of government efforts to contain public concern.

The scientific process itself can be addressed as a social problem. For example, Naomi Aronson (1982, 1984a, 1984b, 1989) examines the operation of nutrition research by conceptualizing science as a claimsmaking activity (Aronson 1982, 1984a, 1984b, 1989). Setting the agenda for later nutrition research, the first generation of nutrition scientists in the United States formed an alliance with the labor reform movement to define nutrition and worker productivity as a social problem to lobby for greater federal support of nutrition (Aronson 1982). In this volume David Smith addresses the development of scientific dietary guidelines in the United Kingdom as a political process involving nutritional scientists, the government, and the medical profession.

Conclusion

The chapters in this book suggest that many food and nutrition problems evoke public concern. The study of food, eating, and nutrition as social problems offers fertile ground for future social science research. At the same time, social problems analysis offers useful tools for people who practice in food and nutrition settings.

References

Allon, N. 1974. "Fat as a Dirty Word: Fat as a Sociological and Social Problem." Pp. 244–247 in *Recent Advances in Obesity Research*, edited by A. Howard. Westport, CT: Technomic Publishing Co.

———. 1975. "Latent Social Services in Group Dieting." *Social Problems* 23:59–69.

Aronson, N. 1982. "Nutrition as a Social Problem: A Case Study of the Entrepreneurial Strategy in Science." *Social Problems* 29:474–487.

———. 1984a. "Social Definitions of Entitlement: Food Needs 1880–1920." *Media, Culture and Society* 4:51–61.

———. 1984b. "Science as a Claims-making Activity: Implications for Social Problems Research." Pp. 1–30 in *Studies in the Sociology of Social Problems*, edited by J. W. Schneider and J. I. Kitsuse. Norwood, NJ: Ablex.

———. 1989. "Why Weren't Vitamins Discovered Earlier?" *Knowledge and Society* 8:87–105.

Ball, R. A., and L. R. Lilly. 1982. "The Menace of Margarine: The Rise and Fall of a Social Problem." *Social Problems* 29:488–498.

Beardsworth, A. 1990. "Trans-science and Moral Panics: Understanding Food Scares." *British Food Journal* 92(5)11–16.

Belasco, W. 1993. *Appetite for Change: How the Counterculture Took on the Food Industry*. Ithaca, NY: Cornell University Press.

Best, J. 1990. *Threatened Children*. Chicago: University of Chicago Press.

Best, J., and G. Horiuchi. 1985. "The Razor Blade in the Apple: The Social Construction of Urban Legends." *Social Problems* 32:488–499.

Conrad, P. 1992. "Medicalization and Social Control." *Annual Review of Sociology* 18:209–232.

Conrad, P., and J. W. Schneider. 1992. *Deviance and Medicalization: From Badness to Sickness*. Philadelphia: Temple University Press.

DeVault, M., and J. P. Pitts. 1984. "Surplus and Scarcity: Hunger and the Origins of the Food Stamp Program." *Social Problems* 31:545–557.

Dodds, J. M., S. L. Parker, and P. S. Haines. 1992. "Hunger in the 80's and 90's." *Journal of Nutrition Education* 24(1):1S–88S.

Ermann, M. D., and W. H. Clements. 1984. "The Interfaith Center on Corporate Responsibility and Its Campaign Against Marketing Infant Formula in the Third World." *Social Problems* 32(2):185–196.

Gerber, J. 1991. "From Bottles to Bombs." *Sociological Focus* 24:225–243.

Gerber, J., and J. F. Short, Jr. 1986. "Publicity and the Control of Corporate Behavior: The Case of Infant Formula." *Deviant Behavior* 7:195–216.

Hilgartner, S., and C. L. Bosk. 1988. "The Rise and Fall of Social Problems: A Public Arenas Model." *American Journal of Sociology* 94(1):53–78.

Laslett, B., and C. A. B. Warren. 1975. "Losing Weight: The Organizational Promotion of Behavior Change." *Social Problems* 23:69–80.

Poppendieck, J. 1986. *Breadlines Knee-deep in Wheat: Food Assistance in the Great Depression*. New Brunswick, NJ: Rutgers University Press.

Troyer, R., and G. E. Markle. 1984. "Coffee Drinking: An Emerging Social Problem." *Social Problems* 31:403–416.

II

Getting Sufficient Quantities of Food

2

Hunger in America: Typification and Response

JANET POPPENDIECK

As a social problem, hunger in America has demonstrated an unusual capacity to command public attention and concern. It has shown an ability to mobilize substantial resources of money, prestige, volunteer time, skilled advocacy, and public policy. Hundreds of thousands of Americans have contributed canned goods to food drives, walked in hunger walk-a-thons, served meals at soup kitchens, delivered meals on wheels, written letters to Congress, or otherwise tried to do something about the problem, and hunger has generated major public programs at the federal, state, and local levels. It has been on the public agenda, in one form or another, for most of the last 65 years. Attention to hunger, however, has not been a steady-state phenomenon. Instead, hunger has undergone periodic "discovery" and "rediscovery"—episodes of claims-making in which claimsmakers succeed in calling attention to the impact of poverty on diet and the unmet nutritional needs of the poor. In this century, hunger has undergone at least three such discoveries. In each, claimsmakers asserted that large numbers of Americans were going hungry and that such deprivation constituted a major moral outrage. The three episodes have differed, however, as to the central focus or content of the problem, the way in which hunger has been typified. This chapter will explore the relationship between the typification of hunger in America as a social problem and the societal response to the problem.

When claimsmakers typify a social problem, they are setting the stage for society's eventual responses to that problem. As Joel Best (1989:xxi) has written, "Claims-makers inevitably characterize problems in particular ways: They emphasize some aspects and not others; they promote specific orientations; and they focus on particular causes and advocate particular solutions." Even when they do not overtly advocate policies or responses, by emphasizing some aspects or images of the problem and ignoring others, they are helping to shape the content of eventual societal responses. This is not to say that all problems that are typified in claims will indeed generate programs and policies: the response is not automatic. But for those that survive the highly contingent selection process to reach what Blumer (1971:302) aptly characterized as "the end of the funnel," the seeds of societal response are planted in the typification or definitional phase.

This crucial role of the definitional phase in shaping eventual policy outcomes was recognized by sociologists and policy analysts long before the language of claims and claimsmakers came into frequent use.[1] What has been less well understood, perhaps, is the reverse proposition, that the available solutions shape the typification of the problem. A simple "life history" model that assumes problem definition, followed by debate, policy choice, and action (Fuller and Myers 1941) or even a more sophisticated model that allows for a new generation of problems derived from the implementation phase of public policy (Blumer 1971; Spector and Kitsuse 1987) fails adequately to represent the ongoing nature of the typification process. A conceptual loop, in which typification and solution are in constant interaction, seems more accurate.

Because of the multiple discoveries of the problem, hunger in the United States provides us with an unusual opportunity to test these assertions. Hunger has been subject to three different episodes of typification, which have led to societal response. The first occurred in the great depression of the 1930s, when hunger was typified by its contrast to agricultural surpluses as the "paradox of want amid plenty." The second took place in the late 1960s, with hunger typified as a failure of federal food assistance programs. And finally, hunger was discovered again in the 1980s, when it was typified as a need for "emergency food." These episodes are separate enough in time to permit substantially independent processes of claimsmaking and typification, but they are close enough together that comparisons of the policies and programs that have constituted society's responses are not spurious; society is not in a dramatically different stage of economic development or human consciousness. Thus hunger in America provides us with a sort of laboratory in which to study the impact of typification upon policy and the impact of policy upon typification. This chapter is confined to the problem of hunger within the United States, rather than U.S. response to global hunger, although the latter is also a phenomenon that has been subject to periodic rediscovery and retypification.

The First Discovery: The Great Depression

The first major discovery of hunger in America as a social problem occurred during the great depression of the 1930s. It was not, of course, the first time that large numbers of people had gone hungry. What was different was the obvious availability of food in huge quantities. When the stock market crash in the autumn of 1929 signaled the onset of the industrial depression, the agricultural sector of the economy had been in crisis for nearly a decade. The European market for American farm products had collapsed at the end of World War I, leaving many U. S. farmers heavily burdened with debt incurred at inflated wartime interest rates to finance expanded production. Faced with reduced demand, industrialists can usually cut costs by laying off workers and reducing production. Farmers, however, heavily mortgaged for capital invest- ment in land and equipment, responded to declining prices by increas- ing production. The result was a sickening spiral of falling prices, mounting surpluses, and farm loss to tax sale and mortgage foreclosure. By the time the full scale depression hit, huge, unmarketable surpluses had accumulated in most storable commodities, and the surplus had become the chief symbol of the farm crisis.

With enormous farm surpluses the primary item on the agricultural agenda and widespread destitution and want in both city and country- side, it is no wonder that the problem of hunger came to be typified by its contrast to the nation's agricultural abundance. "The paradox of want amid plenty" it was called, or "the paradox of scarcity and abundance," or, more colorfully, the "breadline knee-deep in wheat" (see Poppen- dieck 1986). The paradox was dramatized by the occasional instances in which food was intentionally destroyed: piles of California oranges soaked in kerosene to prevent their being eaten by nonpaying custom- ers, or milk poured out across the highways of Wisconsin and Iowa in the course of a farm strike. But even where there was not such dramatic destruction, there was overwhelming waste-crops plowed under or left to rot in the field, piles of grain abandoned at railroad sidings. Depres- sion era memoirs are full of recollections of what one historian has labeled "the plain man's instinctive resentment of poverty surrounded by shops bursting with food and farms smothered under their own productive surplus" (Wecter 1952:36).

The "solution" that flowed from this typification seemed obvious to many observers: use surplus crops to feed the needy. In keeping with the dominant relief ideology of the time, the first efforts to do so were local and voluntary in nature. Boy Scout troops, churches, and local charities collected donations of surplus foods, sometimes establishing elaborate canning operations to preserve fresh produce, and distributed the collected food to the unemployed. The accumulation of huge stores of food in government hands, however, soon moved the question out of the realm of economy in local relief and into the arena of public policy. During the Hoover years, the Federal Farm Board purchased millions of bushels of wheat and bales of cotton in a doomed attempt to stabilize the prices of those two commodities. The Farm Board's intervention may have slowed the price declines, but it did not reverse them, and as prices continued to fall, the Board was unable to justify selling its holdings as it had originally intended. The Farm Board's highly visible stocks of food and fiber grew and grew, leaving the U. S. government sitting on one of the largest commodity reserves in human history. The Farm Board Wheat became the focus of growing demands that the Hoover administration feed the hungry.

Both the Hoover administration and various agricultural interests within the Congress resisted these demands at first, claiming that "no one has starved," that voluntary giving could cope with the needs of the unemployed, and that release of the wheat would further soften grain prices. Eventually, however, the wheat itself became a problem; it was deteriorating, being destroyed, as one Senator put it, by "rats, mice, age, dampness and weevils" and consumed by storage and insurance charges (United States Congress, *Congressional Record* 1932:1191). The symbolism of wheat rotting while people begged for bread became too powerful to resist. On March 4, 1932, Farm Board wheat donated for distribution through the Red Cross became the first federal relief for the unemployed of the great depression. Once the ice was broken, the approach became popular with Congress, and several subsequent measures donated additional wheat and added cotton to the gift. Even Herbert Hoover was eventually converted, claiming credit for the wheat donations during his reelection campaign.

While the President and Congress delayed, however, the underlying typification of hunger had undergone a subtle but powerful transition, linked directly to the availability of the means of solution, the Farm Board Wheat. Over the course of the 15 months that Congress considered a series of wheat distribution resolutions, the wheat had been transformed from a convenient and cheap means to solve the problem of want amid plenty to a morally indefensible waste in the midst of want. Instead of hunger as a problem made intolerable by the ready availability of food to solve it, waste had become a problem made intolerable by the context of hunger. Thus the "problem" would be "solved" if the surplus, the food in jeopardy of being wasted, was applied to the needs of the hungry. This was the solution embodied on a temporary basis in the Farm Board wheat donations, and it was the solution soon to be institutionalized in the New Deal.

The election of Franklin D. Roosevelt brought into office an activist administration committed to bold action to cope with the depression, but 6 months of the New Deal would elapse before the Roosevelt administration would yield to the typification of the hunger problem as the "paradox of want amid plenty." Federal direct relief for the unemployed was enacted quickly in the special session of Congress called to deal with the banking crisis that had come to a head the day before Roosevelt's inauguration, but relief for agriculture was more controversial and more difficult to craft. By the time Congress passed the Agricultural Adjustment Act in May 1933, a new crop was already in the making. The newly created Agricultural Adjustment Agency responded with dramatic action. In June the Secretary of Agriculture offered Southern farmers a cash bonus to plow under a quarter of the standing cotton crop as a means to raise prices by reducing output, and in September, he offered a similar bonus to corn/hog farmers who sent unfinished (small) pigs or piggy (pregnant) sows to slaughter. Farmers in the drought-stricken midwest were short of feed to finish their pigs; they turned the slaughter into a stampede, sending six million baby pigs to market for the account of the Secretary of Agriculture.

The pig slaughter became, for the New Deal, what the Farm Board Wheat had been for the Hoover administration: a public relations disaster that concentrated huge stocks of food in the hands of the United States government while hungry citizens did without. The pig episode was more sudden that the inexorable accumulation of wheat, and it was accompanied by a host of newsworthy sidelights that made it a field day for hostile press. Pigs escaped from stockyard pens built to contain full grown hogs and ran squealing down the streets of Omaha and Chicago, eliciting considerable public sympathy for the piglets, and huge quantities of the pigs, too small for normal processing into meat, were turned into a foul smelling inedible product called "tankage" that clogged gravel pits and rivers throughout the midwest.

The loudest public outcry engendered by the pig project, however, was neither the humane society nor the environmental approach. It was the "wickedness," a word frequently used in letters to the President or the Agricultural Adjustment Administration about the episode, of destroying food while so many people were scraping by on meager relief budgets. "Why, oh why destroy what is so good to eat?" lamented one typical letter, adding that the writer's family had "not had a pork chop or any part of a hog in . . . years" (Biddle 1933). Senator Atlee Pomerene summed it up cogently: "when men, women, and children are hungry, I say that no defense can be made either in law, morals or religion for throwing wholesome meat into a fertilizer vat. I tell you there are some things that are just too much" (Lawrence 1933).

Eventually the criticism was just too much for the Roosevelt administration as well, and on September 21, 1933, a few days after the media outcry over the pigs reached its peak, the White House announced a plan to spend $75 million to procure surplus agricultural products to feed and clothe the unemployed over the coming winter. The President, according to the press release, "considered such action as one of the most direct blows at the economic paradox which has choked farms with an abundance of farm products while many of the unemployed have grown hungry" (Roosevelt 1972:280). Nine days later the President announced a much broader and more permanent surplus procurement and distribution plan, and directed the Federal Emergency Relief Administrator, Harry Hopkins, to establish a nonprofit corporation to manage the program.

The Roosevelt administration, of course, did not link its surplus commodity program to the Farm Board wheat distributions, and indeed the new project was quite different. It would use public agencies, not the Red Cross, to distribute the surplus products. It created an ongoing program rather than a series of single-shot donations, and it would have its own alphabet agency, the Federal Surplus Relief Corporation (FSRC). It would purchase a wide variety of farm products: "We will give them . . . everything necessary for healthful living" promised Hopkins, the President of the FSRC, in an early press conference (*New York Times* 1933b). In the public mind, however, the new program was related to the old and to the underlying paradox that had been the focus of so much attention during the farm board wheat disputes. "In this plan," commented the *Literary Digest*, "is seen a means to end the most tragic and ironic phase of the depression—breadlines knee deep in wheat'" (1933:8). The *New York Times* (1933a) editorial welcoming the announcement of the surplus distribution plan was particularly telling. The new plan would not only relieve the farmer and the unemployed worker, the *Times* declared; it would also "relieve our minds of the distressing 'economic paradox' of unprofitable surpluses existing side by side with extreme want." Noting that the precedent had been set by the Farm Board wheat and cotton distributions, the editor went on to assert that "even if there were not such precedents, the pressing paradox would suggest, if not compel, some such provision."

In short, the typification of the problem as waste amid want engendered a solution: programs to purchase farm surpluses and distribute them to the hungry. This solution was so obvious—"the pressing paradox would suggest, if not compel, some such provision"—that few questioned its wisdom; the critical voices that were raised were drowned out by the general applause for the surplus purchase and distribution plan.[2] In the long run, however, tying food assistance programs to farm surpluses severely limited their capacity to meet the needs of hungry people. When drought, pests, or other unfavorable growing conditions limited the accumulation of surpluses or war or other market opportunities drained them away, poor people did without. Even when surpluses were extensive, they frequently did not occur in the foods that poor people needed most. And tying food assistance to farm income support brought it within both the political and administrative hegemony of American agribusiness; the project that began under the auspices of the New Deal Relief Administration ended up as a division within the marketing arm of the Department of Agriculture (USDA), funded primarily by a permanent appropriation of customs receipts designated to assist farmers as a sort of recompense for the damage done to agriculture over the years by the tariff. The food assistance legacy of the Great Depression was a set of programs dependent upon surplus production, funded from an appropriation regarded by Congress as "farmers' money," administered by a bureaucracy dedicated to promoting the well being of the commercial farmer, and supervised in Congress by Agricultural committees similarly dedicated and notoriously hostile to urban welfare programs.

Between Discoveries

Hunger virtually disappeared from the American agenda during World War II, when shortages replaced surpluses as the primary concern of the agricultural establishment. With the surpluses went most of the federal food assistance for the poor. An innovative Food Stamp Program, created in the later years of the New Deal to direct the farmer's surpluses to the hungry through the "normal channels of trade" (grocery stores), was terminated altogether. Similarly, when the end of the WPA deprived states of the federally subsidized labor that had handled the actual work of distributing surplus foods, both the control and the costs of intrastate distribution were shifted to the county level. Since the volume of surpluses available for distribution was minimal, many of the nation's poorest counties declined to absorb the expense and dropped out of the program.

In the postwar era, hunger at home was completely overshadowed by famine in Europe and Asia, and the USDA, strongly identified with the interests of large scale commercial farmers, resisted attempts by several concerned members of Congress to reestablish the Food Stamp Program. John Kennedy, however, impressed by the suffering he had seen in Appalachia while campaigning in West Virginia, used his first Executive Order to double the number of commodities available through the surplus commodity program and created a pilot Food Stamp Program during his first month in office. Kennedy's actions received little attention, however, and neither the public nor any organized pressure group picked up hunger as a rallying cry. When the Food Stamp Program was moved from pilot to permanent status in 1964, it was characterized as an effort to expand the domestic market for the products of U. S. Agriculture. Even when Michael Harrington's *The Other America* (1962) made poverty a public concern in the early 1960s, many people continued to contrast America's supposedly well fed poor with the starving millions abroad. As George McGovern (1969) put it at the end of the 1960s:

> Hunger is a unique issue in contemporary American politics in that it has only been "discovered" in the late 1960's. Until recently, most Americans assumed that hunger and malnutrition are the afflictions of Asia and other faraway places. How could anyone really be hungry in the world's richest nation—a nation endowed with an agricultural productivity so vast that it has accumulated troublesome surpluses?

The Second Discovery: The 1960s

When events finally did conspire to place domestic hunger on the American agenda once again, the complacency that had marked American beliefs about the diet of the poor—the widespread assumption that the nation's agricultural abundance had automatically trickled down—contributed to the powerful sense of shock and outrage that characterized the public response. Ironically, it was in part a changeover from the surplus commodities program to the food stamp program that provoked the second discovery of hunger. In April 1967, the Senate Subcommittee on Employment, Manpower, and Poverty went to the Mississippi Delta to hold hearings on the Johnson administration's War on Poverty. The situation in the Delta was acute. The mechanization of cotton farming, accelerated in part by a new minimum wage for farm laborers, had combined with a huge cutback in cotton acreage under the federal cotton subsidy program to eliminate the jobs on which many black Delta families—sharecroppers and agricultural wage laborers—had once eked out a marginal living. As county after county in the Delta switched from the surplus commodity program, in which poor people were given free food, to the food stamp program in which participants had to purchase their stamps, desperate Delta families saw even the meager lifeline provided by federal food assistance slip away. When civil rights attorney Marian Wright persuaded Senators Joseph Clark of Pennsylvania and Robert Kennedy of New York to leave the hearing room and accompany her on a tour of Delta homes, they encountered poverty and hunger in their starkest forms.

In the Spring of 1967, nearly anything that Robert Kennedy did was newsworthy, and Kennedy and Clark's discovery of hunger in Mississippi brought the issue briefly into the national limelight. It might have disappeared again, however, as quickly as it had come, had not skilled claimsmakers in a New York-based foundation and a Washington-based citizens organization acted, independently, to keep the issue alive. The Field Foundation responded almost immediately to the press coverage of hunger by sending a team of medical doctors to Mississippi to examine the health and nutritional status of children there, using the credibility of physicians to counter the disbelief with which some Americans had greeted Robert Kennedy's claims of severe poverty-related malnutrition. The Citizen's Crusade Against Poverty, an advocacy group organized to support the war on poverty and chaired by United Auto Workers President Walter Reuther, had already begun looking into Marian Wright's charges of near starvation in the Mississippi Delta when Kennedy made his field trip. The Citizen's Crusade quickly formed a "Citizens' Board of Inquiry into Hunger and Malnutrition in the United States," composed of well respected figures from law, medicine, the academic world, foundations, organized labor, religious organizations, and other social action groups to undertake an examination of government food assistance programs. The Board's report, *Hunger U.S.A.* (1968), was released the following April, just a year after Kennedy's visit to the Delta. It was followed in rapid succession by *Their Daily Bread*, a critique of the National School Lunch Program conducted by a coalition of women's organizations, sit ins at the Department of Agriculture by a contingent of the Poor People's March on Washington, and a major CBS documentary entitled "Hunger in America." In July 1968, the Senate of the United States voted unanimously to create a Senate Select Committee on Nutrition and Human Needs. Hunger had become a public issue (see U. S. Senate 1968 for a chronology).

The dramatic story of the late 1960s rediscovery of hunger has been recounted, ably and in great detail, by journalist Nick Kotz (1969, *passim*). For our purposes, what is important is the typification of hunger that captured public attention and the solutions that proceeded from it. The typification process was not instantaneous. Both the Senate Subcommittee and the Field Foundation medical team returned from Mississippi expressing outrage that people were suffering such privation in the midst of the "richest nation on earth" and calling for immediate government action—emergency assistance—to relieve the situation. It was when the government proved unable to respond quickly, when even the sympathetic Secretary of Agriculture, Orville Freeman, repeatedly reported that his hands were tied by legal, bureaucratic, and political constraints, that the new typification of hunger emerged.

Claimsmakers schooled in the civil rights movement characterized hunger as a failure of government to meet its obligations to citizens, a denial of rights. Hunger became synonymous with the failure of food assistance programs.

There were four major elements in the descriptive critique of food assistance that constituted the primary content of the late 1960s hunger claims. First, the various studies claimed that food assistance programs were failing to reach a majority of the poor; only 18% of the poor were participating in either the Commodity Distribution program or the Food Stamp Program, the federal government's two main family food programs. In many counties, neither program was available, and while food stamps offered greater benefits and convenience to participants, they were too expensive for the poorest Americans, like those Kennedy had discovered in the Delta, to purchase. Second, the programs did not provide sufficient assistance to those whom they did reach to permit them to obtain a nutritionally adequate diet: the food stamp allotments, based on ability to pay rather than nutritional need, were too small, and the commodity bundle, shaped by available surpluses, was never intended to supply a complete diet. Third, those who were helped were often required to pay an excessive price in terms of stigma, humiliation, and inconvenience, especially in places where local officials were hostile to the program. And fourth, the programs did not treat people equally; that is, they did not treat people in similar circumstances the same. Eligibility criteria, the most basic definition of rights under law, varied from locality to locality; in one Indiana township, for example, no family with a dog was permitted to receive surplus commodities (Kotz 1969:46).

When citizens' commissions and members of Congress looked behind these descriptions for explanations, they found, in essence, the legacy of the earlier typification of hunger as waste amid want. They found the link to agricultural surplus disposal that was forged in the Great Depression, the domination by agricultural producers and their representatives in Congress and the Department of Agriculture (USDA) that was the product of New Deal politics, and the local control that was the consequence of the shift of costs to the states and counties in the midst of World War II.

This time, however, claimsmakers were both more organized and more skillful. Informed by and grounded in the civil rights movement of the early and mid 1960s, these reformers knew how to use the power of the courts and were at home with the legislative process. Indeed the primary remedies they foresaw—judicial relief, legislation, and rule-making—helped to shape their characterization of hunger as the failure of government to ensure citizens' rights to food itself and to due process and equal treatment in food programs. With remarkable rapidity, a network of organizations at the local, state, and national levels emerged to wage war on hunger. Known as the "antihunger network" or the "hunger lobby" (Berry 1982), they used an entitlements strategy as the central thrust of their work. Since hunger was typified as an outcome of the failure of government to ensure the citizen's rights to food, the solution was to make such rights legally binding and enforceable in court.

The major tactics that the antihunger advocates used to pursue their goal were research, education, legislation, litigation, and organization. (See Poppendieck, 1985 for a more detailed account of the activities and achievements of the hunger lobby.) The most obvious first step was to make the program available to all poor Americans, regardless of the county in which they lived. Starting with those counties that offered neither Food Stamps nor Surplus Commodities, the Food Research and Action Center, the primary litigation arm of the antihunger network, undertook to sue every county in the nation into offering one of the family food programs. By the end of 1970, the number of counties with no family food assistance program had dropped from 480 to 10. A major step toward the creation of a true entitlement was achieved in the Food Stamp Program by a 1971 law establishing national income and assets eligibility standards, limiting purchase price to 30% of applicants in-comes, requiring states to undertake outreach to notify eligible house-holds of the availability of benefits, and creating a "fair hearing" procedure through which applicants who were denied benefits could contest the decisions of certification workers.

Antihunger advocates worked on issues of adequacy simultaneously with their efforts to guarantee access. In the Commodity program, this was simple enough; the Johnson administration raised the number of commodities by administrative decree when hunger began getting press attention in the late 1960s, although many counties still were unable or unwilling to handle some of the available items. The issue of nutritional adequacy in Food Stamps, however, posed a major challenge. The primary victories were two, one legislative and the other judicial. In 1971, Congress amended the 1964 Food Stamp Act to raise allotments to the level of the USDA's Economy Food Plan. The amended law required that allotments be established so as to "enable recipients to obtain a low cost nutritionally adequate diet," in contrast to the 1964 Act, which had provided that allotments should permit recipients to "more nearly obtain" such a diet. In *Rodway vs U.S. Department of Agriculture* (1975:809, 820), a Federal Court later ruled that the change in wording constituted "a shift from supplementing . . . to *guaranteeing* those households an opportunity for an adequate diet." The Rodway decision became the basis for a series of challenges to the adequacy of the Economy Food Plan, leading eventually to the development of the Thrifty Food Plan upon which allotments are now based. (See Claffey and Stucker 1982:40–46 for further discussion of the steps in reforming Food Stamps.)

As Food Stamp benefits were raised, and prices were lowered, the advantages of the food stamp approach became clearer, and advocates began to put pressure on Surplus Commodity counties to switch to Stamps. A major step toward entitlement status was achieved in 1973 when Congress decreed that the Department of Agriculture must offer the Food Stamp program in every county in the nation, running it directly if the county government declined to do so. The culmination of the drive to create a justiciable right to food came during the Carter years when a number of antihunger activists became USDA insiders. The purchase requirement that had continued to make participation in the Food Stamp Program unaffordable or unattractive to many potential beneficiaries was eliminated. Anticipating that the free stamps would attract many more recipients, budget conscious elements within Congress and the administration crafted a new package that made the stamps free but significantly reduced the gross income eligibility thresholds, strictly limited the deductions that households could claim, and established an overall spending cap for the program.

In a decade, then, Food Stamps were transformed from a struggling pilot program, available only at the discretion of county governments, offering stamps only to those who could scrape together enough cash to purchase them, and providing a standard of assistance based on ability to pay rather than nutritional deficit, to a major national entitlement program, available without charge to recipients in every county in the United States, with standardized eligibility levels and graduated, nutrition-based benefits; the Food Stamp Program had become the closest thing that we have in the United States to a guaranteed annual income, a floor under consumption. Federal expenditure for food assistance grew more than 500% in real terms from the late 1960s to the early 1980s, and participation in the basic family food assistance category (food stamps and surplus commodities) more than quadrupled (Chelf 1992:43).

Food Stamps were not the only federal food program that underwent major reform and expansion during the decade following the rediscovery of hunger. Similar changes occurred in the school breakfast and lunch programs and senior meals programs and the popular WIC (Women's Infants and Children's) Program was created and expanded. As the end of the decade neared, some advocates were ready to claim victory in the war against hunger in the United States. The Field Foundation sent another team of physicians to assess the health and nutritional status of Americans in impoverished areas, and they reported (Field Foundation 1977) that while poverty persisted, hunger was nearly eradicated. Government food consumption data and program evaluations reached similar conclusions. There were dissenting voices, but the dominant mood of the hunger discourse was recalled a few years later in a brief history prepared by the Food Research and Action Center:

> it was clear that the food assistance efforts developed in response to the discovery of hunger in the late 1960's worked. Those programs never ended the problems entirely, but by 1977–78, there was evidence that we were well on the way to eliminating hunger and malnutrition as serious problems in America . . . . It was evidence of a remarkable . . . success story. It is rare in public annals to progress in just a decade from identifying a problem (1967), to putting a response in place, to having evidence that the response works and is eliminating the problem (1977). (Food Research and Action Center 1984:21, 22, 24)

The Third Discovery: The 1980s

The hunger lobby had hardly concluded its victory celebrations when growing discontent with inflation and taxation signaled the beginning of a whole new contest. By the time the Field Foundation doctors reported their findings, as political scientist Carl Chelf (1992:43) has summarized,

> a backlash against Great Society programs, including the food programs, had set in. The programs came in for heavy criticism for spending too much, creating welfare dependency, wasting taxpayers' funds and being corrupt and inefficient. The consensus that had earlier supported these programs disappeared, paving the way for Ronald Reagan and his leadership of a conservative assault on social spending programs, including food aid programs.

The new president lost little time in launching his crusade for reduction of domestic social spending, asking Congress for major cuts in virtually every program designed to aid poor people. In 1981 Congress cut $2 billion from Food Stamps and $1.4 billion from the array of child nutrition programs. Although hunger activists marshaled their forces and forestalled many additional proposed cuts, the Congressional Budget Office estimated that the cuts approved by Congress for fiscal years 1982–1985 would reduce real benefits, adjusted for inflation and unemployment, by $7 billion in the Food Stamp Program, and $5.3 billion for child nutrition. Such food assistance cuts were made more difficult to absorb by parallel cuts in other programs of assistance for the poor: $4.8 billion in the Aid to Families with Dependent Children Program (AFDC), $2.2 billion in housing assistance, over the same period (Kotz 1984:20).

The Reagan-inspired domestic spending cuts occurred in the context of a deep and extended recession, and hunger claimsmakers responded quickly with renewed claims of hunger in America.[3] In the fall of 1982, the U.S. Conference of Mayors reported the results of a national survey of cities and towns, calling hunger "a most serious emergency" (United States Conference of Mayors 1982). Mayors of several large cities called upon the federal government to supply emergency relief, just as it would in a flood or other natural disaster. The mayors' first hunger report was followed by several more extensive studies and a spate of surveys conducted by religious organizations, by advocacy groups, and by the federal government's General Accounting Office. Between the fall of 1982 and the fall of 1984, 15 studies that were *national* in scope were released, along with numerous local and state studies (Physicians Task Force 1985:11–24). The Food Research and Action Center maintains an extensive collection of nearly 250 of these documents released since the early 1970s. The index to this collection suggests the escalation of hunger claimsmaking in the early 1980s: it contains three studies for 1981, 19 in 1982, 31 in 1983, 40 in 1984, and approximately 30 in each of the next three years (Nestle and Guttmacher 1992:19s). Some of these studies reported increases in clinical indicators of compromised nutrition, but the majority relied upon a new index of hunger: requests for assistance from emergency food programs, either soup kitchens or food pantries.

As the studies piled up, a clearer picture of hunger in the 1980s emerged (see, for example, Clancy and Bowering 1992; Kelly et al. 1989). Although the advocates schooled in the hunger contests of the 1960s and 1970s were fond of pointing to the cuts in food assistance benefits as a primary cause, several other factors also played a prominent role in the findings of various commissions and surveys. One was the economy—the combination of unemployment and a shift to lower wage jobs that produced the phenomenon generally called the "new poor": former members of the middle class or comfortable working class whose industrial jobs appeared to be gone forever and who were subsisting on poorly paid service sector work, often part time and without benefits. Some of the first soup kitchens and food pantries to garner national attention were established by labor unions in the "empty smokestack" regions of the country, and studies of food pantry clients frequently identified once comfortable families turning to charitable food programs because all of their income was going to an attempt to hold onto their homes. The recession of the early 1980s accelerated the job loss, but the underlying trends are long term and global in scope.

A second factor contributing to the accelerating use of soup kitchens and food pantries was the erosion of the value of public assistance benefits over the decade of the 1970s. In real terms, AFDC benefits declined in value by approximately one-third between the end of the 1960s and the early 1980s (Kotz 1984:23). By 1984, a House Ways and Means Committee study identified 18 states in which the combined value of food stamps and public assistance equaled two thirds of the poverty threshold or less (Lelyveld 1985:52). Meanwhile, shelter costs rose sharply for almost all Americans in the aftermath of the oil crisis of the early 1970s, forcing many welfare families into a "heat or eat" dilemma. Food stamp benefits are calculated upon the assumption that participating households can allocate a third of their disposable income to food; the stamps are designed to fill the gap between such household food purchases and a minimally adequate diet. As shelter costs rose, however, households began allocating ever larger shares of income to rent and fuel, sharply reducing the amounts available for food. Food pantries across the nation reported that the volume of requests went up sharply in the third and fourth weeks of the food stamp month; the stamps had run out, and the expected household cash allocation for food had gone to the landlord (Cohen and Burt 1989:20).

For some individuals and families, of course, these same factors contributed to the loss of shelter, and homelessness became a prominent factor in the hunger claims arena. The proliferation of soup kitchens and other facilities offering prepared meals was primarily a response to the appearance of large numbers of destitute homeless persons on the streets of cities and towns.

Finally, in an episode remarkably reminiscent of the hunger discovery of the Great Depression, the federal government contributed to the reemergence of the hunger issue by releasing large quantities of surplus agricultural commodities acquired in price support operations for distribution to the poor. The infamous cheese giveaway of the early 1980s (the SDDP or Special Dairy Distribution Program), prompted in part by citizen outrage over the discovery of government owned cheese rotting in warehouses and underground storage caves, led quickly to the development of the Temporary Emergency Food Assistance Program (TEFAP), which allocated a variety of commodities to the states for distribution through voluntary agencies. The cheese supplies lured numerous churches and community centers into the food distribution project, and then lines of people waiting for their share of the nation's dairy surplus attracted the attention of the media and dramatized hunger (Lipsky and Thibodeau 1988:226).

The 1980s typification of hunger was different from either the 1930s paradox definition or the 1960s rights definition. The term that dominated the discourse was "emergency." The soup kitchens and food pantries that proliferated were called "emergency food providers," and local officials, as we have noted, called for emergency assistance from the federal government, which responded with TEFAP.

Several factors appear to have contributed to the use and rapid diffusion of the emergency designation. First, the visibility of homelessness and the prevalence of homeless people among the clientele of soup kitchens prompted an association with "emergency shelter," a term already widely used to distinguish temporary shelters, for which certain categories of federal funds could be used, from more permanent housing arrangements for the homeless. Second, the intent of government and the expectations of many local providers were that the "hunger crisis" would be short-lived and that their responses would be temporary. As Lipsky and Smith (1989:6) pointed out, government officials reacted to growing demand for supplementary food and shelter in the 1980s by accepting the claims of need but defining the need as temporary, an approach that was "facilitated by labeling the needs 'emergencies'." Third, the term "food emergency" was widely used to designate the situation in which a household ran out of food; thus an emergency food provider was someplace to turn in a food emergency. Fourth, the lines of people waiting for cheese and the large congregate feeding sites established by some providers were reminiscent of scenes of disaster relief and reinforced the analogy with natural disasters employed by several of the nation's mayors. And finally, the term was useful to claims-makers who were trying to create a sense of crisis or event that might attract media coverage and provoke action. In any case, the term stuck and began showing up in the titles of reports and public laws and the headlines of newspapers; by 1983, it was in common use.

The emergency typification of hunger has several implications that bear examination here. The analogy with floods and hurricanes seems to suggest the working of unfathomable and uncontrollable forces, as if the deterioration of the economy and the erosion of public assistance were "acts of God" or a massive national case of bad luck. And the hungry, portrayed as the hapless victims of such forces, are profoundly depoliticized. Emergency food providers are overwhelmingly local, voluntary groups that raise major portions of their funds from local donors. The images of hungry people they use to obtain contributions of money and donations of food are the images of dejected poor people waiting patiently in lines. They are a far cry from the hungry poor people of the late 1960s who marched on Washington and sat in at the Department of Agriculture, and they look more like objects of compassion than potential allies.

It is not surprising that the rapid growth of the emergency food system was the primary response to this definition of the problem. Kitchens and pantries grew rapidly in number and capacity. In New York City, for example, the number of emergency food providers rose from approximately 30 before 1980 to 479 by mid decade (Food and Hunger Hotline 1987); the current figure is in excess of 750 (Food for Survival 1993). The growth of emergency feeding operations in New York may be more pronounced than in many other locations, but the trend is clearly nationwide. A recent survey of programs served by a major national food distribution network found that 71% of the 30,000 kitchens and pantries in the network had been established since 1981 (VanAmburg 1994:37).

The kitchens and pantries needed steady supplies of food, and they provided a ready outlet for food salvaged from the general food system. Food banks and food rescue programs were created to procure donations of food, generally edible but unsalable, from manufacturers, wholesalers, retailers, and restaurants and caterers and distribute them to front line providers. Although several food banks date back to the late 1970s, the rapid expansion of food banking in the 1980s is a major part of the emergency food phenomenon. By the early 1990s, Second Harvest, the national food bank network, claimed more than 180 member banks. Once a bank is established in an area, of course, creation of front line emergency food programs becomes easier, both because the banks provide access to a relatively steady supply of food and because they provide advice and know-how.

In the 1980s discovery of hunger an orderly process of problem identification followed by solution is especially difficult to discern. The dominant solution—"emergency food"—was clearly part of the typification process in at least three major ways. First, as noted above, the language of food emergencies and emergency food providers helped to shape the perception of the problem. Second, the fundraising needs and constraints of the providers shaped the images of hungry people that were picked up and communicated by the media. And third, since the measurement of hunger has always been problematic, the growth of emergency food, both the numbers of providers and the numbers of people seeking their help, quickly became a leading index of hunger. Both mayors and advocacy groups made frequent use of statistics on the growing number of meals served or bags of groceries distributed to point with alarm to a growing epidemic.

Despite the expectations of many providers that their emergency food projects would be short lived, and the predictions of numerous observers that a phenomenon so heavily dependent upon voluntary contributions of time and resources would "burn out" in a few seasons, the emergency food network has continued to grow and to develop and reinforce its institutional supports. If the value of food donations is calculated, Second Harvest is the third largest recipient of charitable contributions in the United States, receiving more than the American Cancer Society or the American Red Cross, a remarkable record for an organization that is only 15 years old (Bread for the World Institute 1993:12). Canned goods drives have become a regular feature of the nation's landscape, with the letter carriers collecting in many communities in the spring and the Boy Scouts in the fall. Both churches and schools make efforts to involve youngsters in the emergency feeding project as a way of teaching compassion—or gratitude—and holiday drives allow shoppers to contribute through their charge cards or at their grocery check out counters. Emergency food has become firmly established in the culture as the dominant response to hunger, even though many emergency food recipients, studies repeatedly show, receive far more assistance from food stamps and other public, nonemergency programs. The 1960s response to hunger persists, both in the continued growth of public food assistance programs and in the ongoing efforts of organized advocacy groups, but it is the emergency food phenomenon that has captured public attention.

Any attempt to explain this national fascination with soup kitchens and food pantries is necessarily speculative, but several factors appear as likely candidates. First, emergency food programs are mediagenic and lend themselves to the needs of the media, especially at Thanksgiving and Christmas. Second, these programs are voluntary, and heavily dependent upon volunteers, in an era of voluntarism; in that sense they are in synch with the spirit of the thousand points of light approach. They sometimes make enormous demands upon the dedicated volunteers that supply and staff them, but they require relatively little in terms of tax dollars. Third, the growth of food banking, which transfers edible but unsalable food to the emergency food network via corporate donations, links the emergency food phenomenon firmly with the prevention of waste, a popular cause in a era of environmental awareness. Fourth, the proliferation of canned goods drives, check out against hunger coupons at the supermarket, hunger walk-a-thons, and the like permit many people to participate in small, convenient ways; people feel part of this "solution." One recent poll of registered voters found that 79% claimed to have done something, personally, to contribute to the fight against hunger (Breglio 1992). And finally, participation in emergency feeding programs can be very gratifying, offering people opportunities to comply with the dictates of their religion and the prompting of their conscience without major expense or inconvenience.

Conclusion

The three typifications of hunger and the policies and programs with which American society has responded to each demonstrate the power of typification to shape social action. In the 1930s, the paradox definition, the juxtaposition of hunger with surplus agricultural production, led to programs in both the Hoover and Roosevelt administrations that procured farm surpluses and distributed them to people in need. When the surpluses evaporated, the programs dwindled, leaving poor people with little in the way of food assistance. In the 1960s, the typification of hunger as a failure of government to ensure due process, equal access, and basic survival led to a major reform and expansion of public food assistance and the creation of a legally enforceable entitlement. In the 1980s, the typification of hunger as an "emergency" led to the proliferation of emergency food programs and their institutionalization in an extensive food banking system. Although there are similarities, especially between the 1930s and the 1980s, the marked differences among these typifications and responses lend force to the claim that the definitional phase is the crucial one in shaping a problem's life history.

The relationship between typification and response, however, is neither simple nor consecutive. The three twentieth-century discoveries of hunger in America demonstrate the interactive nature of typification and remedy and suggest some general principles that my apply to this interaction.

1. Awareness of the possibility of "solution" is a precondition for the perception of a problem. This is not a new suggestion. As Spector and Kitsuse (1987:84) note:

> Many writers on social problems have said that the belief that something could be done about a condition is a prerequisite to its becoming a social problem. People do not define as problems those conditions they feel are immutable, inherent in human nature, or the will of God. Nor can it be assumed that dissatisfaction or outrage is either natural or to be taken for granted. Every experience of displeasure and dissatisfaction has its origins in the availability, if not promise, of remedies, cures, reforms, and solutions for such troubles.

This proposition is particularly well illustrated by the history of hunger. Hunger has probably been part of the American experience at least since the first European settlers arrived, but for most of that time, its existence has not been a public issue. This is not to say that communities and their governments accepted no responsibility for its relief. Indeed the colonial Poor Laws, primarily based on the English model, generally set amounts of poor relief in terms of the costs of food and fuel or provided these items directly, in kind. But hunger was not regarded as a public outrage, a shame, a scandal, a blight upon the reputation of the communities in which it was found. Steven Marcus (1975:6–7) has written of the Irish potato famine that "it is in all likelihood the first disaster of its kind in history which was widely responded to, and continues to be thought of, as a moral outrage." It was so regarded, he asserts, because "means had been developed and were at hand to deal with and alleviate both famine and plague, but they were not fully employed." Similarly, hunger in America came to be regarded as a problem, an outrage, only when the food to alleviate it was visibly available.

In the 1930s, the availability of food for solution was so obvious that the problem came to be defined by this contradiction. In the 1960s, the availability of large quantities of food was widely assumed, in part because the Food for Peace program had been shipping substantial quantities abroad, and the capacity of the society to provide food purchasing power to all its citizens was also clear to many in what was routinely referred to as "the richest nation on earth." The situation in the United States was regularly contrasted with that of famine ridden nations abroad. In the 1980s, the huge amounts of waste in the commercial food system played the same function. A major element in the appeal of food banking has been the redirection of this waste toward the hungry.

Throughout the process of discovery and rediscovery, then, the obvious availability of a remedy has been a powerful prerequisite for naming the problem.

2. The nature of the available remedy contributes to the content of the typification. In the 1930s, as we have seen, the food itself—first the wheat and then the pigs—shaped the typification of the problem as "waste amid want." The 1960s rediscovery of hunger provides a particularly interesting example, because the remedy that shaped the problem definition was not so obvious to the entire population as the 1930s surplus; rather, it was the remedy with which the primary claimsmakers, schooled by the legislative victories and judicial relief of the civil rights movement, were able to perceive. In the 1980s, the remedy—emergency food—was so integral a part of the typification as to blur the distinction between problem and response.

3. The typification that "wins" the competition for public attention tends to obscure competing typifications and foreclose the possibility of alternate solutions. Any of the three discoveries could be used to illustrate this facet of the relationship between typification and remedy. In the 1930s, claimsmakers on the left pointed out that the supposed "paradox" of want amid plenty was really the normal working of capitalism, writ large by depression, and called for a more fundamental solution than the artificial reintroduction of scarcity through crop reduction. Their voices, however, were largely obscured by the fascination with the notion of paradox and the relief that both citizens and bureaucrats experienced once the FSRC began purchasing and distributing farm surpluses to the hungry. In the 1960s, an alternative typification of the problem might have focused upon the underlying causes of poverty— joblessness, agricultural displacement, and single parent families, for example, but the remedies that the claimsmakers anticipated shaped their choice of typification. Similarly, in the 1980s and 1990s, the proliferation of small scale, voluntary, points-of-light food programs has relieved some of the pressure for adequate incomes and decent jobs.

The history of U. S. hunger in the twentieth century warrants reflection, both by scholars and by activists. For scholars, particularly social problems theorists, this history points to the need for a more interactive conception of the relationship between typification and response. For activists, the story suggests that advocates and claimsmakers would be well advised to seize the definitional phase of problem identification and to consider with care the implications of the typifications they offer.

Notes

1. While social constructionists have provided the language of claims, claimsmakers, and the claimsmaking process and have drawn our attention to the importance of typification, they are not the only social scientists to notice this phenomenon. Daniel Moynihan (1970), for example, has argued that "the crucial phase in solving a problem is the process by which it comes to be defined." William Ryan (1971:12) made a similar point in *Blaming the Victim*. Much earlier, W. I. Thomas (1966:301, orig. 1931) declared that "if men define situations as real, they are real in their consequences."

2. "If we do not have such obvious 'breadlines knee deep in wheat' as under the Hoover administration," wrote socialist presidential candidate Norman Thomas toward the end of Roosevelt's first term, "it is because we have done more to reduce the wheat and systematize the giving of crusts than to end hunger" (1936:33).

3. It is a matter of interpretation whether the hunger claimsmaking of the early 1980s should be regarded as a "new" discovery, or a continuation of the antihunger activity of the 1960s and 1970s. I have treated it here as a separate

discovery because the typification of hunger was markedly different and because a whole new cast of claimsmakers emerged. The older activity of the antihunger network, however, did not die away, nor was the older definition of hunger as federal food program inadequacy completely superseded. The most accurate portrayal would probably involve two competing conceptions of hunger, each with its own set of claimsmakers, and a gradual but still incomplete convergence of the two.

References

Best, J. (ed.). 1989. *Images of Issues: Typifying Contemporary Social Problems*. Hawthorne, NY: Aldine de Gruyter.

Berry. J. M. 1982. "Consumers and the Hunger Lobby" Pp. 68–78 in *Food Policy and Farm Programs*, Proceedings of the National Academy of Political Science, Vol. 34, edited by D. F. Hadwiger and R. Talbot. New York: the Academy of Political Science.

Biddle, Mr. and Mrs. George to F. D. Roosevelt. letter. August 29, 1933. Hog Emergency Program folder, Files of the Agricultural Adjustment Administration, 1933–1935, Record Group 145, National Archives and Records Service.

Blumer, H. 1971. "Social Problems as Collective Behavior." *Social Problems* 18(3):298–306.

Bread for the World Institute. 1993. *Hunger 1994: Transforming the Politics of Hunger*. Fourth Annual Report on the State of World Hunger. Silver Spring, MD.

Breglio, V. 1992. *Hunger in America: The Voter' Perspective*. Lanham, MD: Research/Strategy/Management Inc.

Chelf, C. P. 1992. *Controversial Issues in Social Welfare Policy: Government and the Pursuit of Happiness*. Newbury Park, CA: Sage.

Citizens Board of Inquiry into Hunger and Malnutrition in the U.S. 1968. *Hunger U.S.A.* Washington, D.C.: New Community Press.

Claffey, B. A., and T. A. Stucker. 1982. "The Food Stamp Program." Pp. 40–53 in *Food Policy and Farm Programs*, Proceedings of the National Academy of Political Science, Vol. 34, edited by D. F. Hadwiger and R. Talbot. New York: the Academy of Political Science.

Clancy, K., and J. Bowering. 1992. "The Need for Emergency Food: Poverty Problems and Policy Responses." *Journal of Nutrition Education* 24(1):12s–17s.

Cohen, B., and M. Burt. 1989. *Eliminating Hunger: Food Security Policy for the 1990's*. Washington, D.C.: The Urban Institute.

Field Foundation. 1977. *Hunger in America: The Federal Response*. 2nd Report of the Physicians Task Force on Hunger. San Francisco, CA: Greenhaven.

Food and Hunger Hotline. 1987. *Report of NYC Poverty, Emergency Feeding and Government Funds*.

Food for Survival. *1993 Annual Report*.

Food Research and Action Center. 1984. *Hunger in the Eighties: A Primer*. Washington, D.C.: Food Research and Action Center.

Fuller, R. C., and R. D. Meyers. 1941. "The Natural History of a Social Problem." *American Sociological Review* 6:320–327.

Harrington, M. 1962. *The Other America.* New York: Macmillan.

Kelly, G., B. Rauschenbach, and C. Campbell. 1989. *Private Food Assistance in New York State: Challenges for the 1990's.* Ithaca, NY: Cornell University.

Kotz, N. 1969. *Let Them Eat Promises: The Politics of Hunger in America.* Englewood Cliffs, NJ: Prentice-Hall.

———. 1984. "The Politics of Hunger." *New Republic* April 30:19–23.

Lawrence, C. W. 1933. "Slaughter of Sucklings Makes Pomerene Angry." Newspaperclipping (source unidentified) attached to letter from C. H. Newkirk to F. D. Roosevelt, September 29. Hog Emergency Program Folder, Files of the Agricultural Adjustment Administration, 1933–1935, Record Group 145, National Archives and Records Service.

Lelyveld, J. 1985. "Hunger in America." *The New York Times Magazine* June 16:20–23+.

Lipsky, M., and S. Smith. 1989. "When Social Problems Are Treated as Emergencies." *The Social Service Review* 63(1):5–25.

Lipsky, M., and M. Thibodeau. 1988. "Feeding the Hungry with Surplus Commodities." *Political Science Quarterly* 103(2):223–244.

Literary Digest. 1933. "The Government Program for Direct Relief." October 14:8.

Marcus, S. 1975. "Hunger and Ideology." Pp. 3–16 in *Representations: Essays on Literature and Society.* New York: Random House.

McGovern, G. 1969. "Forward." Pp. vii–x in *Let Them Eat Promises* by Nick Kotz. Englewood Cliffs, NJ: Prentice-Hall.

Moynihan, D. 1970. "To Solve Problem, First Define It." *The New York Times* January 12:49.

Nestle, M., and S. Guttmacher. 1992. "Hunger in the United States: Rationale, Methods, and Policy Implications of State Hunger Surveys." *Journal of Nutrition Education.* 24(1):18s–22s.

New York Times. 1933a. "Plenty and Want." September 23:14.

———. 1933b. "Roosevelt Decides to Buy Coal, Food and Clothing for the Needy This Winter." October 1:1, 3.

Physicians Task Force on Hunger in America. 1985. *Hunger in America: The Growing Epidemic.* Middletown, CT: Wesleyan University Press.

Poppendieck, J. E. 1985 "Policy, Advocacy, and Justice: The Case of Food Assistance Reform." Pp. 101–131 in *Toward Social and Economic Justice,* edited by D. Gil and E. Gil. Cambridge, MA: Schenkman Publishing.

———. 1986. *Breadlines Knee Deep in Wheat: Food Assistance in the Great Depression.* New Brunswick, NJ: Rutgers University Press.

Rodway vs U. S. Department of Agriculture. 514 F 2d 809, 820 (D.C. Cir., 1975).

Roosevelt, F. D. 1972. *Complete Press Conferences of Franklin D. Roosevelt,* Vol. 2. New York: De Capo Press.

Ryan, W. 1971. *Blaming the Victim.* New York: Vintage.

Second Harvest. 1993. *1992 Annual Report.* Chicago, IL: Second Harvest.

Spector, M., and J. I. Kitsuse. 1987. *Constructing Social Problems.* Hawthorne, NY: Aldine de Gruyter.

Thomas, N. 1936. *After the New Deal, What?* New York: Macmillan.

Thomas, W. I. 1966. "The Relation of Research to the Social Process." Pp. 289–305 in *W. I. Thomas on Social Organization and Social Personality*, edited by M. Janowitz. Chicago: University of Chicago Press.

United States Conference of Mayors. 1982. *Human Services in FY 1982*. Washington, D.C.: U.S. Conference of Mayors.

United States Congress. 1932. *Congressional Record*. 72nd Congress, 1st Session, January 4, 1932, pp. 1181–1194.

United States Senate, Subcommittee on Employment, Manpower, and Poverty of the Committee on Labor and Public Welfare. 1968. *Hunger in America: Chronology and Selected Background Materials*. Washington, D.C.: U.S. Government Printing Office.

VanAmburg Group Inc. 1994. *Second Harvest 1993 National Research Study*. Chicago, IL: Second Harvest National Food Bank Network.

Wecter, D. 1952. *The Age of the Great Depression, 1929–1941*. New York: Macmillan.

3

World Hunger as a Social Problem

WM. ALEX MCINTOSH

Introduction

Researchers have approached social problems from two basically different perspectives. The first considers conditions that harm individuals, groups, or whole societies as social problems. Conventionally, crime, drug use, and family violence serve as examples. The conditions are said to be objective and measurable; thus the objectivist approach evolves out of positivism. Positivists of the nineteenth century tended to view all social conditions as objective and observable. And like the objects studied by the physical sciences, these objective conditions could be changed through applied science. The second approach, social constructionism, argues that a social problem is what individuals or groups select from an array of problematic circumstances. Furthermore, the choices people make in determining problems have less to do with the objective nature of the problem and more to do with subjective assessments (Best 1989). What becomes a social problem has less to do with either the number of persons harmed or the seriousness of that harm for persons and groups and more to do with successful promotion. A condition becomes a social problem if supporters of the view successfully convince others this is so. A third approach, heretofore rarely considered as a means of examining social problems, is what anthropologists refer to as the emic approach (Headland 1990). The strength of the emic perspective lies in its insistence that ultimate validity derives from the subject's point of view. A social problem from this perspective is something that is identified by those who experience it and conclusions that result from the study of social problems must remain consistent with the point of view of the victim. Anthropologists distinguish the emic from the etic epistemology. The etic refers to anthropological theories and concepts an anthropologist brings to bear on a given society and in many cases follows the objectivist epistemology. Sociologists who work in the area of victimology, at first blush, would appear to use an emic perspective. However, most victimologists bring existing theory and concepts to bear on their subject matter, rather than rely on victims' accounts. An emic approach allows individuals to identify the problematic, the harmful, in their own lives in terms that are meaningful to them. Studies of social problems rarely provide victims with a voice.

This chapter explores hunger, famine, and chronic malnutrition from the objectivist, subjectivist, and emic points of view. Hunger, malnutrition, and famine are historical if not prehistoric constants. Their occurrence may vary by time, space, and duration, but they visit human societies with a fair degree of regularity. Ethiopia has a history of famine that stretches far into the past, with the trend accentuated in this century. Like the poor the hungry have always been with us. Some of the earliest writings produced by humankind reference famine, food shortages, and starvation. We tend to think that these terms are interrelated if not a depiction of the same phenomenon. A careful examination of the definitions and contexts in which these and related terms are used demonstrates considerable differences. One interpretation of these differences is that hunger and the related problems of malnutrition and famine are social constructions; that is, a consensus has developed among individuals that hunger is a problematic condition for society and they have convinced others that this is the case. I do not wholly subscribe to this view. Hunger is a problem with an objective reality, regardless of how much consensus has developed over its status as a problem. However, its social definition varies, to a degree, depending on time and place. At the same time, the definition and importance given hunger depend upon the degree to which the definers have political power and have captured adequate resources to pursue their cause. Finally, while conditions of insufficient food have a common objective base, and at the same time, famines and related circumstances undergo social definition at the hands of interested parties, victims experience and react to hunger, malnutrition, and famine in ways not fully captured by either the objectivist or constructionist perspectives. These views must also have a place in the literature. This chapter concludes with an argument for all three perspectives in recognition of the more complete understanding of hunger and other problems that the use of all three provides.

The Objectivist Account of Chronic Malnutrition

Before discussing descriptions of types and prevalence of malnutrition, a few definitions are in order. Famine appears harder than ever to identify as definitions proliferate (Arnold 1988; Devereux 1993; McIntosh 1995). Definitional proliferation has accompanied the proliferation of theoretical explanations for the causes and consequences of famine. Delimiters of famine include insufficient food availability, insufficient food intake, higher than normal mortality, and social disruption. Many of these properties characterize other disasters as well. Furthermore, many of the definitions violate the rules of definitional adequacy in that they contain hypotheses. For example, some have defined a famine as a food shortage that results in an increase in the mortality rate. These are known as "truth-asserting" definitions (Zetterberg 1965). A concept is true by definition; a hypothesis is tested by empirical evidence. Thus, concepts are evaluated for their analytical properties; hypotheses, for truthfulness of their assertions about relationships between objects in the real world. A useful beginning might lie in identifying a famine as a type of disaster in which food intake falls short of minimal standards. Famines could then be further conceptualized by type, including those that involve higher than normal mortality rates. Some select the term "undernutrition" instead of malnutrition. Many have defined these terms as failure to meet some optimum standard such as height for age, weight for age, or food intake; others however, argue that universally applicable "optimums" are difficult to determine and thus such definitions are inadequate (Allan 1993; Payne 1992). Hunger is frequently used synonymously with malnutrition by recent observers (Brown and Pitzer 1989); they are not the same, however, and thus hunger will be defined as a psychological state that includes the experiences one has several hours after eating a meal. These experiences involve the successive phases of "diffuse restlessness, sensations of tension and emptiness, and unpleasant aching, gnawing sensations or hunger pangs. During semi-starvation, hunger is almost a constant companion; in total starvation, hunger ceases after several days" (Keys et al. 1950).

Concerns for definitions and their rigor aside, to discuss issues such as the extent and severity of famine and malnutrition, we must rely on available statistics. Fewer objective data exist regarding the number of persons affected by famine or hunger than chronic malnutrition. Thus, the latter will serve as an example of an objectivist account. Based on a variety of data sources of varying reliability and validity, the World Health Organization (1990) has advised that the principal deficiency diseases prevalent in the Third World consist of anemia and diseases resulting from a deficiency of iodine and vitamin A. Iodine deficiency diseases, including endemic goiter and cretinism, afflict more than 200 million persons, with another 1 billion at risk. As with most deficiency diseases, the bulk of these cases are found in Southeast Asia. Anemia is estimated to prevail in 51% of children between the ages of 0 and 4, and in 60% of pregnant women. Xeropthalmia, vitamin A deficiency, affects nearly 40 million preschool children in 37 countries (WHO 1990). Substantial proportions of these experience blindness and eventual death. Protein energy malnutrition has declined substantially, as have wasting and stunting. However, the latter remain serious enough to merit attention and intervention. Grant (1991) argues, further, that with regards to the world's population of children, 8 million (14%) in the Americas, 30 million (26%) in Africa, and 76 million (47%) in Asia suffer from malnutrition (as defined as 2 standard deviations below desirable weight for age).

More specific data are displayed in Table 1.1, using a sample of low, middle, and upper income countries. These countries were selected in large part by the amount of data available for each. Only the scantiest of nutritional status indicators exist for most countries in the world, including the developed ones. These data suggest that malnutrition in children varies greatly by country and that poor nutrition occurs in places where resources are few. Those countries with the lowest levels of gross national product (GNP) per capita have the highest percentages of children who experience either moderate to severe underweight, stunting, or wasting. However, the relationship between lower income and education and prevalence of iron, iodine, and vitamin A deficiencies is less clear (see the appropriate tables in World Bank 1993).

Using a larger number of indicators than those in Table 1 for those countries for which there are such data permits a more formal investigation of the links between malnutrition and other conditions. The source of these data is the annual World Bank world development statistics (World Bank 1993). Computing zero-order correlation coefficients among these indicators confirms the link between poverty and malnutrition in children, as measured by the prevalence of underweight, stunting, and wasting. Malnutrition in children has no relationship to population variables such as the birthrate, population size, or population growth, and is only weakly related to food availability (calories, protein). However, the chances of malnutrition in children increase with poverty (GNP/capita, percent income spent on food), and lack of modernization (low adult

Table 1.1. Prevalence and Incidence of Chronic Malnutrition and Selected Indicators of Socioeconomic Development for a Sample of Countries[a]

Country	Infants with low birth weight (%)	Underweight (0–4 months) moderate and severe (%)	Wasting (12–23 months) moderate and severe (%)	Stunting (24–59 months) moderate and severe (%)	Iron deficiency (%)	Iodine deficiency (%)	Vitamin A deficiency (%)
Mozambique	**[b]	**	**	14	**	**	**
Sierra Leone	**	**	**	19	50.0	**	**
Ethiopia	20	57	8	**	6.0	34.0	**
Cambodia	17	23	2	3	**	30.0	4.9
Bangladesh	**	38	**	31	66.0	10.5	**
Laos	**	20	3	**	**	**	**
Kenya	28	71	31	**	6.0	15–72	**
El Salvador	39	37	**	**	8.6	48.0	**
Guatemala	15	**	**	8	**	10.6	**
Brazil	15	15	**	**	**	14.7	**
Philippines	14	34	8	2	37.5	14.9	**
Siri Lanka	8	5	**	9	3.8	19.3	**
Thailand	18	33	2	4	11.0	14.7	**
Jamaica	28	38	9	1	76.0	**	**
Egypt	12	26	4	3	22.4	70.0	**
Algeria	8	7	1	**	22.4	70.0	**
Chile	5	13	3	**	20.0	18.8	**
Cuba	9	10	**	**	30.0	30.3	**
Singapore	7	3	14	**	**	**	**
United States	7	14	**	**	**	**	**

[a] Countries are listed in descending order of their 1989 under 5 mortality rates and were selected on the basis of generally available data for illustrative purposes (World Bank 1993).
[b] **Indicates data not available.

literacy, low female literacy, low female school enrollment, and high
percentages of the labor force employed in agriculture). Malnutrition
occurs in a context of overall poor health, in that it increases with higher
rates of low birth weight, infant mortality, under age five mortality,
maternal mortality, and with lower female and total life expectancy
rates.

Big Numbers, Untrustworthy Results

As compelling as the above prevalence and incidence data are and as
sensible as the correlations between child malnutrition and deprivation
appear, use of such estimates requires a great deal of caution. The estimates of the number of malnourished vary a great deal, depending on
the source of data. The differences in the magnitude of these estimates
suggest several things. First, there may be a tendency to exaggerate in
the face of a "good cause." Second, estimators utilize differing methodologies. Some compare the difference in population size and changes
in food availability. Dreze and Sen (1989) infer food insufficiency problems from the decline in per capita agricultural production rates that
have occurred over the past decade in Africa. Others continue to rely on
the differential between worldwide growth rates of population and resources. The World Health Organization (WHO), for example, often must
rely on small-scale sample surveys to obtain country-level estimates for
the number of children who are underweight or who are stunted. In other
cases the data are so sparse that regional estimates are calculated. Such
estimates depend upon available data and statistical modeling. As Mosley and Cowley (1991) observe, both the World Health Organization and
the World Bank utilize the same data sources, but differing statistical
models result in different estimates in country and regional-level vital
statistics.

Presentations of these same data are often problematic. Grant's (1991)
estimates of the extent of iodine deficiency risk in childhood make no
mention of the reference population. Is it all children in the world? If so,
the figure must be based on extrapolation, for not all countries have
generated such data. If the number is based on only those populations for
which iodine deficiency data exist, then Grant should have provided a
baseline. The latter is the more likely explanation, given that the World
Bank tables on health and nutrition provide data only on anemia in
pregnant women and underweight, stunting, and wasting among children. Even these data suggest that not all countries have conducted
health surveys. Focusing on the childhood anthropometric data, the
World Bank publications indicate significant missing data problems. For

example, among the 57 countries with GNP per capita of less than $1,000, only 42 provide information on numbers of underweight children and only 35 have data for stunting. Of the 17 countries with GNP per capita greater than $10,000, only six make stunting data available. The data presented in Table 1 regarding the prevalence of iron deficiency are derived from studies in 37 countries; of iodine, from 60 countries; and vitamin A, from 13 countries (Levin et al. 1993). Perhaps Grant utilized these same data sources as a starting point from which he then extrapolated to the global level. This is only speculation, however, as he makes no mention of his source for the global estimates.

McLaren (1986) provides us with some insights into how global estimates of malnutrition are made. He finds that 73 countries contain populations at-risk of vitamin A deficiency, based on figures provided by the Protein Advisory Group (PAG). The PAG, in turn, utilized cultural, dietary, and economic patterns thought to be associated with vitamin A deficiency. McLaren goes on to say that estimates of prevalence must depend upon local skills and resources and thus vary in scope and quality. "Where facilities are limited these tend to be on small groups of people, unrepresentative of the population as a whole, and may not take into account seasonal variations in prevalence, which tend to be considerable" (1986:2). Of interest is the contrast between the PAG estimate for 73 countries and the 13 countries identified by Levin et al. (1993) as having either local, regional, or societal studies of vitamin A deficiency. Clearly, the PAG engaged in educated guess-work to obtain its estimates.

Problems of a more fundamental nature, however, exist in regards to these numbers (Evers and McIntosh 1977). The first has to do with reliability. It is clear from the collection of both mortality as well as production statistics that those charged with the responsibility for data collection on a particular subject may not use consistent methodology. For example, in some countries, a physician may determine cause of death among mortalities in urban areas while health technicians may do so in rural areas. Furthermore, measurement methodologies regarding the determination of anemia may differ from one country to the next. A great deal of random error may also be introduced into a study by an excessively small sample size. Users of data such as these may have little information regarding the training and supervision of those involved in the collection of data, much less an idea about either the response rate or the representativeness of the sample. A more significant problem, however, lies in the potential invalidity of the available data relative to the uses to which they are put. Until recently, world nutrition problems were determined through the use of food balance sheets that estimate dietary short-falls by dividing the available nutrients in a country's food stocks by the population size. Use of these data to estimate malnutrition requires the assumption that food is equally available to all. In other words, class differences and age and sex differences in the home have no bearing on the distribution of food. The willingness to use such data in this manner led to the serious underestimation of various forms of malnutrition in a number of third world counties (McLaren 1974; Waterlow and Payne 1975). Furthermore, declining food supplies appear to some to represent risk of malnutrition. This may be so, but some studies indicate that hunger and malnutrition may be seasonal in that the quantity of cereals and other crops may exceed national averages during certain times of the year and fall below them at others.

Despite these problems, some researchers continue to utilize data such as available calories and protein per capita as "good" indicators of nutrition (Bradshaw et al. 1993). Turning to anthropometric indicators, serious underweight may be the result of infection, rather than inadequate diet. And underweight and wasting may well reflect either a serious short- or long-term calorie shortfall in the diet, but the presence or absence of other forms of malnutrition cannot be determined by such data. Other forms of malnutrition more likely result from a lack of variety as opposed to quantity in the diet. In the past experts have become convinced on the basis of available data and assumptions they were willing to make about such data that certain forms of malnutrition existed while others did not. In one extreme case, documented by McLaren (1974) and Waterlow and Payne (1975), researchers as policy makers became convinced that protein–calorie malnutrition resulted primarily from a protein shortage. On the basis of this judgment, a great deal of effort was expended to alleviate the problem. Over a decade later, it was discovered that the primary cause of protein–calorie malnutrition (PCM) was not a protein but rather a calorie shortage.

A related concern has to do with the establishment of meaningful reference standards with regard to the very indicators that WHO and the World Bank rely on for comparative data at the nation-state level. Researchers are asking once again whether universal standards that differentiate only in terms of age and sex suffice in the face of intra- and interindividual variations among healthy individuals (Osmani 1992). The assumption underlying the single set of standards approach, referred to as "genetic potential theory," states that all human beings have the same genetic potential in terms of growth. Therefore, significant deviation from the standards suggests that such individuals are unable to function as well as those who come reasonably close to the standards. "Function" here refers to a diverse set of capabilities involving physiological processes such as immune system function, physical capabilities such as work capacity, and psychological abilities such as cognition. Others argue for more relative standards, suggesting that the human body adapts to insufficient diets through the achievement of a smaller body (Payne 1992). Much of the debate revolves around whether this adaptation represents relative optimality or absolute underefficiency. This argument squares nicely with the "relative deprivation" perspective that Chapman (1990) has pursued.

Finally, there is famine itself. Available data on malnutrition may include numbers of individuals experiencing a deficiency disease as a result of famine. However, these are a poor source for estimating the total number of famine victims in a given year. To begin with, many of the data on the prevalence of deficiency diseases worldwide are based on a single collection of data. The figure, usually expressed as a proportion of some population base, is then routinely extrapolated from one year to the next under the ceteris paribus assumption. As famines are irregular and unpredictable, estimates of deficiency prevalence will likely exclude estimates of deficiencies that arose from a famine that occurred in a year different from the one in which the data were collected. Second, as described below, empirical descriptions of the extent of famine often come from relief organizations, rather than host government or United Nations agency studies. These estimates arise in the context of press releases or relief organization reports, frequently with little discussion of potential measurement or sampling errors and bias. And we can surmise that the methodology that generated these estimates varies from one context or organization to the next. In fairness, we should remember that the motivation of these organizations for providing any data lies in the generation of more resources for dealing with the crisis, not in providing precise information for scientific discussion.

The Social Construction of Hunger

The social constructionist approach argues that a condition or event becomes a problem through social activities (Best 1989). Individuals actively engage in calling attention to various conditions and calling for their change or elimination. This requires that these persons make certain kinds of claims about the condition. This may further require organized efforts. Groups may arise to press their case before the public or before legislative or judicial bodies that they define as sources of solution to problems. Social constructionists are less interested in the substantive nature of the problem and instead perceive the sociological problem to be the assessment of the kinds of individuals likely to serve as claimsmakers, the nature and effectiveness of the messages and symbols employed in claimsmaking, and the effectiveness of socially organized efforts in obtaining social problem status for a condition.

Claimants

A variety of claimants from the academic and policy worlds as well as the mass media have helped sustain both public concern and the long-standing debate over the causes of famine and malnutrition and the prospects for the future. The mass media have provided extensive coverage of a number of famines since World War II, and have sometimes purposely attempted to mobilize public involvement in relief efforts. Increasing numbers and types of academics have found famine and chronic malnutrition fertile ground for their theorizing and research. What once was largely the concern of demographers, public health scientists, and nutritionists now has captured the attention of geographers, planners, economists, anthropologists, and sociologists. Finally, an increasing number of governmental and nongovernmental organizations has arisen to tackle problems of emergency relief for famine victims and to improve local circumstances through development activities to alleviate both the threat of famine as well as chronic malnutrition.

Mass Media. Journalists have played a major part in drawing attention to famine, especially to those in a position to provide assistance during such a crisis. The success of famine reporting in this regard lies in television news as opposed to magazine or newspapers. But getting famine into the news has not been easy. Gans (1976) finds that television news devotes only 14% of its broadcasts to foreign news and much of that to events within those nations historically allied with the United States, such as England and France. Print news has much the same character, although more space is provided (28% of column space) for international news. Dramatic events outside Europe take up whatever space remains. Famines are such events, but their frequency in recent years has led editorial personnel to conclude that nothing really new is occurring. For a famine to make much of an impact on an editorial staff, it must be particularly horrendous. And the involvement of American governmental personnel in such a crisis leads to more frequent and widespread television coverage, which declines once those personnel are removed, as in the recent case of Somalia (*Television News Index and Abstracts* 1992–1993). News agencies are frequently unaware that a particular famine is occurring. This is in part due to the fact that most do not routinely station their reporters in those countries in which famines most likely occur. A second reason lies in the lack of an indigenous, independent press corps in those counties. Where such institutions exist, they tend to serve as public relations outlets for their governments (Dreze and Sen 1989; Harrison and Palmer 1986). As a result, only some famines receive any press coverage at all. Turning to related issues, chronic malnutrition, by contrast, receives no attention in the press. It is not a startling, rapidly developing event, but rather a long-term condition that appears to vary little from year to year. The media more frequently report on the resurgence of a chronic disease such as malaria instead of successes in eradication (see, for example, Cowley 1993).

Journalists have aided and abetted these efforts. During the late 1960s, Nick Kotz was particularly effective in drawing attention to hunger in the United States. The wrath expressed by President Nixon toward his reporting clearly indicates the political impact of his stories on poverty and hunger. Less well known in the United States are the names of those mostly non-U.S. journalists who not only awakened the world to famine in Africa, but became active in efforts to intervene with humanitarian aid. Harrison and Palmer (1986) describe the role of both individual reporters and news organizations in three African famines. In each case the famine is said to have been discovered "accidentally," that is, those involved went to Africa in search of other kinds of stories. The famine described to be happening in Kampuchea was discovered as reporters covered First Lady Rosaline Carter's visit to Cambodian refugee camps along the boarder with Thailand (Palmieri 1982). It is clear from these accounts that the reporters had not traveled in search of famine stories. Instead, they intended to cover these conflicts and their aftermath. In each case those involved had to actively promote their stories to get space in the mainstream press. In addition, the mainstream press often becomes interested in a famine story only after exposés published by the tabloids have evoked substantial public outcry. With reference to the Biafran famine, reporters from England had to contend not only with uninterested editors but also with hostile officials who found the stories embarrassing to the British government.

African famine coverage in the United States has also met similar indifference. In 1984, Bill Blakemore of ABC news requested permission to take a crew to Africa to investigate the drought and famine he had been told by sources were occurring (Boyer 1985). His and the editorial staff of the other networks concluded that another famine in Africa was not news because of their frequent occurrence. Furthermore, Africans were afflicted whose plight had no particular public or political importance in the United States. Finally, network executives were reluctant to spend the money required to do the story. Only after the BBC aired a story did network news begin its coverage. Broadcasts continued because of a significant number of phone calls and letters to the networks.

Journalists have often had to engage in arm-twisting to either cover famines or to have their stories published or given air time. Some have done so simply because the event represented "good news," while others developed a sense of moral outrage they wished to express in their communication to their audiences. Both the reporters and the editorial staff with whom they worked often took a further step in calling upon citizens to contribute money to relief efforts or to pressure governmental representatives to act more decisively in providing aid (Harrison and Palmer 1986; Varnis 1990).

The impact of the mass media may increase regarding its ability to alert the public and dramatize conditions in the world (O'Hefferman 1990). The major forms of mass media are owned by corporations with affiliations that extend beyond the boarders of a given country. The increased international interests of these companies as well as advances in technological means have led to the continued globalization of both their coverage of events and their ability to make such news immediately available to a global audience (Lewis 1984). Television has become the leading form of information transmission; as such television's preference for certain types of news suggests that such events will receive greater coverage than others. Many international events such as famine may receive greater attention, as capabilities and audiences grow.

Finally, the role of the indigenous press ought to be given some consideration. Unfortunately, few have undertaken serious study of this. One exception is Ram (1989), who provides information on the press coverage of several famine periods in India. He concludes that the press can actually prevent famine by publishing stories that describe an unfolding crisis. Because such crises reflect badly on governments, this role can be played only by a press that is independent of government control. This most likely occurs within a reasonably democratic culture.

Academics. Academics have recently discovered that maln.itrition and especially famine represent areas in which to apply their ideas and research. Some individual scholars have carved out almost an entire career from their famine work. Others have organized research centers, several of which have outlived the careers of their creators. The Institute of Nutrition of Central America and Panama (INCAP) was founded in the 1950s in Panama to study the effects of malnutrition on children. Francis Moore Lappé and others established the Institute for Food and Development in 1978 (Belasco 1993). More recently Brown University established the Alan Feinstein World Hunger Program, while Tufts has its USDA Human Nutrition Research Center on Aging. In 1975 the Consultative Group on International Agricultural Research (CIGAR) established the International Food Policy Research Institute (IFPRI) to assess various strategies for both increasing food production and improving its distribution. The institute currently employs 45 senior staff members and works collaboratively with approximately 100 institutions mostly located in third world countries (IFPRI n.d.).

Early work by academics concentrated on the role of famine and chronic malnutrition in demographic change, particularly its contribution to mortality. Demographic historians revived this interest in the 1970s, after Peter Laslett (1965) inquired, "Did the peasants really starve?" with regard to whether famine had had much impact on the daily lives of Europeans of earlier times. Appleby (1978), Livi-Bacci (1990), and Walter and Schofield (1989) are among the many reinvestigating the impact of famine on mortality as well as other demographic processes such as marriage and fertility. Others, including economists, have begun to investigate the interrelationship between economic development and improvements in nutritional status, utilizing human capital and other economic models (Cook 1970; Floud 1992; Fogel 1992; Kallen 1973). Still others have argued that famine and chronic malnutrition result from either lack of development, distorted development, or economic dependency (Bennoune 1992; Berg 1973; Mellor and Galvin 1987; Watts 1991; Whit 1994). These divergent approaches have led to debate, much of which has become quite polemical, with some moving beyond description and explanation to assigning blame.

The Malthusians attack the problem from the standard "too many people, too few resources" perspective arguing that food production has not kept up with population growth; when confronted with evidence to the contrary, their fallback position argues that improvements in food production cannot continue indefinitely and population control is needed now. Others have argued that societies develop their way out of chronic food shortages as evidenced by European history. Thus, both agricultural and industrial development provide the way out of the dilemma (Mellor and Galvin 1987).

Relief and Charitable Organizations. Finally, a growing number of organizations have either embraced famine relief as a new activity or arose as an organization designed specifically to deal with famine. At least three types of such organizations can be identified. The first is intergovernmental (referred to as IGOs). These are bureaucratic structures supported by member states and include branches of the United Nations and include the U.N. Relief and Rehabilitation Administration, the United Nations Children's Fund (UNICEF), the World Food Program, and the Office of the United Nations Disaster Relief Coordinator. A second type represents governmental offices established to deal with either development or famine relief. The United States has its Agency for International Development in the State Department and Ethiopia, for a brief period, had the Relief and Rehabilitation Commission (RCC). Nongovernmental organizations (NGOs) differ from governmental in that the former rely on private means, although many accept donations from governmental sources. In

1951 there were 123 IGOs and 823 NGOs; their number had risen to 1,856 and 16,208, respectively, by 1991 (Beigbeder 1991:81–82). Examples of NGOs include the International Committee of the Red Cross (ICRC), Catholic Relief Services, Lutheran World Service, Oxfam, and Save the Children Fund/UK. Finally, there are agencies whose labor force consists primarily of volunteers, referred to as private voluntary organizations (PVOs). Many of these overlap with the category of NGOs. Examples include the Peace Corps and Operation Brotherhood, an organization that stations volunteers from the Philippine medical community in other countries of Southeast Asia.

Religious orders have dedicated a part of their efforts to charitable works as exemplified by the Religious Society of Friends or Quakers, established in the seventeenth century. Charitable organizations such as the International Red Cross have a long history of involvement in health crises. Many organizations, however, appeared after World War II in response to the Cold War. Leaders from both the religious and business communities established International Voluntary Services, Inc. with the expressed purpose of inserting the talents and energy of America's youth into the third world, perceived as threatened by communist domination. Several organizations were created in response to specific famines. Missionaries and others founded Concern, intending to make use of their Biafran experiences in relief efforts in future famines; others who had dispensed relief in Biafra formed the International Disaster Institute (United Kingdom) to provide a more scientific approach to such efforts in future disasters (Harrison and Palmer 1986). Over 20 antihunger groups that focus on nondomestic or international hunger exist in the United States (Knowles 1984). These include organized efforts by various Protestant denominations as well as efforts organized by the Catholic Church and Jewish charities. Some of these specialize in relief only; others, in a combination of relief and evangelicalism; still others mix relief with development. Those emphasizing strictly emergency feeding or that have recently turned away from the goal of long-term development have received criticism for ignoring local institutions and the need for the development of local capacities for long-term sustainable food production (Adam 1993). Others have emphasized the importance of helping the local population to either establish or rebuild local institutions that would engage in both relief and development activities (Charney 1993).

Relief agencies have not only engaged in relief efforts, they historically have warned governments of impending crises. For example, the Friends alerted the British government regarding the impending disaster prior to the onset of the "Great Irish Potato Famine" of the 1740s and Catholic Relief Services drew the attention of the U.N. Relief and Rehabilitation Administration and the Allied military command to likely famine if displaced Balts, Poles, and others were released from holding camps without prior efforts to meet their needs for food and shelter (Egan 1982). Others have lobbied both Congress and the Executive Branch in the United States for increases in food aid during the Biafran, Ethiopian, and Sudanese famines.

Clay (1989) and others argue that relief agencies operate within a political context over which they have little control. It is true that these agencies manage some degree of autonomy from both the donor and recipient governments, as Varnis (1990) suggests. However, during the recent Ethiopian famine some groups found that to function, some degree of cooperation with the revolutionary government was necessary. And as observed by Ruttan (1993:220), these agencies experience continuing problems with donor country government agencies regarding goals. PVOs find agency pursuits of "political or strategic advantage" at loggerheads with their own more humanitarian impulses. PVOs have accomplished varying degrees of compromise. For example,

> CARE, which has limited private financial support, has been driven by both bureaucratic ambition and financial imperatives to suppress whatever misgivings it might have about surplus disposal and security objectives . . . . Catholic Relief Services, mindful of the worldwide evangelical mission of the church, has typically taken the view that more is better, what ever the objectives of its patron . . . . Several other voluntary relief organizations, such as the American Friends Service Committee, have viewed any government support as a corruption of the concept of volunteerism. (Ruttan 1993:220–221)

Claims: Using Numbers

Claims regarding hunger rely heavily on estimates of the magnitude of the problem to draw attention, as do claimants in other problem areas (Best 1989). Two sets of numbers are generated by two different sets of claimants. The first involves representatives of the mass media. These appear in television and print news stories on famine. An article published in the *World Food Program Journal* stated that a "persistent combination of civil war and drought plagues the country. It has rendered some 30 million Africans dependent on food assistance for their survival" (Wolman 1991:16). No source for the figure was provided. Others cite either governmental or relief agencies. In a description of the famine conditions of 1992, Stevenson (1993:138), for example, relies on the International Committee of the Red Cross (ICRC) estimate that 4.5 million Somalis experienced food deprivation and the World Food Program (WPF) estimate that 1 out of the 7 million inhabitants of that country perished. According to *Newsweek*, at the end of 1992 the Red Cross operated 800 kitchens, feeding approximately 1.1 million each day (Bartholet 1992). Although not all such claims are erroneous, there is sufficient precedent of recent origin regarding entirely false claims of excessive deaths and deprivation to render such estimates suspicious. DeWaal (1989) cites convincing evidence that the 100,000 famine deaths said to have occurred in Nigeria during the 1970s never happened. Deng and Minear (1992) note that the Sudanese government claims that sufficient food supplies existed for 1992 were supported by the lack of famine conditions in that year, despite earlier mass media predictions of a looming national tragedy of massive proportions. And the infamous famine deaths said to have transpired in both the former Soviet Union and Kampuchea, once regarded as solid support for criticisms of socialist regimes' inefficiency and cruelty, have lately come under close scrutiny. Again they either never happened or their consequences were far less than once claimed (Watts 1991).

When Numbers Fail: Words and Pictures

Observers have noted that while reports by both activist and journalists utilize estimates, the most effective mechanism remains words and pictures. As Levenstein (1993:151) observed about hunger in the United States, "When all was said and done, it was not the statistics that moved the public, it was descriptions of hungry Americans in the land of plenty." Reports such as the emotional description of famine in Ethiopia have stirred both the public and others in the mass media. The tenor of the programming is caught by titles chosen for special reports. "Seeds of Despair" and "Bitter Harvest" were two such programs aired on the BBC in 1984 .

Pictures play an even greater role than words in the creation of an impact from famine accounts as is true in the portrayal of other kinds of social problems. For such an impact the problem should have several features. First, the problem must have not only visual features, but features that viewers can easily apprehend from still or moving photographs. Second, the features should exhibit emotive quality. If the problem causes suffering, this should be evident in the pictures. The sensation of hunger cannot be photographed nor are pictures of subclinical cases of malnutrition particularly telling. Only the starkness of clinical signs such as severe wasting or edema provides an unambiguous view of the victims. As Loseke (1993:214) observes, "Stated otherwise, if a picture is worth a thousand words, a visual image organized around emotional themes might be worth a thousand word-bound claims."

As an example of the power that pictures can have over editorial decisions, a recent case described in detail by Harrison and Palmer (1986) is instructive. Freelance reporter Paul Harrison returned to England in July 1984 with film of the Ethiopian famine. He contacted several news agencies, only to be turned away. Finally, Channel 4 News decided to run a portion of his film. He was invited to view the final cut version in the studio as it was broadcast. "The news hardened technicians stopped and watched in total silence, something that, Harrison was told subsequently, was practically unheard of" (Harrison and Palmer 1986: 3). ABC news in the United States decided to give this same famine coverage, only after viewing a BBC broadcast. The editorial staff reported that the other news suddenly appeared unimportant; pictures of the famine were "devastating, compelling" (Boyer 1985:21). Once an initial report with emotional descriptions and horrifying pictures received air-time, the public responded to a degree sufficient to persuade other news agencies to provide coverage as well. Ironically, some of these same companies had initially evaluated the event as not newsworthy.

And these stories lead to further media events of a very different sort. An unintended response to the famine film was the televising of live concerts organized specifically to generate charitable contributions for famine relief (Harrison and Palmer 1986). Band Aid, created by Bob Geldof, lead singer in the group Boomtown Rats, brought together such rock and pop entertainers as Sting and Phil Collins. One song from the concert was recorded and sold record numbers. A second concert, Live Aid, followed, which raised over $100 million in donations (Harrison and Palmer 1986:131).

Finally, pictures are most important to that form of mass media from which most people obtain the news. The average television news story is generally no more than several minutes long and easily explained with the aid of pictures. Famines generally meet these requirements well. The story should also fit the sort of values that the mass media prefer to portray, and famines reflect, among others, what are known as "human interest" stories (Medler and Medler 1993).

Irony. In the process of claimsmaking irony abounds, for it grabs the readers' attention. Dreze and Sen (1989), for example, argue that while famine and chronic hunger might have been justifiable in past times because of genuine insufficiencies in food supplies, these are no longer so in a world of relative plenty. Others have observed that this century is characterized by both the greatest increases in food supplies and at the same time the largest number of famine deaths ever (Watts 1991). Whit (1994) begins his chapter on world hunger with a lengthy quote that compares the consequences of the holocaust with the annual starvation death rate. He follows this with the question: "How can the world tolerate this in the midst of plenty?"

Effects of Claimsmaking

The mass media's efforts have numerous consequences, only some of which are intended. Press accounts leave the impression of insufficient agency action, which sometimes results in pressure on government officials to do more. In some situations, reporters purposely criticize such efforts either to increase or redirect them in some fashion.

Press attention to famine and famine relief publicizes the work not only of relief efforts and groups in general, but also of specific agencies. This tends to increase the status of general relief efforts as well as that of particular organizations. More importantly, this publicity leads to an increase in donations (Charney 1993).

Press accounts also have the consequence of rendering victims passive; of making them voiceless. Mass media coverage neglects the efforts of famine victims to cope with their circumstances. Village-level or state-level efforts in dealing with the crisis appear in the news only when they fail. Generally, victims appear helpless, usually during the last stages of their lives. The reporter talks about them rather than to them; they serve as dramatic backdrop for the story. By contrast, the relief workers appear in charge, recounting their heroic struggles in the face of so many victims and so few resources.

Because the Western press expresses the values of concern for not only "social disorganization," but also "rugged individualism" (Gans 1976), only women and children, those considered less able to control events around them, appear as victims. This contrast between legitimate victims and individuals seemingly in control over their own lives (as well as others) was most evident in the early reporting on conditions in Somalia in which the same story juxtaposed dying women and small children with heavily armed men and boys. The men and boys not only avoided starvation through force of arms, but their very acts of self-preservation contributed to the deprivation of others.

The press is not the sole culprit with regards to unintended consequences. Relief organizations often have the responsibility of dispensing aid provided by donor nations. These groups frequently find themselves caught between the policy cracks left by differences between the donor and recipient governments. They sometimes are able to maintain a kind of autonomy, subverting the wishes of the donor and recipient polities. In other cases, they become coopted (from the perspective of others). Relief agencies operating in Ethiopia during the last famine have been accused by some of aiding and abetting the Ethiopian government's resettlement program. Critics have charged this very program prolonged the crisis instead of shortening it (Clay 1990).

A final consequence suggested by DeWaal (1989) is that relief agencies have created "famine tourism." Published accounts of disasters draw the attention of not only the public, but also public officials. Politically concerned government officials and others argue that it is useful to see first hand the nature and extent of a disaster of any type. These same individuals are no doubt aware that their visits will become part of the news, thus increasing their political capital. Famine victims may not complain about such self-serving behavior, but not all victims of disasters are necessarily the unempowered. For example, after the earthquake of 1993, Southern California residents reacted vociferously to numerous visits by hosts of Washington politicians. Many exclaimed when interviewed by the press that they wished that disaster relief would have arrived as quickly as the politicians.

An Emic Approach

The emic/etic approach was first developed by sociolinguist Kenneth Pike in 1947. Pike (1990) designed emics and etics to help distinguish between verbal and nonverbal behavior, respectively. Marvin Harris (1979) began an elaboration and reinterpretation of these terms from a materialist perspective. Although Pike and Harris continue to disagree over the interpretation and use of the approach (Headland 1990), and others have identified serious problems with some of Harris' logical developments (Oakes 1981), the Harris account remains useful. Harris (1979) distinguishes between emics, accounts expressed in the concepts used by the culture under study itself, and etics, accounts in the language of science. A necessary condition of the validity of emic accounts lies within the epistemology of the members of that culture. As Harris (1990) notes, this does not mean that these members would necessarily agree or even fully understand the account, for it was essentially generated for etic reasons. Furthermore, the use of emics is legitimate only to the degree to which it contributes to an etic explanation. A final point is necessary. Etics and emics are not simply synonyms for the object/ subjective dichotomy. A subjective account can meet etic criteria, so long as it adheres to scientific standards. Similarly, some emic accounts meet the standards of objectivity.

Those who make objectivist accounts of famine impose external criteria drawn from the perspective of their profession. In other words, they

prepare etic explanations. As DeWaal (1989) observes, famines are defined by outsiders. Those in the business of relief and/or development
view famines as moral crises whose victims' plight demands immediate
intervention. Others, whose world view begins with technology, define
the crisis in technological terms. Solutions involve the selection of the
proper technology, whether it be early warning systems, nutritional surveillance, food security systems, or logistics (DeWaal 1989:30). Academics define famines from the point of view of their training and
theoretical proclivities. Developmental economists argue that famines
occur only in underdeveloped societies and their banishment can come
only from development (Mellor and Gavian 1987). Others discuss the
consequences of famine and chronic malnutrition in terms of the loss of
human capital, while arguing that insulation from further famine can
result only from investments in such capital (Berg 1984). Sociologists and
other social scientists argue that famines reflect either distorted development, dependency in the world capitalist economy, or socialist dependency (Moon 1991; Varnis 1990; Watts 1991).

The subjectivist accounts ginned up by social constructionists largely
ignore the experiences of victims as well. The subjective experiences of
interest to them consist of what claimants say and do. But claimants
are frequently outsiders; and to the extent they are scientific, these
descriptions are etic or objectivist in nature. They may also be emic
from the standpoint of the claimants' culture. In this case, some of the
claimants are victims. Thus, for example, activists within the gay community and Randy Shilts, a gay reporter with AIDs, successfully created a "crisis" through both greater public awareness and fear as well
as increased National Institutes of Health funding for research on HIV
(Patton 1990). In the case of famine, survivors are not in a position
either culturally or politically to form Famine Victims Anonymous chapters, nor do they write books, appear on talk shows, or testify before
congressional committees.

While social constructionists tend to privilege none of the claims or
claimants, the emic approach elevates the accounts of participants under
study "to the status of ultimate judge of the adequacy of the observer's
descriptions and analyses. The test of the adequacy of emic analyses is
their ability to generate statements the native accepts as real, meaningful, or appropriate" (Harris 1979:32), although as mentioned earlier, the
native might to understand or agree with the purpose of having generated the account in the first place. Emic studies purposely ignore the
cannons of science, and thus for Harris (1979) provide an invalid basis
for understanding social behavior. He suggests, however, that the emic
approach is not necessarily invalid and that "it is possible to be objective
-i.e., scientific- about either emic or etic phenomena" (Harris 1979:35).

This suggests that a set of common famine experiences and meanings might be derived by non-natives as a second order exercise, after researchers gather accurate native accounts.

The academic literature contains a few emic accounts of famine such as Pitrim Sorokin's (1975) personal experiences of hunger in the early days after the founding of the Soviet Union. Anthropological accounts provide the closest approximation to famine accounts currently available. Hunger, malnutrition, and starvation result from increasing degrees of food insufficiency. Those who suffer from these conditions have differing experiences, many of which are conditioned socially and culturally. The definition of hunger varies from one culture to the next, as do explanations for its origins and expectations regarding its consequences. For example, hunger is considered a normal state of affairs among the Hausa of Niger; abnormality involves the inability to control both "literal and figurative" states of hunger (Schmoll 1993). Michael Young (1986:126) describes the Kalauna (Melanesia) definition of hunger as grounded in the experience of food shortages, but representing a "master symbol for all that is deficient, entropic, and anxiety-provoking in the culture." Hunger suggests a state incompatible with the moral basis of society, a state that leads to societal self-destruction. DeWaal (1989) effectively argues that for a number of cultures, the threat of famine lies in the potential destruction to a way of life, not in an increased death rate.

What makes DeWaal's (1989) discussion useful from an emic standpoint, however, is his discussion of the language of hunger and famine in the Sudan. He notes that the term for eating stands for a number of pleasures such as having money, power, or sex. Likewise, hunger stands for almost all types of suffering. Finally, famine is not a single term, but rather famines are given distinct names to reflect their event's particular circumstances. Thus, relatively mild famines are given names that indicate a shortage of grain. More serious famines are indicated by the names of wild foods consumed during food shortages. Finally, famines that render people destitute are considered the worst, for they result in a permanent loss of status in the community. Famines that involve loss of life do not fall into this indigenously constructed continuum. DeWaal (1989) argues that "famines that kill" reflect a qualitatively different phenomena that is beyond classification. Despite this, he argues that the Sudanese perceive the threat of destitution greater than the threat of death.

Devereux (1993) also provides a number of examples of what famine means to local populations. He quite correctly apprehends the difficulties these additional points of view create for those attempting to provide a serviceable definition of famine. Devereux uncovers a further problem: if famine cannot be defined, then how do we know when one is occurring so that we may intervene? The next step is to develop a classification scheme that denotes the varying types of famine by criteria that has cross-cultural relevance. Work along these lines has already occurred.

The theme of "loss of way of life" appears in a variety of emic and etic accounts of community problems. Several sets of meanings seem to underlie this notion. One is the breakdown of the very moral economy said to represent the mechanism that ensures survival during hard times. Scott (1976) and others have argued that peasant societies develop informal social mechanisms that serve as institutions of welfare during hard times. These include social exchanges with extended kin and involvement in patron–client relationships. As Vaughan (1987) suggests, peasants are reluctant to invoke these obligations, for they leave the requester open to social opprobrium. At the same time, under dire circumstances sufferers call forth these obligations. And both Hanks (1962) and Wolf (1969) have observed that as scarcity reaches crisis proportions, kin and patrons have difficulties in meeting their obligations to others. Other observers such as DeWaal (1989) and Webb et al. (1992) argue either directly or indirectly that peasant concerns center on loss of economic and social status within the community. Eating wild foods may ensure physical survival, but the participant pays the price of permanent marginality within the community, much as persons living in the United States who "dumpster dive" (climb into large trash containers) searching for food were they to be observed by family or friends. During times of food deprivation, peasants enact a variety of strategies; these begin with the drawing down of resources set aside for just such an emergency. Once these resources have been depleted, meals are foregone and famine foods are adopted. The family may next sell household goods including kitchenware, furniture, and clothing; once these are gone, productive resources come up for sale (Webb et al. 1992). A certain stigma generally attaches to activities such as eating grass or rats to supplement the family's food supply or selling consumptive and productive assets. The sale of the latter entails not only social disapproval, but a real decline in living standards. The release of the family's hard-earned productive resources represents downward social mobility. Eating wild foods may ensure physical survival, but it also promises what perhaps constitutes a permanent loss of status in the community. Dumpster diving by residents of large cities may afford a certain anonymity unavailable to those in small towns and villages in which identities of most are well-known and gossip serves as a primary means of social control.

The apparent fact that hunger, famine, and malnutrition are differentially defined across cultures should alert us not only to problems of studying these cultures using standard Western notions of these experiences, but also to problems associated with interventions. Agencies that should know better frequently engage in rapid intervention of a charitable nature because of the "crisis" famine represents. The crisis becomes an excuse for ignoring grassroots and bottom-up efforts at dealing with local problems.

It is clear from European history that catastrophes were interpreted in terms of the dominant symbols of the time and placed events such as the plague within the context of the "wrath of God" (Herzlich and Pierret 1987:13). Solutions were found through acts of penitence, offerings, pilgrimages, and invocation of protective saints; famines and other disasters that visited European societies evoked organized acts of charity. Gallant (1991), Garnsey (1990), Yates (1990), Post (1985), and Lindberg (1993) all documented various communal institutions of charity established in ancient Greece, Rome, and China and in Europe during the Middle Ages. What is missing from famine accounts are such actions. Rau (1991) provides evidence that in a number of African countries, villagers have founded development associations and public spirited urban dwellers have founded relief organizations. Few details regarding their operation and effectiveness are available. Emic accounts would be useful here for they would begin to give us an idea of what charity means to both givers and receivers within different cultural settings.

Objectivism Reconsidered

Problems with existing data, differing definitions of hunger, famine, and even malnutrition, and the self-interestedness of organizations whose continued existence depends on these states of affairs should not blind us to the reality of malnutrition. The basis for this claim resides in what is known as the basic needs approach. This perspective argues that certain basic needs exist that require fulfilling for sheer human survival. These needs are biologically given and are thus independent of cultural context or social definition (Dasgupta 1993; Moon 1991). Some attempt to bolster this argument by stating that all known religious and moral philosophies consider charity, to meet the basic needs of those so deprived, a moral imperative (Moon 1991).

Doyal and Gough (1991) and Dreze and Sen (1989) take the more Kantian position that to be human is more than simply to survive, but rather to have the capacity for action and responsibility. To do so the body as well as the mind must be physically capable or competent. As previously mentioned, early work by social scientists on malnutrition and functioning focused on role competence, which includes a constellation of both physical and mental capabilities. This perspective is quite consistent with that of the neo-Kantian.

The problem with the so-called adaptive approach, which permits the view that one person's starvation is another person's acceptable level under the circumstances, is that it permits absolute deprivation. Furthermore, because the adaptive approach permits suboptimal functioning from an absolute standards point of view, it may also consign whole populations to continued poverty and deprivation if a greater than suboptimal level of output in either the classroom or the workplace is needed for persons to take advantage of new opportunities. This adaptive approach does not argue that societal improvements result solely from elevated human capital, but it does embrace the premise that development is not possible without such investments. And without such efforts, resource disparities will likely grow rather than diminish, even in the face of development.

Conclusions

I find no great utility in arguing for the position that there exists only one correct way to study social problems such as famines. The objectivist or etic account has its weaknesses, as discussed previously. Measurement of any condition in essentially imperfect. A certain amount of error will always be present and perfect agreement among objective observers is likely a chimera. Thus, objectivist studies of nutritional conditions will always fall short of perfection. Despite its shortcomings, objectivism can provide the means for a general understanding of hunger, malnutrition, and famine. And many of its problems are not insurmountable. They are not simply different constructions with no hope of resolution. Progress is possible in the area of adequacy of measurement and data on nutritional status will become available for an increasing number of countries as resource constraints are alleviated. I thus tend to privilege the etic point of view. Like Horton (1982), I accept the notion that all cultures desire explanation, prediction, and control over events in their lives, but that the objectivist or etic approach has the best record of achievement in this regard. Having established this, objectivist accounts possess the additional handicap of ignoring the subjective experience of those in particular conditions, partly because it is believed that objective measures of subjective experiences are not feasible and thus are beyond the realm of science. Some social constructionists go so far to as to argue that the objectivist account represents merely the claims made by individuals either in positions of authority or with the power to persuade. This perspective provides a means for a reflexive examination of the problematic and forces a reconsideration of what is truly problematic. It may also lead to the identification of problems that have previously been overlooked. The constructionist evaluation suggests that if what are considered problems depends largely on their promotion as such by interested actors, then there may exist a whole host of troubles yet to be so identified. In other words, there may be problems without champions. The disadvantage associated with adhering to a strict constructionist account is that it encourages us to take seriously only those problems for which champions have stepped forward. It would appear more sensible to consider the constructionist critique as a tool by which problems could be distinguished by the degree to which a broad consensus is possible and those for which such consensus is not. In addition, this approach reminds us that the attention given to social problems is, in part, a function of the power possessed by groups that have aligned themselves both for and against the problem. And finally, the emic account provides the victims' point of view. Without this perspective, a full accounting of deprivation is not possible. The emic approach has the potential for generating whole new taxonomies of famine experiences that can serve as a source for a more universal etic classification of such experiences. And without the emic-based etic approach, many efforts at both short- and long-term relief will fall short of success.

References

Adam, H. M. 1993. "Building Capacity in the Countryside: The Role of Sahelian Voluntary Development Organizations." Pp. 172–204 in *The Challenge of Famine: Recent Experiences, Lessoned Learned*, edited by J. O. Field. West Hartford, CT: Kumarian Press.

Allan, L. H. 1993. "The Nutrition CRSP: What Is Marginal Malnutrition, and Does It Affect Human Function?" *Nutrition Reviews* 51(9):255–267.

Appleby, A. B. 1978. *Famine in Tudor and Stuart England*. Stanford: Stanford University Press.

Arnold, D. 1988. *Famine: Social Crisis and Historical Change*. New York: Cambridge University Press.

Bartholet, J. 1992. "Battlefields of the Food War." *Newsweek* 120 (Dec. 14):36–37.

Beigbeder, Y. 1991. *The Role and Status of International Humanitarian Volunteers and Organizations: The Right and Duty to Humanitarian Assistance*. Dordrecht: Martinus Nijhoff.

Belasco, W. J. 1993. *Appetite for Change: How the Counterculture Took on the Food Industry*. Ithaca, NY: Cornell University Press.

Bennoune, M. 1992. "The Causes and Consequences of Famine in the Third World." Pp. 227–267 in *Civilization in Crisis: Anthropological Prospectives*, edited by C. W. Gaily. Gainesville: University of Florida Press.

Berg, A. 1973. *The Nutrition Factor: Its Role in National Development*. Washington, D.C.: Brookings Institute.

Best, J. (ed.). 1989. *Images of Issues: Typifying Contemporary Social Problems*. Hawthorne, NY: Aldine de Gruyter.

Boyer, P. J. 1985. "Famine in Ethiopia: The T.V. Accident That Exploded." *Washington Journalism Review* January: 19–21.

Bradshaw, Y. W., R. Noonan, L. Gash, and C. B. Sershen. 1993. "Borrowing Aainst the Future: Children and Third World Indebtedness." *Social Forces* 71(3):629–656.

Brown, J. L., and S. T. Pitzer. 1989. "The Paradox of Hunger and Economic Prosperity in America." *Journal of Public Health Policy* 10 (Winter):425–441.

Chapman, M. 1990. "The Social Definition of Want." Pp. 26–33 in *Food in Humanity: Cross-Disciplinary Readings*, edited by M. Chapman and H. Macketts. Oxford: Oxford Centre for the Sciences of Food and Nutrition.

Charney, J. R. 1993. "Coping with Crisis: Oxfam America's Disaster Responses." Pp. 147–171 in *The Challenge of Famine Recent Experience, Lessons Learned*, edited by J. O. Field. West Hartford: Kumarian Press.

Clay, J. W. 1989. "Ethiopia Famine and Relief Agencies." Pp. 232–277 in *The Moral Nation: Humanitarian and U.S. Foreign Policy Today*, edited by B. Nichols and G. Loescher. Notre Dame: University of Notre Dame Press.

Cook, R. 1972. "The Primary Costs of Malnutrition and Its Impacts on Society." Pp. 324–327 in *Proceedings of the 3rd Western Hemisphere Nutrition Congress*. San Diego: Western Hemisphere Nutrition Conference.

Cowley, G. 1993. "A Plague of Global Dimensions." *Newsweek* 121 (January 11):56–59.

Dasgupta, P. 1993. *An Inquiry into Well-Being and Destitution*. New York: Clarendon Press.

Deng, F., and L. Minear. 1992. *The Challenges of Famine Relief: Emergency Operations in the Sudan*. Washington, D. C.: Brookings Institute.

Devereux, S. 1993. *Theories of Famine*. New York: Harvester Wheatsheaf.

DeWaal, A. 1989. *Famine That Kills: Dabur, Sudan, 1984–1985*. New York: Oxford University Press.

Doyal, L., and I. Gough. 1991. *A Theory of Human Need*. New York: Guilford Press.

Dreze, S., and A. Sen. 1989. *Hunger and Public Action*. New York: Oxford University Press.

Egan, E. 1982. "Response to Famine: The Role of the Voluntary Sector." Pp. 123–140 in *Famine*, edited by K. M. Cahill. Mary Knoll, NY: Orbis Books.

Evers, S. and W.A. McIntosh. 1977. "Social Indicators of Human Nutrition." *Social Indicators Research* 4:185–205.

Floud, R. 1992. "Anthropometric Measures of Nutritional Status in Industrialized Societies. Europe and North America Since 1750." Pp. 219–241 in *Nutrition and Poverty*, edited by S. R. Osmani. New York: Clarendon Press.

Fogel, R. 1992. "Second Thoughts on the European Escape from Hunger: Famines, Chronic Malnutrition, and Mortality Rates." Pp. 243–286 in *Nutrition and Poverty*, edited by S. R. Osmani. New York: Clarendon Press.

Gallant, T. W. 1991. *Risk and Survival in Ancient Greece*. Stanford: Stanford University Press.

Gans, H. J. 1976. *Deciding What's News: A Study of CBS Evening News, NBC Nightly News, Newsweek, and Time*. New York: Pantheon Books.

Garnsey, P. 1990. "Response to Food Crisis in the Ancient Mediterranian World." Pp. 126–146 in *Hunger in History: Food Shortage, Poverty, and Deprivation*, edited by L. F. Newman. Cambridge: Bant Blackwell.

Grant, J. P. 1991. *The State of the World's Children*. New York: Oxford University Press.

Hanks, L. 1962. "Merit and Power in the Thai Social Order." *American Anthropologist* 64(December): 1247–1261.

Harris, M. 1979. *Cultural Materialism: The Struggle for a Science of Culture*. New York: Random House.

―――. 1990. "Harris' Final Response." Pp. 202–216 in *Emics and Etics: The Insider/Outsider Debate*, edited by T. N. Headland, K. L. Pike, and M. Harris. Newbury Park, CA: Sage.

Harrison, P., and R. Palmer 1986. *News Out of Africa: Biafra to Band Aid*. London: Hilary Shipman.

Headland, T. N. 1990. "Introduction: A Dialogue between Kenneth Pike and Marvin Harris on Emics and Etics." Pp. 13–27 in *Emics and Etics: The Insider/Outsider Debate*, edited by T. N. Healand, K. L. Pike, and M. Harris. Newbury Park, CA: Sage.

Hertzlich, C., and J. Pierret. 1987. *Illness and Self in Society*. Baltimore: Johns Hopkins University Press.

Horton, R. 1982. "Tradition and Modernity Revisited." Pp. 201–260 in *Rationality and Relativism*. edited by M. Hollis and S. Lukes. Cambridge: MIT Press.

International Food Policy Research Institute. no date. *International Food Policy Institute*. Washington, D. C.

Kallen, D. J. 1973. "Nutrition in the Community." Pp. 33–50 in *Nutrition, Development, and Social Behavior*, edited by D. Kallen. Washington, D. C.: National Institutes of Health, U.S. Department of Health, Education, and Welfare.

Keys, A. J. Brozek, A. Henschel, O. Micklesen, and H. L. Taylor. 1950. *The Biology of Human Starvation Vol. II*. Minneapolis: University of Minnesota Press.

Knowles, L. L. 1984. *A Guide to World Hunger Organizations: Who They Are and What You Should Know About Them*. Decatur, IL: Seeds/Alternatives.

Laslett, P. 1965. *The World We Have Lost*. New York: Charles Scribner's Sons.

Levenstein, H. 1993. *Paradox of Plenty: A Social History of Eating in America*. New York: Oxford University Press.

Levin, H. M., E. Pollitt, R. Galloway, and J. McGuire. 1993. "Micronutrient Deficiency Disorders." Pp. 421–454 in *Disease Control Priorities in Developing Countries*, edited by D. T. Jamison, W. H. Mosley, A. R. Measham, and J. L. Bobadilla. New York: Oxford University Press.

Lewis, J. 1984. "Decoding Television News." Pp. 205–234 in *Television in Transition: Papers from the International Television Studies Conference*, edited by P. Drummond and R. Patterson. London: British Film Institute.

Lindberg, C. 1993. *Beyond Charity: Reformation Initiatives for the Poor*. Minneapolis: Fortress Press.

Livi-Bacci, M. 1990. *Population and Nutrition: An Essay on European Demographic History*. New York: Cambridge University Press.

Loseke, D. R. 1989. "Violence is 'Violence' . . . or Is It? The Social Construction of 'Wife Abuse' and Public Policy." Pp. 191–206 in *Images of Issues: Typifying Contemporary Social Problems*, edited by J. Best. Hawthorn, NY: Aldine de Gruyter.

Loseke, D. R. 1993. "Constructing Conditions, People, Morality, and Emotion: Expanding the Agenda of Constructionism." Pp. 207–216 in *Constructionist Controversies: Issues in Social Problems Theory*, edited by G. Miller and J. A. Holstein. New York: Aldine de Gruyter.

McIntosh, W. A. 1995. *Sociologies of Food and Nutrition*. New York: Plenum (forthcoming).

McLaren, D.S. 1974. "The Great Protein Fiasco." *Lancet* 2(July 13): 93–96.

———. 1986. "Global Occurrence of Vitamin A Deficiency." Pp. 1–18 in *Vitamin A Deficiency and Its Control*, edited by J. C. Bauernfeind. Orlando: Academic Press.

Medler J. F., and M. J. Medler. 1993. "Media Images as Environmental Policy." Pp. 121–132 in *Media and Public Policy*, edited by R. J. Spitzer. Westport, CT: Praeger.

Mellor, J., and S. Gavian. 1987. "Famine: Causes, Prevention, and Relief." *Science* 235: 539–545.

Moon, B. E. 1991. *The Political Economy of Basic Human Needs*. Ithaca, NY: Cornell University Press.

Mosley, W. H., and P. Cowley. 1991. "The Challenge of World Health." *Population Bulletin* 46(4):1–39.

Oakes, G. 1981. "The Epistemological Foundations of Cultural Materialism." *Dialectical Anthropology* 6:1–21.

O'Hefferman, P. 1990. "Television and Crisis: Sobering Thousands on Sound Bites Seen 'Round the World." *Television Quarterly* 25:9–14.

Osmani, S. R. 1992. "On Some Controversies in the Measurement of Under-nutrition." Pp. 121–164 in *Nutrition and Poverty*, edited by S. R. Osmani. New York: Oxford University Press.

Palmieri, V. H. 1982. "Famine, Media, and Geo-Politics." Pp. 19–27 in *Famine*, edited by K. M. Cahill. Maryknoll, NY: Orbis Books.

Patton, C. 1990. *Inventing Aids*. New York: Routledge.

Payne, P. 1992. "Assessing Undernutrition: The Need for a Reconceptualization." Pp. 49–96 in *Nutrition and Poverty*, edited by S. R. Osmani. New York: Oxford University Press.

Pike, K. L. 1990. "On the Emics and Etics of Pike and Harris." Pp. 28–47 in *Emics and Etics: The Insider/Outsider Debate*, edited by T. N. Headland, K. L. Pike, and M. Harris. Newbury Park, CA: Sage.

Post, J. D. 1985. *Food Shortage, Climatic Variability, and Epidemic Disease in Preindustrial Europe: The Mortality Peak in the Early 1740's*. Ithaca, NY: Cornell University Press.

Ram, N. 1989. "An Independent Press and Anti-Hunger Strategies: The Indian Experience." Pp. 146–190 in *The Political Economy of Hunger, Vol. I*. New York: Oxford University Press.

Rau, B. 1991. *From Feast to Famine: Official Cures and Grassroots Remedies to Africa's Food Crisis*. Atlantic Highlands, NJ: Zed Books.

Ruttan, V. W. 1993. "Does Food Aid Have a Future?" Pp. 216–228 in *Why Food Aid?*, edited by V. W. Ruttan. Baltimore: John Hopkins University Press.

Schmoll, P. G. 1993. "Black Stomachs, Beautiful Stones: Soul-Eating Among Hausa in Niger." Pp. 193–220 in *Modernity and Its Postcolonial Africa*, edited by J. Comaroff and J. Comaroff. Chicago: University of Chicago Press.

Scott, J. C. 1976. *The Moral Economy of the Peasant: Rebellion and Subsistence in Southeast Asia*. New Haven, CT: Yale University Press.

Sorokin, P. A. 1975 [1922]. *Hunger as a Factor in Human Affairs*. Gainesville: University Presses of Florida.

Stevenson, J. 1993. "Hope Restored in Somalia?" *Foreign Affairs* (December):138–154.

Television News Index and Abstracts. 1992-1993. Nashville, TN: Vanderbilt Television Archives.

Varnis, S. L. 1990. *Reluctant Aid or Aiding the Reluctant: U.S. Food Aid Policy and Ethiopian Famine Relief*. New Brunswick, NJ: Transaction Publishers.

Vaughan, M. 1987. *The Story of an African Famine: Gender and Famines in Twentieth-Century Malawi*. New York: Cambridge University Press.

Walter, J., and R. Shofield. 1989. "Famine, Disease, and Crisis Mortality in Early Modern Society." Pp. 1–73 in *Famine, Disease, and the Social Order in Early Modern Society*, edited by J. Walter and R. Shofield. New York: Cambridge University Press.

Waterlow, J. C., and P. R. Payne. 1975. "The Protein Gap." *Nature (London)* 258:112–116.

Watts, M. 1991. "Heart of Darkness: Reflections on Famine and Starvation in Africa." Pp. 23–68 in *The Political Economy of African Famine*, edited by R.E. Downs, D. O. Kerner, and S. P. Reyna. Longhorne, NY: Gordon and Breach.

Webb, P., J. von Braun, and Y. Yohannes. 1992. *Famine in Ethiopia: Policy Implications of Copying Failure at National and Household Levels*. Washington, D. C.: International Food Policy Research Institute.

Whit, W. 1994. *Food and Society: A Sociological Approach*. Dix Hills, NY: General Hall (forthcoming).

Wolf, E. R. 1969. *Peasant Wars of the Twentieth Century*. New York: Harper & Row.

Wolman, K. 1991. "Africa: A Cry Unheeded." *World Food Program Journal* 17:2–4.

World Bank. 1993. *World Development Report 1993: Investing in Health*. New York: Oxford University Press.

World Health Organization. 1990. *Global Estimates for Health Situation Assessment and Projections*. Geneva: WHO.

Yates, R. D. S. 1990. "War, Food Shortages, and Relief Measures in Early China." Pp. 147–177 in *Hunger in History: Food Shortages, Poverty, and Deprivation*, edited by L. F. Newman, W. Crossgrove, R. W. Kates, R. Matthews, and S. Millman. Cambridge: Basil Blackwell.

Young, M. W. 1986. "'The Worst Disease': The Cultural Definition of Hunger in Kalauna." Pp. 111–126 in *Shared Wealth and Symbol: Food, Culture, and Society in Oceana and Southeast Asia*, edited by L. Manderson. New York: Cambridge University Press.

Zetterberg, H. 1965. *On Theory and Verification in Sociology*, 3rd ed. Totowa, NJ: Bedminster Press.

III

Avoiding Excessive Food Intake

4

The Medicalization and Demedicalization of Obesity

JEFFERY SOBAL

Introduction

People in contemporary Western societies tend to regard those who are fat as deviant. Judgments about deviance, however, are relative and vary between historical eras and across cultures and subcultures. Most people in the past and the majority of people currently living in traditional cultures consider fatness to be a sign of health and wealth. Present day ballerinas tend to think they are too fat, but Sumo wrestlers rarely think they are too heavy. In modern societies people reject fatness and see it as a major concern, while thinness has become a valued condition that people actively strive to achieve.

When people recognize deviant conditions in society as social problems, they may apply several models of social control to define and deal with those problems. This involves a process of typification that focuses on one aspect of a problem to characterize its nature (Best 1989). Typification can include claims that the problem is best dealt with using moral models, medical models, or political models each of which provides different perspectives about the cause and solution of the problem (Best 1989).

During this century fatness has moved from a moral conception of fat as badness, to the medicalization of obesity as sickness, to the demedicalization of large body size as politically acceptable. This analysis will examine changes in these three conceptions using a constructionist social problems perspective (Blumer 1971; Schneider 1985; Schneider and Kitsuse 1984; Spector and Kitsuse 1987) that examines evaluations of body fat as socially constructed judgments negotiated by several groups in society. Concepts from the social problems and medicalization literature will be used to explain shifting social control over fatness, using examples drawn from the mass media, public and professional literature, and observation in medical and public settings. The focus will be on the medicalization and demedicalization processes, rather than on the social context and natural history of obesity as a social problem. Previous authors have noted that obesity has been medicalized, but have not yet considered the topic in depth (Conrad 1992; Conrad and Schneider 1992; Reissman 1983).

The Rise of the Moral Model of Fatness as Badness

In past historical eras people valued body fat and saw it as a sign of health and wealth (Beller 1977; Brown 1993). Fat stores provided calories in times of uncertain food supplies and protected health against the ravages of infectious disease parasites (Beller 1977). In 85% of traditional cultures for which data exist, a plump body is viewed as desirable (Brown and Konner 1987). Very high levels of body fat in most traditional societies can be attained only by higher socioeconomic groups whose resources provide them with greater access to food and protect them from high levels of energy expenditure (Sobal and Stunkard 1989).

The agricultural and industrial revolutions assured more regular food resources and set the stage for regarding high levels of fatness as an unfavorable condition. The social status relationship for modern societies is expressed in the statement by the Duchess of Windsor that "You can never be too rich or too thin" (Sobal 1991a). In other words, thinness became valued and associated with membership in high social status groups, with a rising emphasis on the value of slimness by the 1920s (Levenstein 1988).

Since the 1950s, shifting social values in the United States have increasingly emphasized the negative social evaluation of fatness (Levenstein 1993). Ideals of female beauty have become based on increasing thinness (Garfinkle and Garner 1980; Wiseman et al. 1992). The rejection of fatness became very powerful. As values supporting slimness began to dominate popular thought, extreme fear of fatness, eating disorders such as anorexia nervosa and bulimia, and exercise addictions emerged (Nichter and Nichter 1991).

Social values abhorring fatness led to frequent stigmatization of the obese. Stigmatization is grounded in the notion that fatness is morally bad and fat people are weak and have no will power (Allon 1973; Kalish 1972; Cahnman 1968; Maddox and Liederman 1969; Tobias and Gordon 1980; Sobal 1991b). Responsibility for being fat was attributed to the fat person (Maddox et al. 1968), emphasizing moral models of fatness as a sin or a crime (Allon 1973). Along with social stigmatization came overt discrimination against the obese in education (Canning and Mayer 1966), rental housing (Karris 1977), employment (Larkin and Pines 1979), marriage (Sobal 1984a), and other arenas of life.

Thus fat had shifted from being evaluated as good and healthy in traditional societies to being seen as being bad, sinful, and ugly. This provided the basis for the moral model of fatness, which suggests that fat people are responsible for their condition and should be punished as a means of social control for being fat.

Medicalization of Obesity as Sickness

Fatness was not viewed as a very serious social problem by the majority of society. Medical claims that obesity was unhealthy had been made for many centuries (Bray 1990). The medicalization of obesity took off in the 1950s with widespread claims that obesity is best dealt with using medical interventions (Levenstein 1993). Best selling popular books such as Wyden's (1965) *The Overweight Society* attracted attention to obesity as a problem. The medical profession viewed success in dealing with obesity as a dismal prospect. "Most obese persons will not enter treatment for obesity. Of those who enter treatment, most will not lose weight, and of those who lose weight, most will regain it" (Stunkard and McClaren-Hume 1958). This call to action for medical science to rectify the situation sparked an intensity of medical involvement with weight that rose dramatically in the 1960s and 1970s (Reissman 1983).

Medicalization is a process by which nonmedical problems become defined and treated as medical problems, usually in terms of diseases or disorders (Conrad 1992). Medicalization of obesity occurred as medical people and their allies made increasingly frequent, powerful, and persuasive claims that they should exercise social control over fatness in contemporary society. Claims supporting medicalization occurred in many forms: naming, defining obesity as a disease, organizational activities, and applications of medical treatments. Claimsmaking about medicalization occurs in many different forums: professional journals, official reports, formation of specialty organizations, development of special clinics or services, organization of hearings and conferences, and statements in the mass media.

Naming: Popularizing the Term "Obesity."   Changing the name of a condition is part of the process of medicalization, with language helping to shift perceptions from badness to sickness (Goode 1969). Use of new labels is not simply euphemism, but instead signifies underlying value shifts. The emergence and use of labels operates to redefine a condition and shape how it is dealt with. Earlier terms for high levels of body fat tended to be derogatory and cast fatness as badness: fat, corpulent, porky, paunchy, plump, chubby, and many others. By contrast, current medical terms portray obesity as sickness using more value neutral and scientifically sounding argot: obese, adipose, and overweight, as did an earlier generation of terms such as pinguedinis and polycsarcia, which physicians later abandoned (Bray 1990). Increasing acceptance of the use of the term "obesity" evoked the prestige of the medical profession (Conrad and Schneider 1992).

Since 1900, the *Readers Guide to Periodical Literature* included both the medical term "obesity" and the moral term "corpulence" as the two primary headings for listings of articles about fatness and body weight (Zada 1977). Prior to 1976–1977, corpulence was the main indexing term, with obesity carrying the footnote: "see corpulence." From 1977 to 1978 onward, obesity was the main term, with corpulence maintained as a term only to refer to obesity for the actual listing of articles. The pattern of usage in the article titles also followed this trend, with the use of corpulence declining and that of obesity rising, indicating a medicalization of fatness in published works.

Language for the two immediate inputs into body weight was also medicalized as the medical community promulgated their terms beyond the clinic and laboratory. High levels of eating moved from gluttony, gorging, and overeating to acoria, polyphagia, or hyperorexia and the designation of binge eating disorders such as bulimia. Low activity level was reframed from sloth, laziness, loafing, dallying, or dawdling to chronic fatigue syndrome, lethargy, and listlessness. Portrayal of the condition itself as well as its immediate causes was medicalized away from personal blame and into a more scientifically neutral portrayal as a condition of illness.

The degree of medicalization is related to the extensiveness of the medical category involved (Conrad 1992). Expansion of categories makes them more inclusive to support more powerful claims about medicalization. The scientific literature and medical practitioners broadened terminology about obesity to include weight disorders, eating disorders, and metabolic disorders. For example, the name of the *International Journal of Obesity* was modified to add the subtitle *And Metabolic Disorders* (Stock 1992). Such expansions involve larger constituencies of medical professionals and lay claim to more extensive audiences of potential patients, making medicalization more pervasive.

Defining Obesity as a Disease.   To successfully medicalize obesity, fatness had to be designated and officially recognized as a disease. Claims that a condition is a disease beyond someone's control permits taking the problem out of the moral realm and putting it under medical responsibility. Underpinning a disease designation is the application of one or more of the various medical models to a condition. Obesity has been fit into several of the variety of available medical models, including genetic deviance (Bouchard 1994; Mayer 1965), endocrinological disturbance (Hoebel and Hernandez 1993), the agent/host/environment conceptualization of epidemiology (Nordsiek 1966), personality disorders (Bruch 1973), and addictions/substance abuse models of psychology (Wilson 1991; Wooley and Wooley 1981). Many medical models exist simultaneously, and the application of each to obesity has its champions.

The presence of a multitude of models for obesity is a double-edged sword for promoting medicalization. Availability of multiple perspectives permits claimsmaking about the medical basis of obesity on many fronts and mobilizes a diversity of health care professionals. Multiple models also provide the ready presence of alternatives to refute publicity for research opposing one particular model. However, the very existence of many models weakens claims based on any given model because so many interpretations, and claims, exist within the medical community about obesity.

The various health professions within the medical community have successfully negotiated a disease designation for obesity that is listed in the *International Classifications of Diseases* (ICD-9-CM 1990). This provided an official sanction of the disease status of obesity. In addition to the idea of conditions being diseases in themselves, the concept of "risk factors" was developed and widely disseminated in the 1970s (Califano 1979). The medical community promoted the concept that obesity was a risk factor for cardiovascular disease, medicalizing obesity as a contributor to the leading cause of death in the United States.

Setting cutoffs for initiating treatment for obesity has been controversial. The most widely promulgated standards are the Metropolitan Life Insurance Company Tables of Ideal Body Weights first published in 1959. The insurance company revised its acceptable body weights upward in 1983 and again in 1990 when they modified the table for the Dietary Recommendations of the U. S. Department of Agriculture. This narrowing of the potential audience for obesity interventions brought some protests by health professionals (Callaway 1984). In the meantime, researchers have challenged the need to attain "normal" body weight to achieve health benefits, claiming that moderate weight reduction in obese people can produce significant health improvement (Goldstein 1992).

Organizational Activities to Medicalize Obesity.   Medicalization typically involves only a small group of individuals and proceeds slowly, often by special organizations within medicine (Conrad and Schneider 1992). These organizations work to convince the public and other professionals that obesity is best dealt with as disease rather than deviance. They aggressively make claims to promote the benefits of slimness (focusing on health justifications more than aesthetic values) and their own ability to treat fatness. This can be seen in the formation of the American Society of Bariatric Physicians (founded in 1949). The Association for the Study of Obesity (1966) has affiliated North American and European Associations, with over 15 countries that also have branches of the group (Howard 1992). To publicize their claims about obesity to the larger medical community, they began to publish journals on obesity, including *Bariatric Medicine, International Journal of Obesity, Obesity Research,* and *Obesity and Metabolism.* These organizations hold professional conferences and training institutes on a regular basis to communicate among themselves, attract and socialize new converts, and publicize their messages on obesity by making public statements to the mass media. Professional events, such as the first International Congress on Obesity in 1974, drew attention to obesity as a problem and encouraged the application of medical models in dealing with obesity (Howard 1992).

Private medical organizations offer support and resources for the portions of the medical community involved in medicalizing obesity. However, medical organizations have limited public recognition. Medical organizations attain greater legitimacy and authority through linkages to official government bodies as forums to sanction medical claimsmaking about obesity. The National Institutes of Health (NIH) is the premier medical research authority in the United States, and offers a series of "Consensus Development Conferences" on various health issues that provide hearings, testimonials by experts, an official publication, and widespread media attention. The NIH chose obesity as a topic for a consensus conference in 1985, resulting in widespread claimsmaking about the role of obesity in health (Burton et al. 1985). A panel of 15 health professionals heard presentations by 19 invited experts, and stated that "In recent years, obesity has become a public health problem of considerable importance in the United States" (NIH 1985:1). Similar conferences occurred in the United Kingdom (Black et al. 1983) and additional government conferences about obesity followed that increased official support for the medicalization of obesity (Kopelman et al. 1994).

Application of Medical Treatments to Obesity. Medicine developed rapidly in the postwar era, and physicians applied existing medical treatments to new problems to reach wider audiences. As obese individuals sought medical treatment and health professionals underwent a division of labor in specialty formation, many existing medical procedures were applied to obesity. Attempts to transfer techniques from established areas of medicine to the problem of obesity occurred as medical professionals expanded their responsibility and jurisdiction for their procedures. This transfer of techniques can be divided into two general areas: technological interventions and psychobehavioral interventions.

Technology played a more important role in medicalizing obesity than in the medicalization of other forms of deviance such as alcoholism or delinquency (Conrad and Schneider 1992). Two forms of medical technology provided mechanical and chemical interventions: surgery and drugs.

Surgery for Obesity. Reissman (1983) suggests that an oversupply of surgeons generated demand for their services by applying their craft to obesity. An early form of eating control was jaw wiring, which required obese patients to subsist on only liquid diets. This procedure gave a physician (with the aid of a dentist) control over the eating of obese patients, producing dramatic weight loss and making physicians medical gatekeepers to the technique. Jaw wiring gained much attention in the mass media as promoting weight loss. However, once jaws were unwired there was typically recidivism back to obesity (Cegielski and Saporta 1978). Physicians lacked enthusiasm for jaw wiring, as evidenced by the relatively small number of publications in the medical literature about the topic (Drenick and Hargis 1978).

The lack of success with jaw wiring led surgeons to seek more lasting medical procedures to control obesity. Permanent surgical procedures that bypassed a part of the digestive process had been around for a long time, and were tried as a solution that allowed eating without the consequences of digestion and consequent fat storage. The intestinal bypass surgical technique was developed by Kremen et al. (1954), leading to the pioneering of jejunoileal bypass surgery for obesity by Payne and De-Wind (1969). In an intestinal bypass a surgeon removes a section of the intestine to prevent absorption of calories. Such surgery involved the highest status specialty of medicine in a dramatic (and hopefully permanent) treatment of deviant behavior that could be claimed as a medical solution. However, a number of complications result from intestinal bypass surgery, including diarrhea, malnutrition, liver disease, renal failure, and arthritis (Bray 1980). The intestinal bypass as a treatment for obesity peaked in the 1970s with published reports on over 10,000 cases by 1980 (Hocking et al. 1983; Joffe 1981). However, the technique lost favor as these side effects received increasing attention, and publicity about the problems associated with the procedure published in prestigious medical journals led to a decline in its use (Hocking et al. 1983).

Mason and Ito (1967) developed the gastric bypass as another surgical solution to obesity. Gastric bypass surgery reduced the size of the stomach to limit the amount of food it would hold (Halmi 1980), avoiding some of the problems of the intestinal bypass while continuing the predominance of surgical intervention as the absolute treatment of chronic obesity problems. As with other surgical means to deal with obesity, the gastric bypass proved to have a number of complications and also has fallen into less use by the medical profession. Physicians have developed few surgical procedures to medicalize other forms of deviance, with the exception of the lobotomy for mental illness. Interest in surgery for the treatment of obesity rose until the late 1970s and then declined (Reissman 1983).

European surgeons developed the surgical technique of suction lipectomy (popularly called "liposuction") to remove fat stored on selected body sites, and it became popularly applied in the United States (Fuerst 1983; *Medical World News* 1983). Such cosmetic surgical treatments are morally ambiguous. Like other forms of plastic surgery, liposuction uses medical technology but deals with appearance rather than disease and does not attach a sickness label to the patient.

Drug Therapy for Weight Loss. Drug therapy is another form of technological intervention applied to exert medical social control over obesity. Drugs had successfully medicalized several other forms of deviance, such as mental illness and hyperactivity (Conrad 1975), and the pharmaceutical revolution in the medical professions (Conrad 1992) paved the way for the application of drug treatment to obesity. Development of pharmaceutical solutions for obesity expanded the applicability of medical treatments more widely than the relatively narrow and heroic social control available through surgery. Drug treatment for obesity opened medicalization to the broader public by expanding the eligible patient population to people who were only slightly as well as extremely fat. Several types of drugs were developed to control obesity, with some of questionable value and some that have negative side effects (Bray 1974; Lasagna 1980). Hypermetabolic drugs increased energy expenditure, expending calories that had already been ingested. Appetite controlling drugs diminished hunger or made foods less tasty, decreasing energy intake. Laxatives and diuretics decrease body weight by increasing excretions, but do not decrease body fat levels. Physicians became gatekeepers for pharmaceutical treatments for obesity using prescription drugs, and medicalization was expanded further by offering over-the-counter drugs as medical means to control fatness.

Psychobehavioral Interventions: Psychiatry and Behavior Modification. As medicine expanded in the postwar era, medical authority increasingly extended into the behavioral realm. This trend was evident in the medicalization of obesity in the application of psychiatric and psychological treatments for weight and eating behaviors.

Psychiatry grew rapidly in the twentieth century, and its application to a number of phenomena enhanced their medicalization. Bruch (1957, 1973) pioneered the study of personality and developmental problems of obese individuals. She used psychotherapy to treat obesity, and described cases of success with that treatment. Others followed the psychotherapeutic path (Crisp 1978), making claims to the public that encouraged them to seek psychiatric treatment for their fatness and treat it as a medical rather than moral problem. Portraying eating as a compulsive urge contributed to the medicalization of obesity by shifting the control of eating from being conscious (and therefore good or bad) to being unconscious (and therefore sick or healthy). The application of psychotherapy as a tool for obesity paralleled its popularity in the wider society, but soon psychotherapy passed out of psychiatric fashion and so did its use for obesity. Use of hypnosis for weight loss was given some attention (Joaquin 1977), but suffered a similar fate of interest and decline.

Other psychologists and psychiatrists have claimed that overeating occurs because people have maladaptive personalities. Schacter (1968, 1971) distinguished between "internal" people who ate only when hungry, and "external" people who ate whenever they saw food. Gluttons became binge eaters and midnight snackers had the "night eating syndrome" (Stunkard 1976).

Like the application of technological procedures to obesity, claims about psychiatric or personality disorders as causes of obesity provide medical professionals with legitimated authority as exclusive gatekeepers for dealing with obesity. Medicalizing obesity by expanding existing psychiatric and psychological theories and procedures creates a monopoly for the source of treatment for obesity.

Behavior therapy provided another application of psychological perspectives to obesity, using another paradigm for psychologists to make claims about medicalization. The behaviorist tradition in psychology has led to the development of the therapeutic procedure of behavior modification. Behavior modification is applied to many other forms of deviance in our society such as mental illness and alcoholism, and was soon extended to obesity in a landmark report of dramatic weight loss by Stuart (1967). Psychologists use behavior modification to change eating habits (Stuart and Davis 1976; Wilson 1980), and it has become a mainstay of treatment of obesity under the medical model. Behavior modification has medicalized eating, and puts people into an extended patient role whenever they are involved with food. On a parallel path with behavior modification is the application of the addiction model, which sees overeating as substance abuse and typically applies behavioral techniques as therapy.

The Medicalization of Dieting.   Most people see changes in eating as the primary way to deal with obesity. The practice of dieting for weight loss has been institutionalized in our society (Schwartz 1986; Seid 1989). Dieting has tended to be more in the realm of popular culture rather than medical practice, although this mix is shifting as medical claims about dieting are more widely made and accepted.

Earlier forms of dieting consisted primarily of restricting the amount of food eaten. Later, the food and pharmaceutical industries developed specialized products and medically supervised regimens for weight loss. Products made "scientifically" for dieting began to gain popularity, as seen in the introduction of "Metrical" in 1959 (Wyden 1965). These drug-like products soon became widely accepted and used. Weight loss products and specially constituted foods support the general medical model of obesity even though they are typically self-prescribed and used without medical supervision. While people who take diet products may not be under the direct control of physicians, these people do enter a patient-like sick role (Twaddle 1981) and approach weight loss using a medical model. Physician-sanctioned diet books (Solomon and Sheppard 1972; Stillman and Baker 1967) extend medical authority over weight control to a larger public than could be done by personal visits to physicians. The major trends in dieting have been toward medicalization, beginning with the medicalization of eating, moving through the development of specially formulated foods, and including medical supervision or prescription of what is eaten.

Weight Loss Organizations and the Medicalization of Obesity.   Dieting organizations have exploded in popularity since the 1960s (Stuart and Mitchell 1980) and they now constitute a 30 billion dollar industry (Berg 1992). The largest and most successful has been Weight Watchers, which was founded in 1963 by Jean Nidetch (1972), a housewife, and has been followed by numerous others. Most weight loss organizations were established by nonmedical groups, but they have moved toward the application of medical models in their treatment of obesity. The medicalization of dieting occurred with the entry of scientific medicine into what had now become a weight loss industry. Medicalization is directly related to profitability (Conrad and Schneider 1992), and people in the medical community quickly realized that the potential profit in terms of money and increased health is large in the field of organized weight loss. The medical community challenges weight loss organizations that deviate from accepted medical models, coopts the ones that are successful, and willingly gets coopted by organizations seeking medical prestige and support.

Weight loss organizations currently apply many regimens, some of which are medical and some of which are not. Calorie control has been the dominant modality, which is a basic nutritional concept grounded in a medical model. Some dietary restrictions have been extremely low calorie, high protein diets that are supervised by physicians. Calorie-restrictive diet organizations clearly operate to medicalize obesity. Weight loss organizations enthusiastically embraced behavior modification, which operates as a medicalized approach grounded in the application of psychological techniques and requires obese people to act like patients.

Other weight loss organizations apply moral rather than medical techniques. Overeaters Anonymous (OA) grew out of the success of Alcoholics Anonymous, emphasizing a spiritual perspective in its morally based twelve step plan to deal with obesity (Millman 1980). Overeaters Anonymous views fatness as a sin, with overeating confessions to the "congregation" at regular meetings. The medical addictions model underlies OA therapies (Wilson 1991). Other weight loss groups also include components of a moral approach, with some using the stigma of obesity as a tool for change (Laslett and Warren 1975) or emphasizing social support rather than medical procedures to cure obesity (Allon 1975).

The Medicalization Process in the Medical Community

The process of medicalization occurs unevenly in the medical community as specialties emerge and segments of medicine become involved, involves specific individuals as crusaders and experts, and operates as alliances are built between medical people and other professions. Each of these will be discussed here as they apply to the medicalization of fatness, and considered later as they operate in the demedicalization of obesity.

Emergence of the Medical Specialty of Bariatric Medicine. An important activity in medicalization is development and designation of medical specialists to deal with specific conditions. A small number of physicians interested in obesity organized themselves into the National Obesity Society in 1949 (Asher 1975a). The purpose and identity of the group vacillated over the decade as they attempted to position and legitimate themselves in the medical world. The name of the group was first changed to the National Glandular Society, then to the American College of Endocrinology and Nutrition, and then reverted back to the National Glandular Society (Asher 1975a). Dietz (1973) introduced the term Bariatrics, based on the Greek root "baros" (weight) and suffix "-trics" (cure). Later, the society became the American Society of Bariatrics, and finally the American Society of Bariatric Physicians (Asher 1975a).

Bariatric physicians were a marginalized group, subject to derogation and challenges as "fat doctors" by both the public and their medical colleagues. To gain professional respectability, the American Society of Bariatric Physicians wrote organizational bylaws, certified members with written and oral examinations, set standards of practice, produced newsletters, and held a series of semiannual meetings and continuing education conferences (Asher 1975a). The group gained some professional recognition within medicine by being first listed in the *Journal of the American Medical Association* as a medical specialty society in 1970 and later granted continuing medical education credits for their conferences by the American Medical Association. By 1972 they began to publish a professional journal, *Obesity & Bariatric Medicine* (Asher 1975b). However, bariatrics never has been strongly accepted within the medical community, with under 100 members during their first decade of existence and barely over 500 by their 25th anniversary. Even more importantly, health professionals who were at the forefront of public and medical work in the obesity arena did not ally themselves with the bariatric movement.

Segmental Medicalization of Obesity within the Medical Community. Conditions are medicalized by small segments of the medical system rather than by universal involvement (Conrad and Schneider 1992), but medicalization proceeds more easily if the entire medical community accepts the condition as a medical problem and acts on it as such. Preventive medicine and nutrition have low status in the world of physicians, and obesity is often ignored in medical education and medical practice. Despite the presence of obesity as one of the 10 most frequent diagnoses by family physicians who make the vast majority of patient contacts in the United States (Marsland et al. 1976), most physicians dislike dealing with the obese and treat them as bad and not necessarily sick (Maddox and Liederman 1969; Maiman and Wang 1979a). General practitioners are not strongly motivated or optimistic about treating obesity (Cade 1991; Price et al. 1987), while specialists in obesity exhibit much more confidence and optimism (Bray et al. 1992).

Reluctance of most physicians to apply the medical model to obesity slows medicalization not only within their own profession, but also in the allied areas that give support necessary for the full medicalization of obesity. For example, the insurance industry is reluctant to provide third party payment for treatment of obesity (ranging from surgical to psychological to exercise programs) partly because of the persistent resistance of the medical community to universally deal with it as a sickness rather than a badness.

Individual Roles in Medicalization: Crusaders and Experts.   Two roles are important for individuals involved in the medicalization process: crusaders and experts.

Crusaders lead the efforts to declare obesity a health problem within the medical domain that can be dealt with using medical interventions. Crusaders work to expand the jurisdiction of the medical model of obesity by seeking attention for the problem, mobilize resources to support medical claims, publicly and privately press medical claims, and work to counter opposing claims made under other models. Leaders in the field of obesity operate as crusaders to advance the acceptance and scope of medical models in science, medicine, and public opinion. Specific activities of crusaders include founding obesity organizations, organizing conferences, making statements to the press and colleagues to gain attention (Garrow 1981), and recruiting new physicians to work on obesity.

The expert is another important role in the medicalization process (Conrad 1992). Experts are invoked as authorities in making claims about obesity, with their support used to document claims and refute opposing claims. The role of expert is socially constructed based on acceptance of experts as knowledgeable and impartial, both of which can be fragile qualities at continual risk of being discredited. The social creation and credentialing of experts make them subject to adversarial techniques as their place is negotiated in the medicalization process. Experts often make claims about the exclusive medical competency to deal with obesity (and other nutritional issue), labeling other approaches as "fraud and quackery" (Short 1994). Physicians claim that medically supervised diets are more successful than those without medical supervision (Blackburn 1993). The American Medical Association's Council on Scientific Affairs has released statements about appropriate treatments for obesity that emphasize the necessity of physician monitoring of very low calorie diet regimens (AMA 1988).

Different experts are invoked by each model of obesity. Moral models may rely upon religious or traditional experts to make claims about fat people being sinful or bad. Medical models use scientific and clinical experts to promote claims about obese individuals being sick and in need of treatment. Shifts in the frequency and influence of experts are indicative of changes in the influence of models of obesity. For example, increased physician sponsorship of popular diets occurred with the rise in the medical model of obesity over moral models.

Vested Interests and Moral Entrepreneurs Involved in Medicalization. Individuals and groups beyond the medical community who advocate medicalization often have vested interests in portraying fatness as a social problem and applying a medical model to obesity. Some interests operate as "moral entrepreneurs" (Becker 1963; Conrad 1975) by advancing claims about obesity to serve their own agendas. A variety of groups have been involved in making claims about the negative attributes of fatness, each having benefits to gain in doing so (Reissman 1983).

The health care industry is at the center of medicalization, making claims about obesity as a problem and their ability to offer particular therapies as treatment for obesity. The pharmaceutical industry promotes thinness as being both beautiful and healthy in its advertising while encouraging people to become thin using medications. The fitness industry emerged as an important voice in promoting thinness and health, offering its services and equipment as routes to prevent and treat obesity in health clubs, spas, and recreational activities as well as in specific products such as Nordic Track ski machines. The food and food-service industries make claims about the value of health and slimness, and offer several product lines of costly weight-loss foods that have a high profit margin as one segment of the overall food market. The apparel industry traditionally promotes thinness using an aesthetic model, but portions of the industry also join the medical model bandwagon to promote fitness apparel sales. The fashion and beauty industry emphasizes slenderness and offers products to help women achieve thin ideals. A separate weight-loss industry has emerged as an independent force in claimsmaking about the importance of fatness as a problem and the use of a medical model, with its entire set of weight-loss services based on the success of such claims.

The insurance industry has carefully balanced claims about obesity as a medical problem. On one hand, the insurance industry has vigorously promoted the concept that overweight is a risk factor for disease. The insurance industry widely promoted the relationship of weight and longevity in its ubiquitous Ideal Body Weight tables. On the other hand, insurance claimsmaking has opposed the designation of obesity as a disease itself that would be included in reimbursements for obesity treatments and prevention.

Medicalization of obesity occurs as various interests jointly make claims to define fatness as sickness. Alliances and coalitions form among various interests to reinforce compatible claims, while other interests may operate independently. Nonmedical organizations often depend on definitions of obese individuals as sick to support the legitimacy of applying their treatments to obese people who enter the sick role and are seeking help that has been socially defined as competent (Twaddle 1981). Vested interests offering products and services to obese people expend a great deal of effort claiming and publicizing their competence to deal with medical aspects of obese people who are entering the role of patient.

The Demedicalization of Obesity

Because of the power of the medical profession and the medical model, demedicalization of obesity required an organized movement (Conrad 1992) and a shift to a different conceptualization of obesity. This movement to accept obesity began as a reaction to the moral model of fatness and its stigmatization and discrimination against fat people. However, the "medical metaphor is not value neutral" (Conrad and Schneider 1992) and the movement also was a reaction to the medical model of obesity. Sickness and disability carry their own stigma and create dependency on medical expertise under the sick role (Twaddle 1981). Advocates of the demedicalization of obesity sought a normalization of large body size as neither badness nor sickness. This led dissatisfied individuals to promote a politicization of obesity in opposition to medicalization. People who identified themselves as "size activists" attempted to politicize weight to demedicalize it, and used political strategies to achieve change. This led to the use of political models that focus on oppression rather than badness or sickness and seek restitution rather than punishment or treatment. Obese people and legal allies use political models in their claimsmaking, in contrast with the health experts used in promoting medical models.

Moral models of obesity continued to be applied by the majority of the public and medical professionals even as the application of medical models became increasingly prevalent. However, the societal context changed greatly in the United States in the postwar era. During the 1950s the rights revolution began to emerge, developing more fully in the 1960s and 1970s, and becoming institutionalized during the 1980s and 1990s. The rights movements (civil rights, womens' rights, elderly rights, and others) used specific tactics to challenge dominant social norms, including protests, formation of organizations, mobilization of victims, conferences, media appeals, legislation, and lawsuits (Baker 1982). These tools were used to make claims to advance their agendas, with a sharing of strategies between different causes.

Obesity was not exempt from the larger rights movement, and a number of individuals and groups attempted to reframe fatness as a political rather than a moral or medical issue. Individuals who were fat began to demand acceptance and use "rights" language to make their claims that weight was a political rather than medical issue. Following the lead of other minority groups, they adopted the concepts, language, strategies, and techniques and other civil rights movements. They claimed that fat people were a mistreated minority group exploited by the rest of society, which practiced fatism, weightism, and sizism under a widespread "Tyranny of Slenderness" (Chernin 1981). Political fat liberation, fat power, and fat pride claims began to be made in the 1960s. These movements promoted the acceptance of large people as normal, rather than bad or sick (Friedman 1974; Grossworth 1971; Louderback 1970; Schoenfielder and Weiser 1983).

Claimsmaking activities for demedicalization paralleled those of medicalization. Those seeking demedicalization renamed the attribute of being fat. Rather than fatness or obesity, neutral or positive terms are used to portray bigness as normal or good, including "large," "ample," and "of size." These labels emerged and were pressed into use to redefine obesity as a neutral condition that does not carry connotations of badness or sickness. As with medicalization, demedicalization also has extended the naming of categories to make more powerful claims by expanding fat acceptance into size acceptance. People involved in demedicalizing obesity have come to label themselves as the Size Acceptance Movement.

Organizations have emerged to play important roles in the demedicalization of obesity. NAAFA was first formed in 1969 as the National Association to Aid Fat Americans, and its focus was on supporting its members as individuals in a minority group. Later, it kept its acronym but changed its name to the National Association to Advance Fat Acceptance to reflect its larger goals of shifting societal treatment of large people away from moral and medical models. Other groups such as the Association for the Health Enrichment of Large Persons, Abundantly Yours, Council on Size and Weight Discrimination, Largesse, National Association of Full Figured Women, Ample Opportunity (Barron and Lear 1989), and the Diet/Weight Liberation Project (Garrison and Levitsky 1993) also emerged as part of the size acceptance movement.

Parallel to the medical journals for those who used a medical model for obesity, magazines such as *Radiance* and *Big Beautiful Woman* emerged to make positive and demedicalized portrayals of large people. An increasing number of articles emerged in the popular press about size discrimination, raising attention to political and legal models of weight in the public consciousness. A spate of books added to the literature, ranging from personal stories to calls to political action (Friedman 1974; Garrison and Levitsky 1993; Grossworth 1971; Louderback 1970).

Experts have been recruited from within the scientific community to assist claimsmaking for the demedicalization of obesity. Sometimes claimsmakers for demedicalization meet medical people on their own "turf" by using data and arguments within the medical model. These claims included statements minimizing the negative health effects of fatness (Ernesberger 1985; Erensberger and Haskew 1987) and focusing on the psychological harms of continued dieting (Wooley and Wooley 1984) in both the professional and popular literature. Other times demedicalization claims rely on a political paradigm, framing their arguments from a completely different perspective than medical claims. This involves experts on discrimination and stigmatization, sometimes using social scientists as experts (Allon 1973; Sobal 1984b).

An antidiet movement has emerged in opposition to the predominant medical model-based intervention for weight control (Bennett and Gurin 1982; Berg 1992; Kano 1989; Orbach 1978). This movement rejects dieting with a goal of weight loss and instead focuses on wellness and self-esteem. However, the antidiet movement differs from the size acceptance movement in that it continues to value slimness and accepts other medical models for obesity than dieting, focusing on exercise and psychological well being.

Litigation has been an important tool in making claims for demedicalization. A number of discrimination cases have been argued on the basis of fatness (Baker 1982; McEvoy 1992; Tucker 1979), with a key part of the deliberation being whether obesity was sickness or badness. The pressing of legal cases expressed the multiple claims about the phenomena of obesity as medical versus normal or criminal. Such cases have usually been decided in favor of the obese person, defining obesity as sickness rather than badness, as an undesired but medically treatable condition. Medical testimony in the trials put physicians into the role of gatekeepers for obese people, helping to medicalize obesity. Social control over the obese has been debated in the courts as a criminal question, but the decisions transfer obesity into the medical model rather than retaining its moral or criminal definition. Part of this claimsmaking about oppression involved documenting stigmatization and discrimination, and social scientists were recruited as experts to make claims on behalf of size acceptance advocates (Allon 1973).

Government bodies have been enlisted to demedicalize obesity. The United States Congress held hearings in 1990 to examine the claims and procedures of the diet industry, revealing abuse and leading to governmental action on weight-loss advertising. The National Institutes of Health held a Technology Assessment Conference in 1992 on weight loss methods, concluding that many weight loss strategies are ineffective and even harmful. These government activities and others like them assisted in the demedicalization of obesity. However, the size acceptance movement remains as a minor voice in public forums about body weight. As a movement it has not had the success of other efforts to promote rights of specific groups, such as women's rights or gay rights.

Conclusion

The models for dealing with high levels of body fat in contemporary society have changed during this century from primarily moral models to an increase in the use of medical models and then an emergence of the application of political models. Most of the time the degree of medicalization and demedicalization has only been partial, with several models competing simultaneously in their claims to typify obesity (Best 1989) and exert "ownership" over the problem.

The continued presence of a moral model of weight loss demonstrates the complexity involved in defining obesity as badness, sickness, or simply difference. Attempts to indict obesity on medical grounds have been somewhat successful. As fatness is medicalized, the moral component of treatment in weight loss may diminish but it will probably not disappear. Moral models of obesity remain as a vestige of the overwhelming interpretation of obesity in the past as a moral and not medical problem. Challenges to medicalization have not exonerated obesity medically, but have achieved some success in demedicalization by reframing the condition as political. While movement toward demedicalization is growing, it is a small yet different voice in the traditional chorus of stigmatization of obesity and the growing bandwagon of medicalization of fatness.

Currently moral, medical, and political models are all being applied to people with high levels of body fat, with a dynamic competition between models permitting multiple definitions of obesity as a social problem. We can anticipate future changes in the social construction of body fat as an issue as competing claims are made to define it as a moral deficit, medical disease, or political discrimination.

References

Allon, N. 1973. "The Stigma of Overweight in Everyday Life." Pp. 83–102 in *Obesity in Perspective Fogarty International Series in Preventive Medicine*, Vol. 2, Part 2, edited by G. A. Bray. Washington, D.C.: U. S. Government Printing Office.

———. 1975. "Latent Social Services in Group Dieting." *Social Problems* 23(1):59–69.

AMA—American Medical Association, Council on Scientific Affairs. 1988. "Treatment of Obesity in Adults." *Journal of the American Medical Association* 260:2547–2551.

Asher, W. L. 1975a. "ASBP's Silver Anniversary." *Obesity & Bariatric Medicine* 4(4):136.

———. 1975b. "ASBP's Silver Anniversary." *Obesity & Bariatric Medicine* 4(5):180.

Baker, J. O. 1982. "The Rehabilitation Act of 1973: Protection for Victims of Weight Discrimination?" *UCLA Law Review* 29:947–971.

Barron, N., and B. H. Lear. 1989. "Ample Opportunity for Fat Women." Pp. 79–92 in *Overcoming Fear of Fat*, edited by L. S. Brown and E. D. Rothblum. New York: Harrington Park Press.

Becker, H. S. 1963. *Outsiders*. New York: Free Press.

Beller, A. S. 1977. *Fat and Thin: A Natural History of Obesity*. New York: McGraw-Hill.

Bennett, W., and J. Gurin. 1982. *The Dieter's Dilemma: Eating Less and Weighing More*. New York: Basic Books.

Berg, F. M. 1992. "Nondiet Movement Gains Strength." *Obesity & Health* 6(5):85–90.

Best, J. (ed.). 1989. *Images of Issues: Typifying Contemporary Social Problems*. Hawthorne, NY: Aldine de Gruyter.

Black, D., W. P. T. James, and G. M. Besser. 1983. "Obesity. A Report of the Royal College of Physicians." *Journal of the Royal College of Physicians* 17(1):5.

Blackburn, G. 1993. "Comparison of Medically Supervised and Unsupervised Approaches to Weight Loss and Control." *Annals of Internal Medicine* 119(7):714–718.

Blumer, H. 1971. "Social Problems as Collective Behavior." *Social Problems* 18:298–306.

Bouchard, C. 1994. *The Genetics of Obesity*. Ann Arbor, MI: CRC Press.

Bray, G. A. 1974. "Treatment of Obesity with Drugs and Invasive Procedures." Pp. 179–205 in *Obesity in America*, NIH Publication No. 70-359, edited by G. A. Bray. Washington, DC: USDHEW, Public Health Service.

———. 1980. "Jejunoileal Bypass, Jaw Wiring and Vagotomy for Massive Obesity." Pp. 369–387 in *Obesity*, edited by A. J. Stunkard. Philadelphia: W.B. Saunders.

———. 1990. "Obesity: Historical Development of Scientific and Cultural Ideas. *International Journal of Obesity* 14:909–926.

Bray, G. A., Barbara York, and James DeLany. 1992. "A Survey of the Opinions of Obesity Experts on the Causes and Treatment of Obesity." *American Journal of Clinical Nutrition* 55:151S–154S.

Brown, P. J. 1993. "Cultural Perspectives on the Etiology and Treatment of Obesity." Pp. 179–193 in *Obesity: Theory and Therapy*, 2nd ed., edited by A. J. Stunkard and T. A. Wadden. New York: Raven Press.

Brown, P. J., and M. Konner. 1987. "An Anthropological Perspective on Obesity." *Annals of the New York Academy of Sciences* 499:29–46.

Bruch, H. 1957. *The Importance of Overweight*. New York: W. W. Norton.

———. 1973. *Eating Disorders: Obesity, Anorexia Nervosa and the Person Within*. New York: Basic Books.

Burton B. T., W. R. Foster, J. Hirsh, and T. B. van Itallie. 1985. "Health Implications of Obesity: A NIH Consensus Development Conference." *International Journal of Obesity* 9:155–169.

Cade, J. 1991. "Management of Weight Problems and Obesity—Knowledge, Attitudes, and Current Practice of General Practitioners." *British Journal of General Practice* 41:147–150.

Cahnman, W. J. 1968. "The Stigma of Obesity." *Sociological Quarterly* 9(3):283–299.

Califano, J. 1979. *Healthy People: The Surgeon General's Report on Health Promotion and Disease Prevention*. Washington, D.C.: U.S. Government Printing Office.

Callaway, C. W. 1984. "Weight Standards: Their Clinical Significance." *Annals of Internal Medicine* 100:296.

Canning, H., and J. Mayer. 1966. "Obesity—Its Possible Effect on College Acceptance." *New England Journal of Medicine* 275:1172–1174.

Cegielski, M. M., and J. A. Saporta. 1978. "Surgical Treatment of Massive Obesity: Current Status of the Art." *Obesity & Bariatric Medicine* 7(4):156–159.

Chernin, K. 1981. *The Obsession: Reflections on the Tyranny of Slenderness*. New York: Harper & Row.

Conrad, P. 1975. "The Discovery of Hyperkinesis: Notes on the Medicalization of Deviant Behavior." *Social Problems* 23:12–21.

———. 1992. "Medicalization and Social Control." *Annual Review of Sociology* 18:209–232.

Conrad, P., and J. W. Schneider. 1992. *Deviance and Medicalization: From Badness to Sickness*. Philadelphia: Temple University Press.

Crisp, A. H. 1978. "Some Psychiatric Aspects of Obesity." Pp. 336–343 in *Recent Advances in Obesity Research*, edited by G. Bray. London: Newman.

Dietz, R. E. 1973. "What's in a Name . . . Revisited." *Obesity & Bariatric Medicine* 2(5):138.

Drenick, E. J., and H. W. Hargis. 1978. "Jaw Wiring for Weight Reduction." *Obesity & Bariatric Medicine* 7(6):210–211.

Ernsberger, P. 1985. "The Death of Dieting." *American Health* 4:29–33.

Ernsberger, P., and P. Haskew. 1987. "Rethinking Obesity: An Alternative View of Its Health Implications." *Journal of Obesity and Weight Regulation* 6(2):2–81.

Friedman, A. I. 1974. *Fat Can Be Beautiful: Stop Dieting, Start Living*. New York: Berkeley Publishing.

Fuerst, M. L. 1983. "Suction-Assisted Lipectomy Attracting Interest." *Journal of the American Medical Association* 249:3004.

Garfinkle, P. E., and D. M. Garner. 1980. "Cultural Expectations of Thinness in Women." *Psychological Reports* 47:483–491.

Garrison, T. Nicholetti, and D. Levitsky. 1993. *Fed Up! A Woman's Guide to Freedom from the Diet/Weight Prison.* New York: Carroll and Graf.

Garrow, J. S. 1981. *Treat Obesity Seriously.* London: Churchill Livingstone.

Goldstein, D. J. 1992. "Beneficial Health Effects of Modest Weight Loss." *International Journal of Obesity* 16:397–415.

Goode, E. 1969. "Marijuana and the Politics of Reality." *Journal of Health and Social Behavior* 10:83–94.

Grossworth, M. 1971. *Fat Pride: A Survival Handbook.* New York: Jarrow Press.

Halmi, K. 1980. "Gastric Bypass for Massive Obesity." Pp. 388–394 in *Obesity,* edited by A. J. Stunkard. Philadelphia: W. B. Saunders.

Hocking, M. P., M. C. Duerson, P. O'Leary, and E. R. Woodward. 1983. "Jejunoileal Bypass for Morbid Obesity: Late Follow-up for 100 Cases." *New England Journal of Medicine* 308:995–999.

Hoebel, B. G., and L. Hernandez. 1993. "Basic Neural Mechanisms for Feeding and Weight Regulation." Pp. 43–62 in *Obesity: Theory and Therapy,* edited by A. J. Stunkard and T. A. Wadden. New York: Raven Press.

Howard, A. N. 1992. "The History of the Association for the Study of Obesity." *International Journal of Obesity* 16(supplement):S1–S8.

ICD-9-CM. 1990. *International Classification of Diseases-Clinical Modifications.* Washington, D.C.: U.S. Department of Health and Human Services.

Joaquin, A. H. 1977. "Brief Group Treatment of Obesity Through Ancillary Self-Hypnosis." *American Journal of Clinical Hypnosis* 19:231–234.

Joffe, S. N. 1981. "Surgical Management of Morbid Obesity." *Gut* 22:242–254.

Kalish, B. J. 1972. "The Stigma of Obesity." *Journal of the American Dietetic Association* 72(6):1124–1127.

Kano, S. 1989. *Making Peace with Food.* New York: Harper & Row.

Karris, L. 1977. "Prejudice Against Obese Renters." *Journal of Social Psychology* 101:159–160.

Kopelman, P. G., N. Finer, K. R. Fox, A. Hill, and I. A. MacDonald. 1994. "ASO Consensus Statement on Obesity." *International Journal of Obesity* 18:189–191.

Kremen, A. J., J. H. Linner, and C. H. Nelson. 1954. "An Experimental Evaluation of the Nutritional Importance of Proximal and Distal Small Intestine." *Annals of Surgery* 140:439–448.

Larkin, J. C., and H. A. Pines. 1979. "No Fat Persons Need Apply: Experimental Studies of the Overweight Stereotype and Hiring Preference." *Sociology of Work and Occupations* 6(3):312–327.

Lasagna, L. 1980. "Drugs in the Treatment of Obesity." Pp. 292–299 in *Obesity,* edited by A. J. Stunkard. Philadelphia: W.B. Saunders.

Laslett, B., and C. A. B. Warren. 1975. "Losing Weight: The Organizational Promotion of Behavior Change." *Social Problems* 23(1):69–80.

Levenstein, H. 1988. *Revolution at the Table: The Transformation of the American Diet.* New York: Oxford University Press.

————. 1993. *Paradox of Plenty: A Social History of Eating in Modern America*. New York: Oxford University Press.

Louderback, L. 1970. *Fat Power: Whatever You Weigh Is Right*. New York: Hawthorne Books.

Maddox, G. L., and V. Liederman. 1969. "Overweight as a Social Disability with Medical Implications." *Journal of Medical Education* 44(3):214–220.

Maddox, G. L., K. W. Back, and V. R. Liederman. 1968. "Overweight as Social Deviance and Disability." *Journal of Health and Social Behavior* 9(4):287–298.

Maiman, L., and V. Wang. 1979. "Attitudes Toward Obesity and the Obese Among Professionals." *Journal of the American Dietetic Association* 74:331–336.

Marsland, D. W., M. Wood, and F. Mayo. 1976. "Content of Family Practice. I. Rank Order of Diagnosis by Frequency; II. Diagnosis by Disease Category and Age/Sex Distribution." *Journal of Family Practice* 3:38–68.

Mason, E. E., and C. Ito. 1967. "Gastric Bypass in Obesity." *Surgical Clinics of North America* 47:1345.

Mayer, J. 1965. "Genetic Factors in Human Obesity." *Annals of the New York Academy of Science* 131:412–421.

McEvoy, S. A. 1992. "Fat Chance: Employment Discrimination against the Overweight." *Labor Law Journal* 43:3–14.

Medical World News. 1983. "Removing Fat by Suction: New Surgery Works but Misuse Feared." March 14:6–11.

Millman, M. 1980. *Such a Pretty Face: Being Fat in America*. New York: W. W. Norton.

Nichter, M., and M. Nichter. 1991. "Hype and Weight." *Medical Anthropology* 13:249–284.

Nidetch, J. 1972. *The Story of Weight Watchers*. New York: Signet.

NIH (National Institutes of Health). 1985. *Health Implications of Obesity*. Bethesda, MD: National Institutes of Health.

Nordsiek, F. W. 1964. "An Epidemiological Approach to Obesity." *American Journal of Public Health* 54:1689–1698.

Orbach, S. 1978. *Fat Is a Feminist Issue: The Anti-Diet Guide to Permanent Weight Loss*. New York: Paddington Press.

Payne, J. H., and L. T. DeWind. 1969. "Surgical Treatment of Obesity." *American Journal of Surgery* 118:141–147.

Price, J., S. Desmond, R. Krol, F. Snyder, and J. K. O'Connell. 1987. "Family Practice Physicians' Beliefs, Attitudes and Practices Regarding Obesity." *American Journal of Preventive Medicine* 3:339-345.

Reissman, C. K. 1983. "Women and Medicalization: A New Perspective." *Social Policy* 14:3–18.

Schacter, S. 1968. "Obesity and Eating." *Science* 161:751–756.

————. 1971. "Some Extraordinary Facts About Obese Humans and Rats." *American Psychologist* 26(2):129–144.

Schneider, J. W. 1985. "Social Problems Theory: The Constructionist View." *Annual Review of Sociology* 11:209–229.

Schneider, J. W., and Kitsuse, J. I. (eds.). 1984. *Studies in the Sociology of Social Problems*. Norwood, NJ: Ablex.

Schoenfielder, L., and B. Weiser (eds.). 1983. *Shadow on a Tightrope: Writings by Women on Fat Oppression.* Iowa City, IA: Aunt Lute Book Company.

Schwartz, H. 1986. *Never Satisfied: A Cultural History of Diets, Fantasies, and Fat.* New York: Free Press.

Seid, R. P. 1989. *Never Too Thin.* New York: Prentice-Hall.

Short, S. H. 1994. "Medical Quackery: Our Role as Professionals." *Journal of the American Dietetic Association* 94:607–611.

Sobal, J. 1984a. "Marriage, Obesity, and Dieting." *Marriage and Family Review* 7:115–139.

———. 1984b. "Group Dieting, the Stigma of Obesity, and Overweight Adolescents: The Contributions of Natalie Allon to the Sociology of Obesity." *Marriage and Family Review* 7:9–20.

———. 1991a. "Obesity and Socioeconomic Status: A Framework for Examining Relationships between Physical and Social Variables." *Medical Anthropology* 13:231–247.

———. 1991b. "Obesity and Nutritional Sociology: A Model for Coping with the Stigma of Obesity." *Clinical Sociology Review* 9:125–141.

Sobal, J., and A. J. Stunkard. 1989. "Obesity and Socioeconomic Status." *Psychological Bulletin* 105:260–275.

Solomon, N., and S. Sheppard. 1972. *The Truth about Weight Control: How to Lose Excess Pounds Permanently.* New York: Stein and Day.

Spector, M., and J. I. Kitsuse. 1987. *Constructing Social Problems.* New York: Aldine de Gruyter (originally 1977).

Stillman, I. M., and S. S. Baker. 1967. *The Doctor's Quick Weight-Loss Diet.* Englewood Cliffs, NJ: Prentice-Hall.

Stock, M. J. 1992. "Editorial." *International Journal of Obesity and Metabolic Disorders* 16:719–720.

Stuart, R. B. 1967. "Behavioral Control of Overeating." *Behavioral Research and Therapy* 5:357–365.

Stuart, R. B., and B. Davis. 1976. *Slim Chance in a Fat World: Behavioral Control of Obesity.* Champaign, IL: Research Press.

Stuart, R. B., and C. Mitchell. 1980. "Self Help Groups in the Control of Body Weight." Pp. 345–354 in *Obesity,* edited by A. J. Stunkard. Philadelphia: W. B. Saunders.

Stunkard, A. J. 1976. *The Pain of Obesity.* Palo Alto, CA: Bull Publishing Co.

Stunkard, A. J., and M. McClaren-Hume. 1958. "The Results of Treatment for Obesity." *Archives of Internal Medicine* 103:79–85.

Tobias, A. L., and J. B. Gordon. 1980. "Social Consequences of Obesity." *Journal of the American Dietetic Association* 76:338–342.

Tucker, D. H. 1979. *Report on the Study of Weight and Size Discrimination.* Baltimore, MD: The Maryland Commission on Human Relations.

Twaddle, A. C. 1981. *Sickness Behavior and the Sick Role.* Cambridge, MA: Schenkman Publishing Company.

Wilson, G. T. 1980. "Behavior Modification and the Treatment of Obesity." Pp. 325–444 in *Obesity,* edited by A. J. Stunkard. Philadelphia: W. B. Saunders.

———. 1991. "The Addiction Model of Eating Disorders: A Critical Analysis." *Advances in Behavioral Research and Therapy* 13:27–72.

Wiseman, C., J. J. Gray, J. E. Mosimann, and A. H. Ahrens. 1992. "Cultural Expectations of Thinness in Women: An Update." *International Journal of Eating Disorders* 11(1):85–89.

Wooley, S. 1984. "Should Obesity Be Treated at All?" In *Eating and Its Disorders*, edited by A. J. Stunkard and E. Steller. New York: Raven Press.

Wooley, S., and S. Dyrenforth. 1979. "Obesity and Women." *Women Studies International Quarterly* 2(1):69–72.

Wooley, S., and O. W. Wooley. 1981. "Overeating as Substance Abuse." In *Advances in Substance Abuse*, Vol. 2. Greenwich, CT: JAI Press.

Wyden, P. 1965. *The Overweight Society*. New York: William C. Morrow.

Zada, L. (ed.). 1977. *Readers Guide to Periodical Literature*. New York: H. W. Wilson.

5

Never Too Rich . . . Or Too Thin: The Role of Stigma in the Social Construction of Anorexia Nervosa

KAREN WAY

Introduction

For decades, the media and popular culture have equated thinness with "glamour," something for "normal" Western women to emulate. Yet the lines have become blurred in recent years as to what is "desirable" thinness. What is "normal" dieting behavior and weight concern and what is anorexia?

Research suggests that "normal" and "anorexia" lie on the same continuum in our society. However, I argue that physical and character stigmas have been employed in the medicalization of eating disorders to differentiate between what is "normal" and what is "anorexic." These stigmas have been legitimated by mental health professionals, popular media, corporate operatives (e.g., fashion and beauty industries, women's magazines), and other vested interests. Ultimately, stigmas create social distance and apathy, and in the case of eating disorders, lessen the likelihood that audiences will respond to eating disorders as social problems worth "doing something" about.

The Social Climate: Pressures toward Thinness

Feminist psychotherapist Susie Orbach argues that for decades, people have considered it "normal" for women to be vigilant about their weights and sizes, to diet and to count calories and fat grams, and to make thinness a priority. Orbach (1986:64–65) believes that women have a paradoxical relationship with food, and cites the cultural message a woman learns: that "the food she prepares for others as an act of love and an expression of her caring is somehow dangerous to the woman herself."

In describing the pressures women feel to vigilantly strive for thinness, Orbach (1986:65) argues:

> Diet, deprive, deny is the message women receive, or—even more sinister— they must pretend that cottage cheese and melon is as pleasurable as a grilled cheese sandwich for lunch. For a woman, then, food is an object of an entirely different character. It is a potential enemy and a threat. A cardinal rule of femininity, from young women in their teens through women in their fifties, is that they should be desirable. Desirability is linked with an ever-diminishing body size, which is attainable by most women only through severe restrictions on their food intake. And because the "right size" for women has been decreasing yearly since 1965, so women have been encouraged to decrease their food intake yearly.

Psychologists and social researchers contend there has been a 30-year trend toward a feminine ideal of ever-increasing slenderness. Garner et al. (1980) documented a dramatic rise in dieting articles published in women's magazines from 1959 to 1978. The obsession appears to be gender-specific: in their comparison of 48 men's and 48 women's magazines, Silverstein et al. (1986) find 63 advertisements for diet foods in women's magazines and only 1 in men's magazines.

This trend also emerges in studies that have analyzed the heights, weights, and measurements of Miss America Pageant contestants and *Playboy* centerfolds. Garner et al. (1980) report that Miss America Pageant contestants and *Playboy* centerfolds got smaller from 1959 to 1978, while average women became heavier. An update by Wiseman et al. (1992), consistent with the earlier findings, reports a significant decrease in body weight for Miss America contestants and continued low weights for *Playboy* centerfolds from 1979 to 1988. Wiseman et al. (1992) also claim that 69% of the *Playboy* models and 60% of the Miss America Pageant contestants had weights at least 15% below an acceptable minimum for their ages and heights—therefore meeting the American Psychiatric Association's (1987) first diagnostic criterion for anorexia nervosa.

For the overwhelming majority of women in Western societies, chronic dieting has become a way of life (Rodin et al. 1985). Rosen and Gross (1987) report that dieting behaviors are widespread among adolescent females. They found that 63% of high school girls were on diets the day they were surveyed, compared with 16.2% of the boys. Some studies report that children are becoming concerned about weight at younger and younger ages—as early as seven or eight (Bordo 1993:61).

"A woman can never be too rich or too thin." Susie Orbach, Kim Chernin, Marlene Boskind-White, and Marcia Millman would argue that this widely quoted statement, originally attributed to Wallis Warfield Simpson, the Duchess of Windsor (Brumberg 1988:33), has been an enduring theme in our culture. There has been no shortage of literature touting the claim that "society" is responsible for the "surge" in cases of anorexia nervosa and eating disorders over the last two decades. Journalists, psychologists, and other social commentators have blamed beauty and thinness ideals, "waif" models, the media, fashion industry, and other related concerns for fueling anorexia nervosa and eating disorders.

In 1984, the beauty magazine *Glamour* surveyed 33,000 women about their perceptions of their weight and body image. Nearly 75% of the respondents claimed they were "too fat" (30% of these respondents were judged to be *below* the norm for their weights) and a majority reported they were "dissatisfied" or "ashamed of" their stomach, hips, thighs, and buttocks. In her analysis of the survey, Boskind-White (1985) notes a "steadily growing cultural bias—almost no woman, of whatever size, feels she's thin enough." Similarly, Kevin Thompson (1986) concludes that 95 out of 100 women "free of eating-disorder symptoms" overestimate their body size by at least 25%.

These claims are the usual banter on television talk shows that focus on eating disorders. For instance, large-size model Christine Alt (sister of supermodel Carol Alt), who struggled with anorexia nervosa early in her career, claims:

> Our society does this to us. We look at magazines and we see paper thin women. And the males in our society look at these beer commercials with these women in string bikinis who are ultra-thin, and they're going, "Wow, look at this girl!" And we see this, and we think that we have to be this thin. They are the thin ones, we are the normal-sized ones. (*The Maury Povich Show* 1992a)

A teen on a *Geraldo* talk show touted as "Teen Diet Horror Stories" similarly remarks:

> Everyone thinks they are too fat; the skinniest people think they are fat. Because we have models and they're like Christie Brinkley and stuff;

they're perfect. And the guys will go, "Oh Christie Brinkley's beautiful."
So you think, I have to look like that too, I have to lose my weight so when
I put on my bikini I'll look like they do. (*Geraldo* 1989)

Studies report that without exception, females appear to be more condemning of their overweight peers than males (Richardson 1977, quoted
by DeJong and Kleck 1986). This is evident in a recent poll of 18- to 25-
year-old women in *Esquire* magazine (January 1994), in which half of the
women said they would "rather be dead than fat." Even Ann Landers
(1994) recently remarked in her daily advice column: "excess weight is
unsightly and unhealthy and can rob one of some precious years."

Sociologist Edwin Schur (1984:77) states that females are socialized to
have a *fear of visual deviance* in our culture. He argues that "nearly *all*
women in our society feel compelled to make continuous efforts not to
'violate' appearance norms." As a stigmatized condition, being overweight may lead to social rejection (Crocker et al. 1993; Goffman 1963).
Studies report that overweight people are attributed numerous negative
characteristics—being morally and emotionally impaired, socially hand-
icapped, lazy, and less intelligent (Crandall and Biernat 1990; DeJong
and Kleck 1986; Miller et al. 1990). A recent study in the *New England
Journal of Medicine* (Gortmaker et al. 1993) reports that being overweight
reduced a woman's life chances, earning potential, and likelihood of
marrying.

But stigmatization of the overweight is nothing new. Social historian
Maud Ellmann (1993:8–9) notes that during World War I, women who
were 40 pounds overweight were said to be "hoarding sixty pounds of
sugar" in their extra girth, thereby "depriving European allies of their
rations." Ellmann argues that fat women became scapegoats for the guilt
America felt at its begrudgingly late entry into the war; doctors claimed
"that fat people were unpatriotic, because the energy required to support their corpulence demanded calories that other people needed."

In their study documenting prejudices toward overweight children,
Maddox et al. (1968:15) observe that definitions of weight are socially
constructed—"a function of *best* weight and tolerable deviations from
that standard." The question of who establishes and aids in reinforcing
these standards is an issue to be taken up next.

The Business of Thinness

Many vested interests (e.g., the corporate beauty industry, manufacturers of dieting products, the fashion industry, women's beauty maga-

zines) fuel the cultural obsession with thinness. These interests all profit from the perpetuation of beauty and thinness ideals.

Of course, this has been a part of our cultural heritage since the early nineteenth century, when astute capitalists realized the great lucrative potential in exporting French fashions to America. A surge of entrepreneurs arrived on the scene: dressmakers, hairdressers, cosmeticians, and department store owners (Banner 1983:3), who realized that they could sell nearly any product with enough hype, puffery, and advertising. The economic benefits were evident, as Banner (1983:28) quotes a commentator of that time: "Who makes fortunes faster among the working classes than those who minister to the desire for beauty?"

In *The Beauty Myth*, Naomi Wolf (1991:17) argues that today's profits are just as astounding, that selling beauty—like selling dreams—is extremely lucrative. According to her estimates, the dieting industry grosses some $33 billion annually, the cosmetics industry $20 billion, and over $300 million goes to cosmetic surgeons.

Media researcher Kathryn Weibel (1977:161–163) criticizes corporate interests and advertisers for manipulating the self-image of females with the idea that consuming of beauty and fashion products will meet basic emotional needs—all for the almighty dollar: "Entire product lines have been built up and marketed around insecurities and the need for approval . . . . The cosmetics industry has grown rich by exploiting female insecurities regarding youth and glamour."

Women's fashion and beauty magazines are in a category of their own, as the primary purveyors of beauty standards and thinness ideals. Media researcher Christianne Miller (1987:2) observes that women's magazines speak in a strange language all their own—a language seemingly designed to create anxiety. Typical phrases contain the word "should," usually preceded by "you" and spoken by a third-person or otherwise anonymous expert who offers the same general message: "there is something wrong with 'you.' . . . Most often, the author or editors will stimulate the reader's insecurity in the introduction to a piece, and then give her the advice she needs to allay it."

Naomi Wolf (1991:49) claims that women's low self-esteem and poor self-image developed in response to the needs of the marketplace. Another 1990s icon of the liberal feminist movement, former *Wall Street Journal* reporter Susan Faludi (1991:202), agrees with Wolf, arguing that the formula that has succeeded for more than a century is still in place: undermine a woman's self-esteem, induce high anxiety in respect to a "feminine" appearance—and the product sells itself. The emphasis on "light" and "slim" is even evident in product *names*—for example, "Ultra Slim Lipstick," "Miller Lite," and "Virginia Slims" (McLorg and Taub 1987).

Doctors in the business of treating anorexics often chastise corporate interests for their commoditization of thinness and beauty when they appear on television talk shows. Dr. William Rader, founder of the Rader Institute, a treatment center for disorders, recently remarked on *Geraldo*:

> Look at that next commercial. The person on there doesn't even look that way. They work out hours a day, weeks to months to look that way, and that's what our kids think they should be. Marilyn Monroe today would be considered to be fat, chubby. So what's scary is our kids are trying to emulate an abnormal figure, and in the process are getting caught in the trap of compulsive overeating, or bulimia, where they eat large quantities of food and vomit, and also anorexia. (*Geraldo* 1989)

William Davis, clinical director of the Renfrew Center, an eating disorder treatment facility in Philadelphia, similarly criticized corporate interests for their manipulation of the "young and vulnerable" in a recent news report: "If a kid takes Kate Moss seriously . . . no matter how the kid looks, the kid is going to feel fat compared to the way Kate Moss looks—that's a set-up" (*The Bulletin with Larry Kane* 1993).

Spector and Kitsuse (1987:148) observe that claims made by groups, agencies, or individuals that certain situations are "intolerable and must be changed" can produce outcries from those with a vested interest in maintaining the status quo, who may react by launching campaigns of their own. The industries cited above could be said to have a "vested interest" in protecting their assets and in ensuring that charges that they are "causing" anorexia and eating disorders don't stick.

Such interests typically side-step claims that young girls are being driven to starvation by the dictates of fashion and beauty, by the culture of women's magazines and corporate profits. In fact, corporate interests most commonly counterattack by claiming that pursuing thinness is "normal"; only "sick" people have anorexia. Those vested interests avoid being blamed for causing anorexia by invoking character stigmas and blaming the victim—issues arising from the medicalization of eating disorders, to be discussed in the next section of this chapter.

To offer an example of this type of counterattack, a recent *People Magazine* cover story devoted to the question of whether Kate Moss and other "waif" models were sending "a dangerous message" to "weight obsessed teens" took the fashion industry off the hook by concluding:

> Fortunately, most eating-disorder experts agree that merely admiring waif models is not enough to bring on anorexia or bulimia. "There has to be a predisposing vulnerability," says [Dr. Michael] Strober of UCLA. A real anorectic "suffers from extreme self-doubt, inadequacy concerns and self-

esteem anxieties that are far more extreme than other people's. The average person will not be induced into anorexia because they see Kate Moss." (Lague et al. 1993:80)

In the same magazine article (1993:80), and in a classic psychology-driven "blame the family" claim, Dr. John Mead, director of the eating disorders clinic at Rush-Presbyterian-St. Luke's Medical Center in Chicago, states that a "good family" will inoculate a daughter from developing an eating disorder: "Girls who have a healthy self-image and come out of a good parent–child relationship do not fall victim to eating disorders, yet they all want to be thin."

Nina Blanchard, head of a successful L.A. fashion modeling agency for 32 years, casts aside the "trivial" concerns with Kate Moss: "It would be better if people would stop saying that this is the downfall of Western civilization." In Blanchard's mind, it would be far more productive for people to "worry about the mental health of [their] children and look into their problems in terms of self-esteem, instead of worrying that they're not eating because they want to look like Kate Moss" (Lague et al. 1993:80).

The "Epidemic" of Eating Disorders

Leading researchers of anorexia nervosa have remarked on the "growing consensus" that the incidence of anorexia nervosa has increased over the last several decades. Many attribute the apparent increase to sociocultural factors and the trend toward a thinner ideal of female beauty (Gordon 1990:37; Polivy et al. 1986:103–105).

High-profile anorexics first captured the public's attention. In the preface to her best-selling book *The Golden Cage*, Houston psychiatrist Hilde Bruch (1978) describes anorexia nervosa as "a disease that selectively befalls the young, rich, and beautiful." She adds, "The puzzling question is why such a cruel disease should affect young and healthy girls who have been raised in privileged, even luxurious circumstances."

This portrayal of anorexia as a "disease of the rich and privileged" was reinforced in stories about Pat Boone's daughter Cherry Boone O'Neill in 1982, Karen Carpenter's death in 1983, and in rumored innuendoes throughout the 1980s about Princess Diana. Words like "epidemic" emerged in 1980, when John Sours (1980:3) proclaimed that anorexia "now affects tens of thousands of high school and college age and appears to be increasing rapidly in most countries where there is an affluent, well-educated segment of society." The revised message portrays anorexia as not just an affliction of the "rich and famous," but *of* middle-class girls—even from "good homes."

According to social historian Joan Brumberg (1988:14–18), anorexia became "in" among affluent adolescent girls and young women in the 1980s. In a circuitous loop of media hype, claimsmakers expanded their population of concern by implying that eating disorders were occurring in "epidemic proportions" among middle- and upper-class young women and girls. The anorexic became an icon, according to feminist Kim Chernin (1981:46–47), who states: "if our will were sufficient to accomplish our desire, many of us would begin to look like our anorexic sister. The anorexic girl has become our present cultural heroine."

In her posthumously published book, *Conversations With Anorexics*, Hilde Bruch (1988:4) stated that anorexia had "acquired a fashionable reputation" and that it wasn't uncommon for girls to "express interest in 'trying it' after they have been exposed to a movie on anorexia." There were talks of "copy-cat" anorexia, in which females mimicked behaviors they saw on made-for-TV movies, like *The Best Little Girl in the World* (1981), written by Steven Levenkron, Karen Carpenter's psychologist (Brumberg 1988:14–18). Psychologist Richard A. Gordon (1990:2–3) notes that anorexia, described as the "psychiatric disorder of the 80s" in the popular press, was "widely publicized, glamorized, and romanticized."

But how common is—or was—anorexia? Gordon (1990:37–39) observes that although the incidence of anorexia has "clearly increased," it is still not common—particularly in its severe form. Gordon identifies the "population at risk" to be young women in their teens and twenties; the prevalence of anorexia is estimated to be about 0.5 to 1% of these at-risk populations in the United States and England. Yet Gordon (1990:37–39) believes the actual incidence of anorexia and eating disorders may be underestimated because only severe cases are brought to the attention of medical and mental health authorities. Research suggests that eating disorders have a spectrum of severity, that many college women exhibit borderline conditions (Hesse-Biber 1989), and that the spectrum of anorexia and eating disorders merges with realms of "normal" weight-concerned behaviors.

Then why the media hype? Joel Best (1988) has documented the use, misuse, and manipulation of statistics as persuasive tools in constructing social problems. As he notes, the rule seems to be the bigger the number—especially an "official" number—the better, in estimating the magnitude of a particular problem. In the case of anorexia, claimsmakers lump together estimated occurrences of anorexia nervosa with another more common eating disorder, bulimia (or binge–purge syndrome). This larger number tends to make claims sound more urgent and alarming. For instance, in its 1986 program literature, ANRED (Anorexia Nervosa and Related Eating Disorders, Inc.), a hospital-affiliated private organization founded to treat eating disorders, offered this substantial claim: "Researchers estimate that eating disorders now affect as many as 20% of young women between 12 and 30."

This process of legitimation through statistics and other "facts" is crucial, for as Blumer (1971:303) observes: "A social problem must acquire social endorsement if it is to be taken seriously and move forward in its career . . . . If a social problem does not carry the credentials of respectability necessary for entrance into these [public] arenas, it is doomed . . . it flounders and languishes outside the arena of public action." By the mid-1980s, claimsmakers cast the widest possible net of vulnerability. The claim became: "Today . . . researchers find self-starvation in women of all ages, all ethnic backgrounds, and all socio-economic groups" (ANRED 1986). In 1992, the number of "eating-disorder afflicted" persons was boosted to "an estimated 8 million Americans" (Sporkin et al. 1992:93). Six months later in another article, the number jumped to "about 11 million women and 1 million men" (Dunn 1992:74).

In 1993, the claims took on a more urgent tone: "for 1-in-25 American females, that obsession with thinness turns into a life-threatening eating disorder, such as bulimia or anorexia nervosa" (*CNN Newshour* 1993). We do not know *whose* estimates these are, but as Best (1988:86) observes: "As long as some source actually gave these figures, the press report is accurate: it is true that authorities gave statistic X, even if X is wildly wrong."

Today, talk show hosts and journalists typically claim that nearly all women are vulnerable to eating disorders. When Larry King devoted a segment on his TV program to "older anorexics" (in their 30s), he stressed that his guests "are not youngsters," yet struggle with eating disorders (*Larry King Live* 1991). Similarly, talk show host Maury Povich, summarizing his thoughts after a show segment on eating disorders, offered this insight: "I think we have shed some light on the fact that eating disorders can strike anyone; it's not only the rich and famous. Regular folks, please be aware" (*The Maury Povich Show* 1992a).

The Stigmatization of Anorexia Nervosa

Anorexia nervosa was first recognized as an independent clinical entity 100 years ago in France, although reports of "self-starvation" as "nervous consumption" appeared as early as 1689 by Richard Morton (Bruch 1973:211). From the very beginning, the nature of what was said in medical literature about anorexia—what it was and what caused it—

fueled a stigmatizing portrait: Morton described his patient "like a Skeleton only clad in Skin"; Gull, who has been credited with identifying anorexia in 1874, attributed the ailment to "a morbid mental state" (Bruch 1973:211–213).

Sociologist Erving Goffman (1963:4–5) identified three types of stigma—two of which have been salient in claims made about anorexia nervosa. *Physical stigmas* refer to physical deformities, extremes in weight or lack of height. *Character stigmas* are "blemishes of individual character," such as mental disorders, addictions, alcoholism, sexual deviances, possessing a criminal record, a weak will, "unnatural passions," a rigid belief system, or dishonesty. Finally, *tribal stigmas* are generalizations about a person based on his or her race, ethnicity, or religion.

Besides physical stigmas, which will be discussed below, claims made about anorexia often impute character stigmas. This is rooted in the medicalization of eating disorders, as anorexia nervosa has been defined in medical literature as a "psychiatric syndrome" for more than 100 years (Williamson 1990:8). And as Conrad and Schneider (1980:247) observe, mental illnesses are stigmatized illnesses.

When medical perspectives define the problem and its solutions become dominant, they overshadow competing definitions (Conrad and Schneider 1980:242). In this process of medical social control, norms are constructed to define what is "healthy." Medical operatives enforce "norms," defining behavior outside of established norms as "deviant" and needing to be medically controlled.

In efforts to further legitimate claims that anorexia is a psychiatric illness, medical operatives have aligned anorexia nervosa with obsessive–compulsive disorder and other anxiety disorders, fueling the stigmatized portrait of anorexics. In *Assessment of Eating Disorders*, clinical psychologist Donald Williamson (1990:80–98) compiles a laundry list of "common secondary psychopathology associated with eating disorders," including depression, anxiety, obsessive–compulsive behavior, social anxiety, interpersonal and family problems, personality disorders, and substance abuse (e.g., cigarettes in regard to anorexics). Similarly, Craig L. Johnson (1991) claims that recent research indicates "approximately one-third of the patients who present with disordered eating also have significant personality disorders," which accounts "for most of the poor outcome in the brief treatment literature. They are difficult to treat and usually require longer-term, informed individual psychotherapy."

Such claims exemplify the "individualization of social problems"—the tendency to look for causes within the individual—even blaming the victim for her psychopathology (Conrad and Schneider 1980:250). But then, it could be said that there are interests to protect. Medical, psychiatric, and psychological operatives have carved out a niche in eating disorders, establishing specialized journals such as *International Journal of Eating Disorders* and *Eating Disorders* and organizing conferences and societies. Medicalization keeps the problem contained within the realm of medicine.

Besides being stigmatized personally as "psychiatrically ill," the behavior and mental processes of anorexics are often itemized and stigmatized. In their literature review of "characteristics of females who exhibit anorexic or bulimic symptoms," researchers Kerr et al. (1991:847) conclude that anorexics have overcontrolling egos, and display a greater degree of social conformity and impaired cognitive functioning. As they summarize, "anorexics think simply and concretely with irrational logic. Information that does not fit into the anorexic's simple conceptual framework may cause immobilizing stress or rejection."

Similarly, psychiatrist Hilde Bruch (1988:6) characterized the mental processes of anorexics as follows:

> Deep down, every anorexic is convinced that basically she is inadequate, low, mediocre, inferior, and despised by others. She lives in an imaginary world with an assumed reality where she feels that people around her— her family, her friends, and the world at large—look down on her with disapproving eyes, ready to pounce on her with criticism . . . . All her efforts, her striving for perfection and excessive thinness, are directed toward hiding the fatal flaw of her fundamental inadequacy.

Character stigmas are evident in much literature geared to the general public on anorexia as well. One typical claim in a brochure distributed by the Department of Health and Human Services (n.d.) is that anorexics tend "to be childish in their thinking, in their need for approval, and in their lack of independence." The brochure reinforces medical definitions of anorexia, noting: "Psychological symptoms such as social withdrawal, obsessive–compulsiveness and depression often precede or accompany anorexia nervosa. The patient's distorted view of herself and the world around her are the cause of these psychological disturbances."

Eating disorder "help" organizations also fuel the character stigmatization of anorexia nervosa. In a 1990 newsletter, AA/BA (American Anorexia/Bulimia Association, Inc.) outlines the following "danger signal" behaviors for anorexics:

- develops unusual interest in food
- develops strange eating rituals and eats small amounts of food, e.g., cuts food into tiny pieces or measures everything before eating extremely small amounts
- becomes a secret eater

- becomes obsessive about exercising
- appears depressed much of the time
- begins to binge and purge
- becomes obsessive.

The behavioral definitions cited above create social distance between the suspected "deviant" and the evaluator. The greater the social distance between the individual and the evaluator, the greater the likelihood that the individual will be labeled "deviant" and devalued (Schur 1984:197–198). Mental health professionals tend to have rigid definitions of mental illness and believe their primary task is a circuitous one: to uncover signs of mental illness to support their presumptions that individuals referred to them are mentally ill (Jones et al. 1984:106–107). The dramatic physical appearance of severe anorexics often reinforces their evaluations.

The media frequently highlight the physical stigma of anorexia nervosa. In their quest to demonstrate and define "what *is* anorexia nervosa," television talk shows and journalists typically showcase sensational cases (e.g., "Anorexic Twins" on *The Maury Povich Show* [1993]) and/or elicit claims that will provide titillating commentary on "freakish" aspects of appearance from recovering anorexic guests.

Christine Alt, sister of model Carol Alt, was solicited for this kind of commentary by talk show host Maury Povich, who asked, "I had heard, for instance, in the worst periods, your color would change?" She responded:

> Oh, yeah. You would—you would get the color of a corpse, almost. You'd get the gray pallor [audible encouragement from Maury] . . . . Yeah, it was just—and you would get dark circles under your eyes, and your eyes would look almost sunken. Just like a skeleton would look. (*The Maury Povich Show* 1992a)

Because of time constraints in news reports, in a typical example, CNN (Cable News Network) capsulized the conveyance of physical stigma into a soundbite. After flashing a picture of anorexic "Margie," who at 65 pounds "couldn't ignore the disorder any longer," CNN reporter Linda Champa immediately cut to the "now healthy Margie," who disparagingly described what being anorexic was like: "You get extremely dry skin. Your hair starts to fall out. Your eyes become so dry that you can't wear contact lenses. You basically become a mess" (*CNN Newshour* 1993).

Attention-grabbing claims that focus on unpleasant aspects of appearance are not the lone provinces of journalists and talk show hosts. In 1978, psychiatrist Hilde Bruch offered an extremely stigmatizing account of anorexia, perhaps even setting the stage for future talk show portrayals. Describing her first encounter with an anorexic named "Alma," Hilde Bruch (1978:2) recounted:

> When she came for a consultation she looked like a walking skeleton, scantily dressed in shorts and a halter, with her legs sticking out like broomsticks, every rib showing, and her shoulder blades standing up like little wings. Her mother mentioned, "When I put my arms around her I feel nothing but bones, like a frightened little bird." Alma's arms and legs were covered with soft hair, her complexion had a yellowish tint, and her dry hair hung down in strings. Most striking was the face—hollow like that of a shriveled-up old woman with a wasting disease, sunken eyes, a sharply pointed nose on which the juncture between bone and cartilage was visible. When she spoke or smiled—and she was quite cheerful—one could see every movement of the muscles around her mouth and eyes, like an animated anatomical representation of the skull.

Such sensational claims—packed with drama, novelty, and emotion—make their way into the public foray because an entire population of claimsmakers is vying for the public's attention to their particular social problem. Prime space and prime time for presenting claims are limited commodities—whether in the media or the medical community. Thus, the competitive process of constructing social problems encourages such dramatic and sensational appeals (Hilgartner and Bosk 1988).

Examples abound—for instance, the emotional account of TV star Tracey Gold's mother Bonnie, who said she almost fainted when she saw her daughter change out of street clothes in her dressing room. Tracey's mother said she was "horrified by the skeletal apparition before her" and both mother and daughter "stood there crying" (Sporkin et al. 1992:92–93).

I encountered another dramatic claim while publicizing my book on anorexia. When the radio host G. Gordon Liddy asked for a definition of eating disorders, my fellow guest, Caroline Miller, a recovering bulimic, seized the moment to "differentiate" between anorexics and bulimics:

> Anorexics are hard to miss. They're skeletal, their skin often becomes yellow, they exercise compulsively, often 5 or 6 hours a day. Their hair starts to fall out. I mean, the usual description is like a concentration camp victim. And they don't eat much food. Bulimics, on the other hand, are 10 to 12 times more common. You're far more likely to know a bulimic than you are to know an anorexic. And bulimics are often the perfectionistic, attractive, outgoing achievers, quite often athletes in sports where weight is considered important. (*G. Gordon Liddy Show* 1993)

In this claim, Miller seems to be creating an eating disorder hierarchy, in which one eating disorder is deemed to be "better" and one "worse," perhaps in an effort to minimize the stigma associated with bulimia. For as Erving Goffman (1963:4–5) noted, the end result of a stigmatizing condition is that it creates distance, an "undesired differentness" from a so-called "normal." A stigmatized person is perceived as "not quite human" and is typically imputed to possess a wide range of imperfections on the basis of the original stigma.

It is important to note that claimsmakers and other actors in the social construction of problems may be operating under a number of goals— for example, television producers may be seeking ratings; medical professionals may be seeking to fill inpatient beds; mental health workers may be seeking clients and reputation enhancements; "experts" may be seeking to sell books. Certainly, there are enormous profits to be made in the "treatment" of anorexia nervosa and eating disorders. In reading the fine print of eating disorder literature, some eating disorder "help" organizations are affiliated with hospital treatment programs, networks of treatment professionals, or are selling their own training and programs.

For instance, the National Anorexic Aid Society, Inc. (NAAS) offers— for a fee—educational programs, professional training seminars, and an "Annual National Conference for professionals." NAAS, which maintains a network of "professionals and support groups worldwide," supports the medicalization of eating disorders: "Eating disorders must be diagnosed and treated by qualified professionals. . . . Treatment may include physical assessment, nutritional counseling, medication therapy, individual psychotherapy, family therapy, marital therapy, and group therapy" (1989). The most common method of medically controlling anorexics has been inpatient hospital treatment programs. Early on, most programs were based on B. F. Skinner's brand of behaviorism, with positive reinforcement schedules (e.g., increased freedom and privileges) for eating and weight gain. Critics charge that these programs are "too authoritarian," that they focus on weight gain, rather than underlying problems (Romeo 1986:54–55), and that their long-term success is questionable (Way 1993:74–81).

With the growth of specialized medicine and medical technology, prescription drugs have become the most common method to medically control deviance (Conrad and Schneider 1980:242–243). This has been evident in proposed treatments of anorexia nervosa and eating disorders as well. Social historian Joan Brumberg (1988:26) notes that throughout the twentieth century, anorexics have been treated with thyroid extracts, testosterone, lithium carbonate, L-dopa, calf pituitary implants, insulin, and among other treatments, shock therapy and prefrontal lobotomy. In the Spring 1990 issue of the American Anorexia/Bulimia Association newsletter, Diane Mickley, M.D., F.A.C.P., wrote of Prozac as an "exciting" treatment option: "This new anti-depressant can play a role not only in the treatment of depression, but also may be used for bulimia, anorexia, obesity, obsessive–compulsive disorder, and even panic disorder."

To some, particularly the friends and family of eating disordered patients, the uses of prescription drugs and biochemical explanations for anorexia nervosa and eating disorders are welcomed, as they believe this reduces the person's responsibility for her or his condition, and, therefore, the stigma associated with it. In Conrad and Schneider's (1980:247) terms, they are no longer "bad"; they are "sick"—it is not their fault.

This is a sentiment that MTV News reporter Tabitha Soren (1993) noted in a recent newspaper column: "Some recent studies suggest that eating disorders are not something people 'do' to themselves; that, depending on their biochemical makeup, some people may actually have a propensity for binge-eating. In other words, the eating disorder may not be their fault."

Yet Susan Bordo (1993:50–53) believes that this claim is misguided. In looking to biological causes to explain why the vast majority of eating disorder sufferers—90%—are female, Bordo says the medical community ignores the obvious: that the overwhelming majority of those who purchase weight loss products and attend weight loss centers are women, that this is a cultural phenomenon. The persistency of such medical models requires no leap of logic, says Bordo (1993:53), who argues that "the medical model has a deep professional, economic, and philosophical stake in preserving the integrity of what it has demarcated as its domain."

Still, removing the blame from the anorexic or eating disordered patient via biochemical explanations is a relatively new phenomenon. Yet another "blameless victim" claim has been around for decades: most common in psychiatric and "family systems" circles, the blame is taken away from the individual and placed squarely on the shoulders of the family—or in true psychoanalytic tradition, the mother.

Italian psychiatrist Mara Selvini Palazzoli (1974) blames the anorexic's mother for the daughter's anorexia. Describing "the monotonous behaviour of the mothers of anorexics," Palazzoli (1974:39–40) writes:

> They foster ambition and assertiveness in their children, but, in so doing, distinguish sharply between their sons and daughters. The boys are more immune to the mother's wiles and demands, largely because their experience and prospects make it more difficult for them to identify themselves with her. The girls, by contrast, are more easily subdued: they become the model children of a domineering, intolerant and hypercritical woman, who prevents them from standing their own ground and stunts their

emotional development. The daughters grow up in the shadow of the maternal super-ego.

Using a psychoanalytic framework, feminist Kim Chernin (1981:152) also claims anorexia and eating disorders are a way "to express towards our own flesh whatever angers we have acquired toward woman, our mother, throughout our life." In their literature review summary, Kerr et al. (1991:847) also conclude that anorexics and their mothers tend to be "hostile-dependent" and the mothers of anorexics "overinvolved in their daughters' lives."

Family systems theorists Minuchin et al. (1978) extend the blame to the family as a whole for a daughter's anorexia. He contends that the families of anorexics are "highly enmeshed" and overly involved in each other's affairs. Other studies report that women having families with "unhealthy functioning" (e.g., conflict resolution, empathy, clarity of expression, interpersonal distrust) are more likely to exhibit eating disordered attitudes and behaviors (Reeves and Johnson 1992; Kerr et al. 1991).

Recent "blame the family" claims also have centered on child abuse, parental addictions, and psychological problems. In her media appearance on a recent Larry King show, psychiatrist Dr. Virginia Codello stated: "There is a statistical significance of childhood physical, sexual, and other psychological abuse [and] statistical evidence of . . . either one or two parents having a history of obesity and/or other substance abuse and/or other psychiatric illnesses, such as major depression" (*Larry King Live* 1991).

Regardless of whether the eating disorder is blamed on the family, on chemical imbalances, or on the anorexic herself, the stigma associated with eating disorders persists. McLorg and Taub (1987) observe that in being labeled "anorexic" or "bulimic," a person is ascribed a deviant status—a master status identified before all others. This deviant identity affects social interactions, as the labeled deviant is scrutinized carefully— particularly in regard to eating and other behaviors.

Such stigmatization creates distance and indifference. It also, I believe, increases public apathy and lessens the likelihood that audiences will respond with conviction that eating disorders are a social problem we must "do something" about.

The Feminist Model of Eating Disorders

The feminist movement has included eating disorders and anorexia nervosa under its rubric of concern, viewing eating disorders as the consequences of women's lower status as objectified pawns in a patri-archal, male-dominated society (Bordo 1993; Chernin 1981, 1985; Orbach 1986). This view was also infused with mainstream energy in the early 1990s, through best-selling books such as *Backlash* (Faludi 1991) and *The Beauty Myth* (Wolf 1991).

Feminist claims have drawn attention to cultural factors contributing to eating disorders. For instance, Kim Chernin (1981:99–100) states that "anorexia nervosa began to be a widespread social disease among wom-en" in the 1960s, and links the resurgence of the women's movement in the 1960s to an "epidemic" of eating disorders. She claims that the women's movement, "asserting woman's right to authority, develop-ment, dignity, liberation and above all, power," threatened the fashion and diet industries, which responded by promulgating slimmer stan-dards of beauty. Chernin metaphorically equates thinner beauty stan-dards to pressuring women "to make themselves *smaller*, to *narrow* themselves, to become *lightweight*, to lose *gravity*, to be-*little* themselves." Chernin (1981:102) also believes that out of anger and rage at seeing what it means to be a woman in contemporary society, the anorexic is rejecting womanhood.

Moreover, Chernin (1985:188) believes that women were being forced to emulate men to achieve power, citing women's adoption of the male business uniform in the workplace. This corporate manipulation, in the midst of a struggle for liberation, had devastating consequences: "the present epidemic of eating disorders must be understood as a profound developmental crisis in a generation of women still deeply confused, after two decades of struggle for female liberation, about what it means to be a woman in the modern world" (Chernin 1985:17).

Susan Bordo (1993:23–42) greatly expands these themes, exploring in depth the complex intersections and crystallizations of culture that are present in the phenomena of eating disorders. Such elements include general cultural attitudes—the valuation of thinness in our culture and the role of consumer culture, as discussed earlier, cultural representations of female hunger and eating, the medicalization of eating disorders and other "female" disorders (hysteria, anxiety disorders such as agorapho-bia, obsessive–compulsive disorder), the common ground between eating disorders and "normal" female experiences, and so on. Bordo's analysis is an ongoing dialectical process, identifying crystalizations and interac-tions, in sharp contrast to the dualistic causal models that typify medical perspectives.

To Bordo (1993:58–60), stigmatizing the minds of anorexics as "faulty," "flawed," and displaying "invalid logic, poor reasoning, or mythological thinking," is pointless and misguided. These processes naturally follow when a person is deprived of food: "the diet" is itself a precarious, unstable, self-defeating state for a body to be in—a reality that the "disorder cognitions" of bulimics and anorectics are confronting all too clearly and painfully . . . each of these "distorted attitudes" is a fairly accurate representation of social attitudes toward slenderness or the biological realities involved in dieting.

Bordo (1993:32–33) also defends the work of Kim Chernin and Susie Orbach from attacks made by such critics as Joan Brumberg, who misread the feminist/cultural model as reducing eating disorders as a simple pursuit of thinness. These authors have "always stressed the intersection of culture with family, economic, and historical developments and psychological constructions of gender," the crux of the feminist/cultural model of eating disorders, according to Bordo.

Perhaps Bordo's (1993:56–57) strongest critique of the medical model is her contention that "normal" women's weight and dieting-conscious behaviors lie on the same continuum with those of "eating-disordered" women: "Most women in our culture, then, are 'disordered' when it comes to issues of self-worth, self-entitlement, and comfort with their own bodies; eating disorders, far from being 'bizarre' and anomalous, are utterly continuous with a dominant element of the experience of being female in this culture."

Apathy about Anorexia and Eating Disorders

Anorexia nervosa and eating disorders remain "minor league" social problems. The point we have reached now is public apathy. There has been no official response to the problem of eating disorders by a governmental agency, institution, or other influential group; no "official investigation," and no proposals for reforms—Spector and Kitsuse's (1987:148–151) criteria for progression to a second stage in a four-stage "natural history" of a social problem.

Perhaps public apathy is due to the overexposure of eating disorders in the 1980s (Brumberg 1988:14–40; Gordon 1990:2–3). Hilgartner and Bosk (1988:63) note that flooding can lead to a reduction in the impact of messages and increased apathy. This lack of public recognition may also relate to the types of claims that have been made and their (lack of) effectiveness. Spector and Kitsuse (1987:144) hypothesize that the more vague the sense of dissatisfaction, the more diffuse and general the claim will be, and the more unlikely that the claim will be recognized or responded to. Blaming society for eating disorders—as perceived by critics of the feminist/cultural model—may fall into this amorphous category. The alternate view—blaming the individual—as typically espoused in medical models—may be more palatable to the general public, because of its dualistic nature, offering concrete, black-and-white explanations for the causes of eating disorders.

Susan Bordo (1993:53–54) argues that the feminist/cultural perspective on eating disorders has deeply threatened the medical model. According to Bordo, the feminist/cultural model, shaped by the work of Kim Chernin, Susie Orbach, and Marlene Boskind-White, (1) challenges the designation of eating disorders as psychopathology, emphasizing the learned and addictive aspects of these behaviors; (2) recasts the roles of culture and gender as primary factors in the onset of eating disorders, rather than "triggering" or "contributory"; and (3) forces the "reassignment" of individual dysfunctional causes to social factors.

Critics of the feminist/cultural model are well-documented, as noted above, and include medical and mental health concerns, corporate operatives, the beauty and fashion industries, and other vested interests. Their response to the feminist/cultural model is the same: females become eating disordered because there is something wrong with them—they are "crazy" (or at least "mentally defective"), or deficient biochemically. For example, social historian Joan Brumberg (1988:38) also attacks the feminist/cultural model, arguing that "current cultural models fail to explain why so many individuals *do not* develop the disease, even though they have been exposed to the same cultural environment."

Bordo (1993:61–62) retorts, "of course we are *not* all exposed to 'the same cultural environment,'" but one that is tempered by unique factors such as race, class, age, education, religion, sexual orientation, family, genetic makeup and so on, that affect a person's interactions with cultural images. In a similar counterattack, Becky Wangsgaard Thompson (1992:558) observes that reducing eating disorders solely to cultural, appearance-based factors of women trying to attain certain beauty ideals is problematic to all women:

> The construction of bulimia and anorexia as appearance-based disorders is rooted in a notion of femininity in which white middle- and upper-class women are portrayed as frivolous, obsessed with their bodies, and overly accepting of narrow gender roles . . . . This construction of white middle- and upper-class women is intimately linked to the portrayal of working-class white women and women of color as their opposite: as somehow exempt from accepting the dominant standards of beauty or as one step away from being hungry and therefore not susceptible to eating problems. Identifying that women may binge to cope with poverty contrasts the notion that eating problems are class-bound. Attending to the intricacies of race, class, sexuality, and gender pushes us to rethink the demeaning construction of middle-class femininity and established bulimia and anorexia as serious responses to injustices.

Bordo (1993:64) criticizes Michael Strober, editor of the *Journal of Eating Disorders*, for suggesting that "the intensifying preoccupation with body shape and dieting so common in nonclinical adolescent populations" may be "indicative of a symptomatically milder or partial expression of the illness." Bordo observes that the medical model of eating disorders as "illness" and "disease" is so entrenched that Strober is "willing to 'medicalize' the majority of adolescent women into the bargain."

And so the arguments go, back and forth. Yet when we peel them away, one question remains: how successful has the feminist/cultural model been in countering medical claims of individual dysfunction, deviance, and stigma—claims that have been legitimated by the media, corporate operatives, the beauty and fashion industries as "objective truth"?

Spector and Kitsuse (1987:143–144) have observed that the more powerful the group, the more effective it is in pressing (and countering) claims. So who wins this public foray, this tug-of-war between opposing claims, the medical vs. the feminist/cultural? Well, I ask you: who has the most power?

References

AA/BA Newsletter. 1990. Teaneck, NJ: American Anorexia/Bulimia Association, Inc. Summer.

American Psychiatric Association. 1987. *Diagnostic and Statistical Manual of Mental Disorders, Third Edition - Revised*. Washington, D.C.: American Psychiatric Association.

"Ann Landers." 1994 *The Philadelphia Inquirer*, April 1.

ANRED (Anorexia Nervosa and Related Eating Disorders, Inc.) 1986. *Anorexia Nervosa and Bulimia*. Eugene, OR: ANRED.

Banner, L. W. 1983. *American Beauty*. New York: Alfred A. Knopf.

Best, J. 1988. "Missing Children, Misleading Statistics." *The Public Interest* 92:84–92.

Blumer, H. 1971. "Social Problems as Collective Behavior." *Social Problems* 18:298–306.

Bordo, S. 1993. *Unbearable Weight: Feminism, Western Culture, and the Body*. Berkeley: University of California Press.

Boskind-White, M. 1985. "Bulimarexia: A Sociocultural Perspective." In *Theory and Treatment of Anorexia Nervosa and Bulimia: Biomedical, Sociocultural, and Psychological Perspectives*, edited by S. W. Emmett. New York: Brunner/Mazel.

Bruch, H. 1973. *Eating Disorders: Obesity, Anorexia Nervosa, and the Person Within*. New York: Basic Books.

———. 1978. *The Golden Cage: The Enigma of Anorexia Nervosa*. New York: Vintage Books.

————. 1988. *Conversations With Anorexics*, edited by D. Czyzewski and M. A. Suhr. New York: Basic Books.

Brumberg, J. J. 1988. *Fasting Girls: The Emergence of Anorexia Nervosa as a Modern Disease*. Cambridge, MA: Harvard University Press.

The Bulletin with Larry Kane. 1993. KYW-TV3, Philadelphia. November 5.

Chernin, K. 1981. *The Obsession: Reflections of the Tyranny of Slenderness*. New York: Harper & Row.

————. 1985. *The Hungry Self: Women, Eating and Identity*. New York: Times Books.

CNN Newshour. 1993. "Anorexia Plagues Many Image-Conscious Young Women." Cable News Network, April 26.

Conrad, P., and J. W. Schneider. 1980. *Deviance and Medicalization: From Badness to Sickness*. St. Louis: C. V. Mosby.

Crandall, C., and M. Biernat. 1990. "The Ideology of Anti-Fat Attitudes." *Journal of Applied Social Psychology* 20(3):227–243.

Crocker, J., B. Cornwell, and B. Major. 1993. "The Stigma of Overweight: Affective Consequences of Attributional Ambiguity." *Journal of Personality and Social Psychology* 64(1):60–70.

DeJong, W., and R. E. Kleck. 1986. "The Social Psychological Effects of Overweight." Pp. 65–87 in *Physical Appearance, Stigma, and Social Behavior: The Ontario Symposium Volume 3*, edited by C. P. Herman, M. P. Zanna, and E. T. Higgins. Hillsdale, NJ: Lawrence Erlbaum.

Dunn, D. 1992. "When Thinness Becomes Illness." *Business Week* 3277(August 3):74–75.

Ellmann, M. 1993. *The Hunger Artists: Starving, Writing, and Imprisonment*. Cambridge, MA: Harvard University Press.

Faludi, S. 1991. *Backlash: The Undeclared War Against American Women*. New York: Crown.

The G. Gordon Liddy Show. 1993. "Eating Disorder Panel." August 30.

Garner, D. M., P. E. Garfinkel, D. Schwartz, and M. Thompson. 1980. "Cultural Expectations of Thinness in Women." *Psychological Reports* 47:483–491.

Geraldo. 1989. "Teen Diet Horror Stories." January 10.

Goffman, E. 1963. *Stigma: Notes on the Management of Spoiled Identity*. Englewood Cliffs, NJ: Prentice-Hall.

Gordon, R. A. 1990. *Anorexia and Bulimia: Anatomy of a Social Epidemic*. Cambridge, MA: Basil Blackwell.

Gortmaker, S. L., A. Must, J. M. Perrin, A. Sobol, and W. H. Dietz. 1993. "Social and Economic Consequences of Overweight in Adolescence and Young Adulthood." *New England Journal of Medicine* 329:1008–1012.

Hesse-Biber, S. 1989. "Eating Patterns and Disorders in a College Population: Are College Women's Eating Problems a New Phenomenon?" *Sex Roles* 20(1/2):71–89.

Hilgartner, S., and C. L. Bosk. 1988. "The Rise and Fall of Social Problems: A Public Arenas Model." *American Journal of Sociology* 94(1):53–78.

Johnson, C. L. (ed.). 1991. *Psychodynamic Treatment of Anorexia Nervosa and Bulimia*. New York: The Guilford Press.

Jones, E. E., A. Farina, A. H. Hastorf, H. Markus, D. T. Miller, and R. A. Scott.

1984. *Social Stigma: The Psychology of Marked Relationships.* New York: W. H. Freeman.

Kerr, J. K, R. L. Skok, and T. F. McLaughlin. 1991. "Characteristics Common to Females Who Exhibit Anorexic or Bulimic Behavior: A Review of Current Literature." *Journal of Clinical Psychology* 47(6):846–853.

Lague, L., A. Lynn, L. Armstrong, G. Saveri, and L. S. Healy. 1993. "How Thin Is Too Thin?" *People Magazine* 40(September 20):74–80.

Larry King Live. 1991. "The Agony of Eating Disorders." October 9.

Maddox, G. L., K. W. Back, and V. R. Liederman. 1968. "Overweight as Social Deviance and Disability." *Journal of Health and Social Behavior* 9:287–298.

The Maury Povich Show. 1992a. "Starving for Attention." March 13.

———. 1992b. "Dying to be Thin." April 27.

———. 1993. "Twins with Eating Disorders." November 16.

McLorg, P., and D. E. Taub. 1987. "Anorexia Nervosa and Bulimia: The Development of Deviant Identities." *Deviant Behavior* 8:177–189.

Miller, C. 1987. "Who Talks Like a Women's Magazine? Language and Gender in Popular Women's and Men's Magazines." *Journal of American Culture* 10:1–9.

Miller, C., E. D. Rothblum, L. Barbour, P. A. Brand, and D. Felicio. 1990. "Social Interactions of Obese and Nonobese Women." *Journal of Personality* 58(2):65–80.

Minuchin, S., B. L. Rosman, and L. Baker. 1978. *Psychosomatic Families: Anorexia Nervosa in Context.* Cambridge, MA: Harvard University Press.

NAAS Newsletter. 1989 (spring). Columbus, OH: National Anorexic Aid Society, Inc.

Orbach, S. 1986. *Hunger Strike: The Anorectic's Struggle as a Metaphor for Our Age.* New York: Avon.

Palazzoli, M. S. 1974. *Self-Starvation: From Individual to Family Therapy in the Treatment of Anorexia Nervosa.* Northvale, NJ: Jason Aronson.

Polivy, J., D. M. Garner, and P. E. Garfinkel. 1986. "Causes and Consequences of the Current Preference for Thin Female Physiques." Pp. 89–112 in *Physical Appearance, Stigma, and Social Behavior: The Ontario Symposium Volume 3,* edited by C. P. Herman, M. P. Zanna, and E. T. Higgins. Hillsdale, NJ: Lawrence Erlbaum.

Reeves, P. C., and M. E. Johnson. 1992. "Relationship Between Family-of-Origin Functioning and Self-Perceived Correlates of Eating Disorders Among Female College Students." *Journal of College Student Development* 33:44–49.

Rodin, J., L. Silberstein, and R. Striegel-Moore. 1985. "Women and Weight: A Normative Discontent." Pp. 267–307 in *Nebraska Symposium on Motivation: Vol. 32. Psychology and Gender,* edited by T. B. Sonderegger. Lincoln, NE: University of Nebraska Press.

Romeo, F. 1986. *Understanding Anorexia Nervosa.* Springfield, IL: Charles C. Thomas.

Rosen, J. C., and J. Gross. 1987. "Prevalence of Weight Reducing and Weight Gaining in Adolescent Girls and Boys." *Health Psychology* 6:131–147.

Schur, E. M. 1984. *Labeling Women Deviant: Gender, Stigma, and Social Control.* New York: McGraw-Hill.

Silverstein, B., L. Perdue, B. Peterson, and E. Kelly. 1986. "The Role of the Media in Promoting a Thin Standard of Bodily Attractiveness for Women." *Sex Roles* 14(9/10):519–532.

Soren, T. 1993. "New Hope for Eating Disorders by Keeping Chemicals in Balance." *The Philadelphia Inquirer* October 26:B3.

Sours, J. A. 1980. *Starving to Death in a Sea of Objects: The Anorexia Nervosa Syndrome*. New York: Jason Aronson.

Spector, M., and J. I. Kitsuse. 1987. *Constructing Social Problems*. New York: Aldine de Gruyter.

Sporkin, E., J. Wagner, and C. Tomashoff. 1992. "A Terrible Hunger." *People Magazine* 37 (February 17):92–94.

Thompson, B. W. 1992. "A Way Outa No Way: Eating Problems among African-American, Latina, and White Women." *Gender and Society* 6:4):546–561.

Thompson, K. 1986. "Larger Than Life." *Psychology Today* April:20:38–44.

U.S. Department of Health and Human Services Public Health Service. n.d. "Facts About Anorexia Nervosa." Bethesda, MD: National Institutes of Health.

Way, K. 1993. *Anorexia Nervosa and Recovery: A Hunger for Meaning*. Binghamton, NY: Haworth Press.

Weibel, K. 1977. *Mirror, Mirror: Images of Women Reflected in Popular Culture*. Garden City, NY: Anchor/Doubleday.

Williamson, D. A. 1990. *Assessment of Eating Disorders: Obesity, Anorexia, and Bulimia Nervosa*. New York: Pergamon Press.

Wiseman, C., J. J. Gray, J. E. Mosimann, and A. H. Ahrens. 1992. "Cultural Expectations of Thinness in Women: An Update." *International Journal of Eating Disorders* 11(1):85–89.

Wolf, N. 1991. *The Beauty Myth: How Images of Beauty Are Used Against Women*. New York: Morrow.

IV

Contested Quality of Food

6

The Management of Food Ambivalence: Erosion and Reconstruction?

ALAN BEARDSWORTH

Introduction

The interplay of the ecological, economic, cultural, psychological, and physiological factors that shape the act of eating provides a seemingly inexhaustible source of challenging questions and fascinating puzzles. Moreover, possibly some of the most fascinating of these puzzles arise from the fact that where there are multiple significances (and, indeed, multiple layers of meaning) there is also the likelihood of conflict, uncertainty, and ambivalence. Where there is conflict, uncertainty, and ambivalence, there is also likely to be anxiety. In the not too distant past, the overriding anxiety relating to food, for all but a privileged minority, was the fear of shortage, or even actual starvation. In the developed Western economies such fears (in their most extreme form) have now receded for the vast majority of the population (although they may persist for certain vulnerable or marginal groups). Increasingly, however, more subtle anxieties, nutritional and ideological, that have always been present, but that may have been partially masked by more pressing concerns, have surfaced and found expression. These anxieties, and the ambivalences that underpin them, have had a profound effect on the ways in which food-related social problems in modern societies have been constructed and construed. What is more, while historically it has been the usual pattern for food anxieties to be projected downward through the social hierarchy (middle class concerns about the food expenditure habits and nutritional standards of the poor, and adult concerns about the food intake of children, for example), this is now no longer so clearly the case. In contemporary western societies it is now much more acceptable to exhibit concern about one's own nutritional status, as well as that of one's offspring or social inferiors.

In view of the foregoing discussion, this chapter will address itself to four main issues:

1. What is the nature of the underlying ambivalence of food and eating, and what are the characteristic anxieties generated by such ambivalence?
2. What are the traditional confidence-generating cultural devices that serve to manage and control such anxieties?
3. In what sense have these traditional cultural devices been eroded or attenuated, and what are the processes involved?
4. What are the consequences of this erosion, and are novel processes and forms emerging to replace these older modes of confidence maintenance?

To cast light upon these questions, I employ a deliberately eclectic approach, unashamedly plundering the insights of such scholars as the sociologist, the social anthropologist, and the social historian.

On The Nature of Food Ambivalence

There can be little doubt that the omnivorous inclination of *Homo sapiens* has been one of the crucial factors behind the current success of our species and its global distribution. However, while the omnivore's strategy offers potentially important advantages such as adaptability, versatility, and the capacity to respond rapidly to novel opportunities, it also carries potentially significant risks. Rozin (1976), for example, discusses what he terms the *omnivore's paradox*. This paradox emerges out of the contradiction between *neophilia* (the omnivore's drive to sample possible new food sources) and *neophobia* (the omnivore's fear of the hazards that may involved in consuming previously untried food items). The tension between neophilia and neophobia is one that all omnivores, humans included, must cope with, along with the concomitant stress and anxiety such tension may induce. Interestingly, Fischler has argued that, for the human omnivore "modern society develops in such a way

Table 6.1.   Positive and Negative Aspects of the Three Paradoxes[a]

Positive	Negative
1. Food provides gustatory pleasure, satiety, etc.	Food can produce gustatory displeasure, dyspepsia, nausea, vomiting
2. Food is required for vigor, energy, and health	Food can introduce illness and disease
3. Food is required for the continuation of life	Food entails the death of the organisms consumed

[a] Adapted from Beardsworth and Keil (1992a).

that it tends to increase the anxiety of the paradox instead of regulating it" (1980:945). It is this crucial proposition that this chapter sets out to explore, examining various explanations of this effect along the way.

Eating is a profoundly ambivalent activity, and the human individual's relationship to food is inevitably imbued with a certain tension. Indeed, this ambivalence has many more dimensions than the neophilia/neophobia paradox discussed above. It is, of course, impossible in this chapter to focus attention on anything more than a limited selection of these dimensions. In their discussion of contemporary vegetarianism Beardsworth and Keil (1992a) identify three particular paradoxes that can be seen as generating food ambivalence, and I employ these examples illustratively to advance the present argument (see Table 6.1). Each of the three paradoxes consists of a contradiction or an opposition between a positively valued and a negatively valued aspect of the intake of food. In turn, each contradiction can be seen as giving rise to its own characteristic forms of eating-related anxiety.

Paradox 1 (the pleasure/displeasure paradox) refers to the fact that while food can provide intense pleasure and a welcome sense of fullness and satisfaction, it can also produce sensations and reactions ranging from mildly unpleasant to severely distressing. The anxieties produced by these possibilities include fear of experiencing unpalatable tastes or flavor combinations and the resulting sense of revulsion, fear of experiencing digestive distress ("indigestion," "dyspepsia," "bloatedness," etc.), and fear of experiencing nausea or even actual vomiting. Such concerns are likely to be particularly significant in relation to a neophobic response to a novel food item. In addition, individuals may also be nervous about possible effects of food intake that are perceptible to others. These include short-term effects like flatulence and belching and long-term effects like cosmetic overweight or obesity, which can sometimes undermine what Goffman (1969) has described as the performance required for the presentation of a socially competent self in the course of everyday social interaction.

Paradox 2 (the health/disease paradox) refers to the fact that food can be conceived of as the primary source of energy, vitality, and good health, but at the same time clearly carries the potential to introduce disease-inducing substances or organisms into the body. These possibilities give rise, on the one hand, to anxieties about acute effects (e.g., rapidly acting toxins or infections) and, on the other, to anxieties about chronic effects (e.g., slow acting toxins or disease-causing agents and long-term nutrient deficiencies).

Paradox 3 (the life/death paradox) refers to the fact that while eating is an absolute and unavoidable necessity for the maintenance of life, it frequently involves the dissolution of some other organism in the process of its being consumed. There are, of course, some exceptions to this rule in the human diet (for example, the use of milk produced by domesticated mammals, although dairy production does usually involve the slaughter and consumption of surplus males and older, less productive females). Although, typically, the ingestion of plants or their fruits gives rise to little concern in this connection, the eating of animals is another matter. Here anxiety may be generated as a result of moral concerns about inflicting physical suffering on, and taking the life of, a food animal. However, not all animals are accorded the same concern in this respect, there being a fairly distinct hierarchy with large mammals at the top (Midgley 1983:90). The work of Beardsworth and Keil (1992a) indicates that vegetarians (who are usually particularly sensitive to such issues) often explicitly recognize such a hierarchy.

Although, as has been emphasized above, these paradoxes are only selected examples, they do serve to illustrate the kinds of food-related anxieties that have to be managed, regulated, or controlled. From the point of view of the social scientist, such management is not something that can be achieved simply by individuals acting and thinking in isolation. Solutions or coping strategies must emerge and be sustained at the cultural level. What, then, are the kinds of cultural adaptations that exist to regulate these anxieties? To attempt to answer this question, attention must turn first to traditional societies.

Traditional Modes of Managing Food Ambivalence and Anxiety

In addressing the issue of the ways in which traditional societies manage food-related anxieties, it is, of course acknowledged that in such societies all too often the overriding nutritional concern may be the avoidance of malnutrition or starvation. Nevertheless, lurking beneath episodic or cyclical shortages, or even chronic deprivation related to structural, economic, or ecological factors, the kinds of nutritional paradox discussed above still exist. Broadly speaking, however, it can be argued that a heavy sedimentation of belief, custom, and ritual, laid down over many generations, provides a stable and taken-for-granted frame of reference within which the anxieties generated may be effectively neutralized. Returning to the three specific paradoxes already discussed, it is worth examining in some detail how their associated anxieties are coped with.

· *Paradox 1 (Pleasure/Displeasure) Anxieties*

Anxieties concerning the possibility of experiencing gustatory displeasure or even a severe sense of revulsion in relation to particular tastes can be very immediate ones, as can fears about the risk of becoming nauseous or vomiting. However, in traditional societies, where what Beardsworth and Keil (1992a) have referred to as the "alimentary totality" of food items defined as suitable for human consumption tends to be relatively stable over time, sheer familiarity with the aliments in question, and their modes of combination, is in itself reassuring. Indeed, in this connection Rozin and Rozin (1981:246) have argued that many traditional cuisines are based upon distinctive "flavor principles," and that the principles operated by such major "cuisine groups" as India, China, and Mexico exhibit an impressive long-term stability. These characteristic combinations of flavoring elements, the authors suggest, may have significance at a number of levels, but one of their purposes may be to reinforce the eater's sense of familiarity with what is being consumed. In fact, Fischler (1980), developing a point made by Rozin (1976), reminds us that well-established flavor principles can effectively mediate between neophilia and neophobia, since new food items can be incorporated into an existing cuisine by being made to taste familiar and hence less threatening. More generally, the entire corpus of a long established culinary culture can be seen as providing a reassuring effect, with its rules and norms concerning food combinations, meal patterning, and commensality, food preferences and taboos, eating etiquette, food preparation techniques, and gender and status-related forms of nutritional differentiation.

In traditional societies, the digestive distress produced by overeating may not be regarded as a particularly important hazard. Opportunities for overindulgence in terms of food intake are usually relatively rare, at least for most individuals. Indeed, recurring acute food crises may be the norm, as well as the possibility of chronic food shortages. For example, as Mennell (1985:24–27) points out, harvest failures and famines were common features of the early modern period in Western Europe, and the fear of hunger was a constant theme in European popular consciousness. Additionally, Mennell argues, the insecurity of the food supply may lead to a state of oscillation between fasting and feasting, with occasional (often ritual) gorging as a welcome relief from an anxious preoccupation with the unpredictable availability of one's next meal. Such extreme oscillations of mood and activity are seen by Elias (1982:237–288) as characteristic of earlier medieval attitudes. It is also Elias' view that the medieval personality, largely unfettered by the internalized constraints that are seen as the result of what he terms the "civilizing process," was less likely to be inhibited about the physiological processes of digestion, and about their auditory and olfactory manifestations (Elias 1978:129–143). This point can be taken even further by noting that in many traditional cultures what would be seen in contemporary western society as an embarrassing prandial *faux pas*, can actually be a required expression of politeness. For example, Grimble (1952:35–36) records that among the inhabitants of the Gilbert Islands of the Western Pacific, a guest given food is expected to produce a sonorous belch to demonstrate enjoyment and appreciation of the hospitality provided.

What is more, the fear of weight gain, or of obesity, which may dominate the nutritional attitudes and practices of many individuals in western societies, leading to varying levels of commitment to weight controlling or weight-reducing diets, may be largely irrelevant in traditional societies. Where the threat of food shortage is always a reality, a substantial covering of body fat may provide both a welcome insurance against future privation and a very visible symbol of high social status.

Thus, overall, it seems plausible to suggest that in traditional or premodern societies the anxieties associated with paradox 1 are of relatively low visibility, or are rendered irrelevant by long established custom and practice.

Paradox 2 (Health/Disease) Anxieties

The possibility that the intake of food may introduce disease-inducing agents into the body is one of particular relevance to the human omnivore. Counteracting the fears associated with this possibility we have the full force of a society's nutritional culture. In the case of a traditional society, this culture, as well as its powerful expressive and symbolic elements, will consist both of an extensive body of detailed empirical knowledge, and a component of what western thought would regard as "magical" beliefs and ideas. Empirical knowledge concerning the production, preparation, and consumption of food builds up over many generations to provide an extensive body of ideas and techniques based upon experience and trial and error. While such knowledge may be formulated in terms that appear somewhat exotic to the western observer, he or she would probably be prepared to recognize the validity of, for example, the causal relationships being described. On the other hand, magical thinking (which is also essentially oriented toward achieving practical ends) is based upon conceptions of cause and effect that would no longer be accepted in terms of modern western rationality. Thus, attempts may be made to control people, animals, objects, or processes through "sympathetic" magic (which is based upon the idea that manipulating some object similar to the target object will produce the desired effect). Similarly, "contagious" magic seeks to manipulate the target object by contact with it, or with some part of it.[1]

However, the sympathetic/contagious dichotomy does not exhaust all the possibilities of magical thinking in relation to nutrition and the avoidance or treatment of disease. In many traditional societies foods are classified according to a hot–cold dimension, and this may be closely associated with beliefs concerning health and illness (Manderson 1987; Messer 1987; Pool 1987). For example, the people of the fishing villages of the east coast of the Malay Peninsula studied by Wilson (1981) classify all food items as either "hot" or "cold" (these properties being unrelated to the physical temperature of the food itself). They believe that after giving birth a woman is in danger of becoming "cold," which could pose a serious threat to her health. Strenuous efforts must be made to keep her "hot" for 40 days to avoid such risks. Hence she may eat only foods defined as "hot" (e.g., rice, dry roasted fish, salt, coffee, manioc, peppers). The ingestion of "cold" foods (e.g., vegetables and most fruits) is something to be avoided at all costs. While such a view of the dietary requirements of newly delivered mothers might be viewed with some skepticism by western experts, and does seem to be very vulnerable to straightforward refutation, magical knowledge is highly elastic and therefore extremely resilient. As Gluckman (1965) points out, magical thought copes with awkward cases or pieces of discrepant evidence by stretching its principles to accommodate them. What is more, empirical knowledge and magical ideas tend to become interwoven with each other, and in general the line between the two is blurred or has little or no common sense significance. Empiricomagical knowledge evolves slowly and imperceptibly over long periods of time, and is not, by its very nature, subject to rapid revolutionary changes, or to the "paradigm shifts" that Kuhn (1970) has argued are crucial, if occasional, features of scientific thought and discourse. For these reasons empiricomagical nutritional knowledge and practices seem natural, taken-for-granted features of everyday experience for the individuals who employ them. The authority of such ideas, and their apparent immutability, means that they operate as very powerful devices for generating a robust, unquestioning confidence in existing foodways and nutritional patterns, effectively neutralizing paradox 2 anxieties, or providing ready made modes of responding to them.

However, it should be noted that the foregoing argument is not intended to imply that the magical component of nutritional ideas can ever be completely arbitrary. Empiricomagical knowledge usually works well enough for practical purposes, although it may be more effective at recognizing short-term or acute outcomes than identifying long-term processes or chronic effects. As Fischler (1980:941) remarks, a culture could not sustain positively harmful features indefinitely, but would be compelled to adjust toward a better fit between environment, society, and the human organism.

Paradox 3 (Life/Death) Anxieties

While the consumption of plant foods engenders little or no concern about the welfare or interests of the organisms concerned, animal-derived foods pose humans with an altogether different problem. Since most of these foods (although, of course not all) entail the killing of the donor animal, questions concerning the moral acceptability of taking the life of an entity with a nervous system and the ability to experience pain and apprehension inevitably surface. This is not to suggest that all species of animal are likely to stimulate equal levels of ethical interest. Forms perceived as remote from humanity (arthropods of all species, for example) are likely to elicit scant concern, whereas forms perceived as close to humanity (large mammals, for example) present altogether more worrying issues for their would-be consumers. However, in traditional societies, the anxieties generated by the practice of dining upon such ethically challenging creatures are dealt with in a number of imaginative and ingenious ways.

In cultures in which the hunting of game represents a significant contribution to food resources, rituals aimed at the propitiation of prey animals killed are common (Frazer 1936, Part V, Vol. II:204–273, Kent 1989:12–13). Coon (1976:140–141) describes the elaborate apologies made to a slain elephant by the Akoa Pygmies, the content of the ceremonial incantation performed being perfectly clear in its implications:

Our spear strayed from its course,
O Father Elephant!
We didn't mean to kill you,
We didn't mean to hurt you,
O Father Elephant!
It wasn't the warrior who took your life,
Your hour had come,
Don't come back to trample down our huts,
O Father Elephant!
Don't be angry with us,
From now on your life will be better,
You live in the land of the Spirits,
Our fathers will go with you to renew their bond,
You live in the land of the Spirits.

The author also describes an analogous rite of appeasement carried out on the body of a dead elephant by the Mbuti Pygmies (Coon 1976:142–144). On the other hand, Sharp (1988) demonstrates that specific rituals may not be necessary to salve the uneasy conscience of the hunter, since reassuring beliefs can actually be inherent features of a traditional society's entire cosmology. Thus the Chipewyan, a people of the Canadian Boreal forest with a still active hunting culture, believe that a prey animal can be killed only with its own consent. Animals may be willing to die because they "like" the hunter, or because they "pity" him. Animals are simultaneously natural and supernatural, renewing themselves by becoming young again each spring. Great care must be taken not to offend them, lest they withdraw their consent to offer themselves up to the humans who depend upon them (Sharp 1988:187). In a rather different vein, Guenther (1988:198–199) notes that Bushman hunters, while regarding their prey with a sense of affection and aesthetic and symbolic appreciation, maintain a strong sense of the "otherness" of animals in relation to humans, a sense that balances their perceived "sameness." Thus animals do not come to be seen as surrogate humans, and the hunter is protected from any feelings of guilt that might arise out of the acts of killing and consuming them.

Pastoralist or agricultural peoples may justify the slaughter of domesticated species with the idea that human beings have been granted a divine license to exploit animals (and, indeed, the natural world in general). This concept finds one of its clearest and most explicit expressions in the Judeo-Christian tradition, although the permission granted by God to Noah and his descendants to eat flesh was conditional on the observation of elaborate prohibitions and rituals, most notably the draining of the blood from the animal so that its spirit could flow into the earth (Farb and

Armelagos 1980:134–141). Even where a system of religious belief is explicitly opposed to the taking of animal life, customarily approved modes of accommodation can emerge. Harris (1986:23–24) points out that although Buddhists are forbidden to slaughter or to witness the slaughter of animals, they are permitted to consume flesh as long as they did not participate directly in the taking of the animal's life. Thus Buddhists typically consume a wide range of animal products, and "blame" for the killing involved may be passed down the social hierarchy, or transferred to specialist castes or pariah groups (Simoons 1961:11–12). Similarly, Harris (1986:60–61) notes that Hindu farmers may rid themselves of unwanted cattle by selling them to Moslem traders, whose religion does not place upon them the absolute prohibition on the killing of cows that is such a central feature of Hinduism. The resulting meat is consumed by Moslems, Christians, and even lower caste Hindus, although it is commonly labeled as "mutton" in deference to Hindu sensibilities.

At this point it is worth attempting to summarize the overall effects of the cultural devices discussed above: In traditional societies the multi-generational sedimentation and slow evolution of nutritional cultures give foodways and cuisines a sense of being "natural," largely unquestionable, and hence essentially unproblematic. Long established flavor principles may exist to reinforce this effect, and to provide a familiar and reassuring culinary vocabulary of taste sensations. Furthermore, traditional cultures typically embody respected ritual, cosmological or theological complexes that legitimate the killing of animals for food and absolve the perpetrator from personal blame (or, alternatively, devices exist for transferring that blame to others). In addition, these features usually exist in circumstances in which exposure to, or intrusion of, foreign or exotic foodways is relatively rare (such foodways, if encountered, appearing "unnatural" or bizarre). The cumulative effect of all these features is that, in general, individuals experience a high level of nutritional confidence, in the specific sense that the three paradoxes chosen for examination, and their accompanying anxieties, are not salient features of everyday thought and discourse. On the other hand, concerns about food shortage, nutritional deprivation, or the broader symbolic or ritual significance of food may well be the focus of considerable attention.

The Erosion of Traditional Modes of Anxiety Management

Increasingly, these traditional modes of anxiety management are in decline as a result of a complex of interlocking changes. Of course, modern developed societies have witnessed far reaching and fundamental transformations of their entire food system, so that by the late twentieth century a number of deep-seated trends have become apparent. These include a shift away from the local and the insular in terms of culinary cultures and the establishment of a highly reliable food supply, whose abundance has effectively eliminated shortages and serious malnutrition (although there may persist certain disadvantaged groups that remain at risk). Accompanying this abundance is a veritable explosion of choice, insofar as the boundaries of the alimentary totalities of modern societies (i.e., the range of food items or aliments offered) continue to expand at an impressive rate. The underlying factors that have contributed to these transformations in food systems are sufficiently familiar to require only broad summarization. Perhaps the most important of these are the long-term process of rationalization and industrialization that has had as revolutionary an effect on the food system as upon the rest of the structures and relationships of the advanced societies. The impact has been felt not only in the sphere of food production, but also in processing, preservation, transportation, and retailing. Innovations in these areas have facilitated the globalization of the food supply, which has produced substantial benefits for consumers in the industrialized societies. Within these societies, rising real incomes, changes in household structure, and the increasing movement of women into the labor market have all introduced changes into nutritional practices and patterns of food consumption (see Goodman and Redclift 1991).

A series of factors operating at the cultural level has also reinforced these effects. Not least of these is the ideological potency of consumerism, with its emphasis on open-ended material aspirations, heavily influenced by fashion and the pursuit of "style." This is compounded by the globalization of culture itself, driven by migration, mass tourism, and the creation of worldwide mass communications networks. The mass media themselves, most obviously through the impact of advertising, have also been deeply involved in these changes. All these factors, whether material or cultural, have contributed directly to the erosion of traditional foodways by providing a plethora of novel ideas, food items, dishes, flavor principles, and nutritional opportunities. Further, these effects can be placed in the broader context of the widespread decline of customary practices and traditional beliefs associated with the processes of secularization and rationalization at the heart of the development of modernity. Indeed, as Gofton (1990) has pointed out, the very fact that the processes of food production and food processing are becoming increasingly divorced from the household setting, and increasingly beyond the view of everyday experience, can give rise to concerns about food quality and food safety. What is more, Gofton argues, if we accept the idea of emerging postmodern cultural forms, the new flexibility of the postmodern household means that eating becomes a much more individualized and loosely organized activity. As tightly structured meal patterns and habitual household commensality become increasingly unusual, yet another feature of traditional foodways can be seen to be in decline.

The development of scientific thought has played a particularly prominent role in the decline of traditional modes of maintaining nutritional confidence. Scientific discourse and practice (and their technological applications) have, of course, had an ever expanding influence upon many aspects of everyday life from the beginning of the early modern period onward. Food and nutrition have received an enormous amount of scientific attention. For example, Turner (1982) examined the increasingly elaborate medical discourse on diet and health from the seventeenth century onward. Burnett (1989) provides a detailed account of the impact of the work on food adulteration carried out in the early nineteenth century by Frederick Accum (a professor of chemistry), and Mennell (1992) examined the complex interaction, throughout the nineteenth and twentieth centuries, of lay and professional medical beliefs concerning the "digestibility" of various food items, and their suitability for given age groups. Perhaps the most useful overview of the development of the science of nutrition in relation to its influence on popular attitudes and state policy is provided by Levenstein (1988), who seeks to document the way in which professional opinion has undergone significant transformations in its views concerning dietary requirements and priorities. The power and prestige of modern science, and the great advances in understanding it has achieved, mean that its ideas now exert a potent influence not only upon "official" or "expert" discourses on diet, but also upon "common sense" views of food and eating. The ideas and pronouncements of nutritionists, dietitians, physicians, microbiologists, toxicologists, and food technologists have now largely (but not entirely) supplanted empiricomagical forms of knowledge.

However, inevitably and unsurprisingly, by its very nature science constantly raises what Weinberg (1972) has termed "trans-scientific" questions. These are questions that can be posed quite rationally as matters of "fact," open to scientific examination, yet to which science itself cannot provide satisfactory and unambiguous answers, at least in the short to medium term (and sometimes even in the long term). As Tracey (1977) indicates, certain aspects of human nutritional requirements exhibit trans-scientific features. I have argued elsewhere (Beardsworth 1990) that many current issues concerning the links between diet and health (e.g., connections between eating patterns and heart disease, possible threats posed to human health by beef products from herds infected with bovine spongiform encephalopathy, and the long-term effects of chronic exposure to pesticide residues in food) also raise trans-scientific questions that may prove stubbornly resistant to satisfactory resolution. This may be due in part to ethical restrictions on work involving human subjects, and in part to the enormous difficulties involved in linking given disease outcomes with specific causal agents, given the extremely complex interactions of the many factors that may potentially be implicated. The nature of scientific doubt and uncertainty, and the essentially provisional nature of scientific pronouncements and explanations, on the other hand, may not be readily understood by the public at large. Indeed the public, often relatively poorly equipped to assess the practical significance of statistically expressed risks to health, may experience exaggerated levels of anxiety, or demand economically impracticable risk-free guarantees (Paulos 1988). Thus questions relating to food and nutrition raised by the life sciences may generate public uncertainty and anxiety while at the same time offering no clear cut answers or straightforward short-term remedies. At this point we have arrived at another paradox. Science exerts an authoritative (albeit usually indirect or mediated) influence on public opinion, yet at the same time it is provisional and often rapidly changing. In this latter sense, it is the exact opposite of the empiricomagical thinking at the foundations of traditional forms of nutritional confidence. There is, of course, a peculiar irony inherent in this situation. Scientific discourses may act to elevate levels of food anxiety at the same time as scientific insights and their applications are achieving significant advances in areas such as productivity and hygiene standards.

The erosion of nutritional confidence can be seen as having direct consequences for the extent to which the three paradoxes intrude into everyday consciousness and generate a sense of unease or concern. In relation to paradox 1 (pleasure/displeasure), Mennell (1992) demonstrates that in England from the early nineteenth century onward both medical and lay opinion becomes increasingly preoccupied with the uncomfortable, unpleasant, or embarrassing aspects of food ingestion. Foods became more and more likely to be classified according to their perceived tendency to cause unwanted effects like indigestion, constipation, and flatulence. Mennell (1992:7–8) notes that not only did this lead to the sometimes excessive and potentially harmful use of interventions like laxatives, but also to the progressive exclusion of suspect foodstuffs from the worried individual's diet. The concerns analyzed by Mennell can, in a sense, be seen as manifestations of the broader "civilizing" process that Elias (1978, 1982) sees as involving, among other features, a shift from an emphasis on external constraints on the individual's actions toward an emphasis on internalized constraints. Thus, as has already been argued, the medieval and early modern enthusiasm for feasting and gorging can be seen as a response to external constraints on food intake imposed by cycles of shortage and abundance largely outside the individual's own control. Conversely, once the reliability of the food supply becomes more assured, the expectation is that individuals will exercise self-restraint in eating, and anxieties over the effects of, and the reactions of others to, perceived overindulgence come to the fore. What is more, these changes take place in the context of an increasing sense of shame concerning the bodily functions associated with ingestion and elimination (Elias 1978:135–139).

The effect of these processes on paradox 1 anxieties is also compounded by the fact that the reassuring sense of gustatory familiarity provided by the existence of a long established flavor principle can easily be lost. The globalization of culinary culture means that in modern industrial societies an array of alternative flavor principles is on offer. These principles are often associated with particular ethnic or national groups, but their use is by no means restricted to their original owners. Flavor principles may no longer act as forces for stabilizing and constraining gustatory experiences, but have become commodities among a host of other commodities for sale in restaurants, supermarkets, or bookshops. Along with the commoditization of flavor principles, whole customary culinary cultures may find themselves in decline, with a loosening of their previously binding rules governing food selection, preparation, and consumption.

Paradox 2 (health/disease) anxieties, focused upon the possibility of links between diet and illness, also intensify with the attenuation of customary modes of managing them. On occasions, such fears may give rise to dramatic collective effects, such as the so-called "food scares" that have occurred several times on the British scene in recent years. These have included acute rises in anxiety concerning the risks associated with consuming eggs infected with *Salmonella*, beef from cattle exhibiting the symptoms of bovine spongiform encephalopathy (BSE), and pâté, cook-chill foods, and soft cheeses contaminated with *Listeria* (Mitchell and Greatorex 1990). In certain respects these food scares are analogous to what Cohen (1973) has termed "moral panics" in connection with social deviance. The mass media clearly play an important role in drawing public attention to, and sustaining, such food related panics (Beardsworth 1990; Gofton 1990), although as Hilgartner and Bosk (1988) observed, such issues compete with others for attention in public arenas, and once saturation occurs interest falls and media attention shifts (perhaps only temporarily) elsewhere. Nevertheless, such anxiety-amplifying news spirals may induce significant changes in food consumption patterns and consumer attitudes.

As well as these relatively sudden and dramatic eruptions of collective disquiet, questions about the links between diet and disease can establish themselves as long running issues in the public eye. For example, the British government's concern about the relatively high levels of coronary heart disease observed in the United Kingdom has led to a series of health education campaigns to modify the British diet. There is clear evidence that these campaigns have raised the public's level of awareness of the idea that food consumption patterns play some role in the etiology of this disorder (Evans and Durant 1989), even though awareness of nutritional guidelines does not necessarily imply that they are actually adopted in practice. Similarly, the possibility that many of the numerous additives used in food processing and manufacturing may pose health risks is also a continuing focus of public debate.

Ethical doubts about the acceptability of the use of animals or animal products for food (related to paradox 3, the life/death paradox) also seem to become much more important in modern developed societies. An intense philosophical debate has emerged in relation to the exploitation of animals (not only for food, but also for experimentation, product testing, entertainment, etc.). Thus, from varying philosophical positions, authors such as Singer (1976), Midgley (1983), and Regan (1984) have argued that the killing and consumption of animals is morally indefensible. Indeed Fiddes (1991) suggests that the current decline in red meat consumption in the United Kingdom is a reflection of underlying changes taking place in western cultures in attitudes toward the relationship between humans and the natural world. The consumption of red meat was traditionally seen as an act that symbolized the dominion over nature granted to human beings, and thus red meat was viewed as a highly prestigious and desirable food item. Fiddes maintains that significant increases in awareness of environmental issues in developed societies, and the emergence of environmentalist movements and lobbies on a substantial scale, are symptomatic of the decline of the long standing western world-view that sees nature essentially as a cornucopia of resources for exploitation. In these circumstances, he argues, meat consumption (especially red meat) is likely to engender feelings of guilt, and is increasingly likely to be avoided. Indeed, this effect is likely to be compounded by increasing secularization and the consequent dilution of the theological justifications of meat consumption. The rising popularity of vegetarianism (in its various forms) is seen as evidence supportive of this proposition. More generally, attitudes relating to eating and specific food choices in western societies are more likely than ever to be influenced by qualms about ethical issues, whether these be related to the use of animals, to the possibilities of environmental damage as a result of food production techniques, or, indeed, to the dramatic nutritional inequalities that divide the average western consumer from his or her third world counterpart.

Erosion and Reconstruction?

In the foregoing section I have argued that western societies have undergone a shift that has seen the replacement of relatively stable and reassuring food ideologies (albeit set against the backdrop of a decidedly insecure food supply) with a set of circumstances characterized by a relatively secure food supply, open-ended choice resulting from abundance, chronic uncertainties concerning health issues and burgeoning moral misgivings. Fischler (1980:947–948) uses the term *gastro-anomy* to describe the situation in which consumers find themselves when freed from the constraint and reassurance of the customary rules, norms, and meanings associated with food. Gastro-anomy results from a crisis in *gastronomy* itself (this term being used by Fischler in its literal sense to refer to the whole corpus of food rules and representations in a society). In such circumstances, anxiety is likely to be the response to a lack of clear criteria for nutritional decision making. Fischler's use of the term gastro-anomy, with its explicitly acknowledged derivation from Durkheim's (1952) concept of anomy, clearly involves the proposition that food-related anxiety is an inherent and inevitable feature of the individualistic and anomic tendencies of modern urban society.

The view put forward by Warde (1991) is basically compatible with the overall argument that has been developed so far in this chapter, although it is expressed in somewhat different terms. Warde's position is that there are now three competing forces pulling in contradictory directions within the food systems of modern societies. The first is made up of professional nutritional discourse and the official health-oriented advice that is aimed at the public at large, the second consists of the body of customary practice and belief that makes up a culinary culture, and the third is what Warde refers to as the taste for novelty (a taste that has been seen as a feature not only of eating choices, but of consumption patterns in general, particularly in relation to the pursuit of style, and to the expression of social difference). Warde characterizes the contemporary situation as a "mire of uncertainty" (Warde 1991:9), an uncertainty generated by the contradictions between custom, a "disciplinary" discourse on nutrition, and the modernist cultivation of novelty. Given his own theoretical orientations, Warde is not willing to conceptualize these processes in Durkheimian terms, nor indeed to see them as symptoms of postmodern tendencies. Rather he views them as typically modern, or hypermodern, in the sense implied by Giddens (1990).

The positions adopted by Fischler and Warde both entail the view that food-related uncertainties and anxieties (over and above the straightforward fear of shortage or starvation) are features built into the very foundations of modern societies. This rather pessimistic vision of contemporary eating, which this chapter so far has also subscribed to, does have alternatives, of course. Indeed, Fischler himself argues that there exist pressures to reintroduce order and a normative logic into everyday eating (1988:290). It may well be that it is possible to identify novel devices for handling conflict and uncertainty, and alternative modes of either masking the paradoxes discussed earlier, or of generating a sense that they have been resolved for all practical purposes. Sellerberg (1991) uses the term "strategies of confidence" to refer to these devices that individuals use to establish what she calls their trust in food in the context of a confusing background of scares, reports, and a welter of nutritional information, suggesting that the most effective ones will be those exhibiting a resonance with fundamental "cultural narrations" (Sellerberg 1991:196–197). With specific reference to the views of Fischler and Warde, Beardsworth and Keil (1992b) suggest that we may be witnessing the gradual emergence of a new kind of coherence in the contemporary food system. The term *menu* is used to describe the sets of selection principles that individuals use to make choices from the alimentary totality that their society makes available to them (given their age, gender, position in the social hierarchy, etc). The argument put forward is that what may be emerging out a somewhat anomic and confused set of circumstances is the new phenomenon of *menu-pluralism*. Having witnessed the breakdown of the unquestioned authority of one overarching master menu (or what Fischler would term the weakening of the traditional rules of gastronomy), modern societies may be moving through a transitional phase toward a situation where, within a framework of broad overall consensus, a whole range of menu principles can legitimately compete with each other. Individuals, households, or broader social groupings may, therefore, increasingly be in a position to draw upon these alternative menus as resources (according to situation, mood, purchasing power, etc.) to construct highly personalized diets. It is feasible to describe a whole series of such menus that appear to be emerging and establishing themselves currently. For example, *rational menus* are aimed at specific ends (disease avoidance, weight loss) and may be based upon scientific or pseudoscientific principles, and often involve a quantitative element (weighing food, weighing the body, calorie counting, and the like). *Moral menus* involve selection criteria based upon ethical principles (e.g., related to animal welfare or environmental issues). *Hedonistic menus* are aimed purely at gustatory satisfaction, whereas *expressive menus* are concerned with display and social differentiation, and *convenience menus* are designed to minimize the time and labor involved in food preparation.

A pluralistic framework should be able to accommodate potential conflicts between particular principles, and some individuals may apply different menu principles to different situations (e.g., hedonistic or expressive principles when eating out, and rational or convenience principles when eating at home). Such situational selectivity will be gradually absorbed into nutritional culture. On the other hand, some individuals may opt for one principle as the overriding one (say rational or moral) and attempt to adhere to it in all or most situations. Such a stance will increasingly be seen as the result of a legitimate personal "lifestyle" choice. Of course, this is not to say that menu pluralism implies complete individual nutritional autonomy and equality. Quite clearly, powerful pressure groups and entrenched vested interests may employ a whole range of strategies to advance their own causes and to persuade the public that their interpretations and priorities are valid and should be adopted.

It is certainly interesting to speculate upon the emergence of a new pluralistic setting that offers choice within a coherent framework, as opposed to a situation approximating an anomic free-for-all. However, for such a framework to establish itself and become stabilized, the kinds of food ambivalence to which this chapter has devoted a good deal of attention still have to be dealt with. It is certainly feasible to detect in modern societies specific features or processes that appear to indicate the emergence of innovatory ways of coping with the anxieties created by one or more of our three paradoxes. Perhaps one of the most striking of these processes is the development of a range of alternative dietary ideologies, most notably in relation to "wholefoods" and "health foods." The analysis by Kandel and Pelto (1980) of what they term the "health food movement" in the United States identifies a number of motifs that run through these ideologies: an emphasis on "natural" foods, an emphasis on foods seen as "organic" as opposed to "chemical" or "artificial," stress laid upon the importance of certain key nutrients, and a mystical element that judges foods by their symbolic properties (e.g., the idea that the consumption of raw foods is particularly beneficial since they contain "life energy"). The authors seek to classify the different levels of involvement in the movement, noting the roles played by cult leaders and by the authors of widely read books and articles. They see information as diffusing into the various levels of the movement through the television appearances and publications of its leaders, through proselytizing tours by leaders and their apostles, through healthfood stores, restaurants, etc., which bring adherents together and act as clearing houses for ideas, and through face to face communication along lines of kinship and friendship. As well as discussing what they call "revitalization cults," Kandel and Pelto (1980:357–359) also suggest that health food use may constitute a kind of alternative medical system, and go so far as to make a direct comparison with traditional beliefs concerning the significance of particular foods in maintaining health or introducing disease. Taking their arguments one step further, it seems plausible to conclude that the health food movement, diverse as its components may appear to be, does exhibit an underlying coherence and can be seen as a series of interconnected, collective strivings to construct food ideologies that exhibit the reassuring and confidence-generating features of traditional forms of belief and practice. In this sense, such a movement can be seen as offering the means for coping with paradox 2 (health/disease) anxieties and, to some extent, with paradox 1 (pleasure/displeasure) anxieties. This view receives some support from the conclusions drawn by Atkinson (1980) who, in examining the symbolic significance of health foods, maintains that they have come to stand for a more "natural," "rural" mode of existence, conceptualized as in opposition to the perceived negative aspects of "urban" and "civilized" modes of life.

Similarly, vegetarianism, a dietary option of increasing significance in the United Kingdom, for example, can be seen as offering its devotees a sense that their dietary stance provides them with access to pure foods, full of vitality that promotes the retention of health and youthfulness (Twigg 1979). Conversely, the avoidance of meat, a food seen as redolent of death and decay, is also regarded as an act that is positively health promoting. The work of Beardsworth and Keil (1992a) tends to support this picture of the vegetarian world-view and goes on to argue that a vegetarian diet (whether fairly loosely conceived or strictly vegan) can provide, for some individuals, at least, a way of reducing many of the ethical misgivings associated with paradox 3. Paradox 2 anxieties may also be effectively assuaged, insofar as fears concerning the ability of food to introduce disease into the body appear to become much more narrowly focused for vegetarians, concentrating on the dangers of the "corrupting" or "putrefying" nature of "dead flesh." Hence the avoidance of meat (especially red meat) can, at a stroke, provide at least a partial resolution of a range of anxieties. This may even apply to paradox 1 anxieties, as vegetarians often report a strong sense of disgust in relation to the taste and texture of meat (Beardsworth and Keil 1992a:273–274).

In considering the mechanisms for the reconstruction of nutritional confidence, the possibility must also be considered that the commercial, profit-oriented dynamic of capitalist food systems may also play a role in this connection, despite the fact that capitalism is classically seen as inherently anomic, dependent on the constant creation of new wants. Atkinson (1983) points out that large-scale food manufacturers and re-tailers can, and do, make extensive use of concepts such as tradition, nature, and the appeal of rural life to market their products, drawing upon a retrospective reference to the supposed virtues of an older order to legitimate their products. This is particularly the case for mass pro-duced and mass marketed health foods. The wide availability and acces-sibility of such products, due to the increasing commercialization of their marketing, mean that an even broader public can routinely have access to foods charged with comforting, albeit somewhat spurious, symbols of reassurance. Similarly, Beardsworth and Keil (1993) advance the proposition that although vegetarianism, in certain of its forms, can be seen as posing an explicit challenge to existing food ideologies, it is in the process of being absorbed into the developing pluralist framework discussed above. This absorption, while operating partly at the cultural level, is also going on at the commercial level, as more and more prod-ucts, publications, and services are provided for the expanding vegetari-an market. The variety and increased availability of such products and services mean that the threshold of entry into some forms of vegetari-anism has been appreciably lowered (although this is less the case for stricter forms like veganism). Thus many individuals who might for-merly have been deterred by social and practical barriers, can now much more readily resort to vegetarianism as a way of alleviating the strains of one or more of the paradoxes.

As well as these rather specific instances, the commercial logic of western food systems can have broader confidence-generating effects. The creation of brand loyalty is an end to which corporations devote enormous amounts of advertising and promotional resources. While the existence of a reservoir of brand loyalty is a highly prized asset for any business, such loyalty also has, in one sense at least, an advantage for the consumer. The purchasing of familiar branded products is one way of alleviating paradox 1 anxieties (reducing the likelihood that the tastes experienced will be unwelcome or disgusting) and paradox 2 anxieties (the safety of the products is seen as assured by the fact that large corporations need to guard their reputations to avoid commercial disas-ter). Even paradox 3 anxieties may be relieved (e.g., by buying food products labeled as produced using humane or environmentally respon-sible methods). The familiarity of nationally or internationally known branded food products can act as a substitute for the familiarity of foods or dishes guaranteed by custom and tradition. In this fashion, some of the taken-for-granted nature of eating, once derived from traditional foodways, can be reinstated. The potency of this effect is attested to by the fact that some of the most revered icons of western consumerism are, indeed, the brand images of food (and drink) products.

In this context, the concept of "McDonaldization" employed by Ritzer (1993) is of obvious relevance. Ritzer maintains that the fast food restaurant (such as McDonald's and its numerous clones) has effectively replaced the bureaucracy as the most appropriate contemporary exemplar of the relentless process of rationalization, seen by Weber (1968) as a fundamental driving force in modern western societies. Ritzer contends that the principles of the fast food restaurant (paralleling those of rationalization in general, i.e., efficiency, control, quantification, and predictability), are not only spreading internationally, but also into numerous spheres of life outside the catering industry. Whatever may be the limitations of Ritzer's McDonaldization thesis (and he admits, for example, the applicability of the process may vary greatly from sector to sector, and that certain postmodern countertrends may also be evident) one aspect is of particular interest. This is the issue of predictability. Whatever other factors contribute to the appeal of fast food chains like McDonald's, predictability is surely the key. The standardization of products means that the consumer eating away from home, no matter where the outlet is located, can have a high degree of confidence that paradox 1 and paradox 2 anxieties will not need to be confronted. Thus, geographically and socially mobile individuals have available, should they feel the need to fall back on it, a ready made source of familiarity. (It is perhaps worth noting in passing that McDonald's may also offer reassurance in relation to certain environmental extensions of paradox 3 anxieties, as many restaurants now display statements concerning the ozone-friendly nature of the packaging employed, and denying the use of beef produced using methods damaging to tropical rainforests.)

Perhaps less obviously, the rationalization and intensification of food production and processing, coupled with long-term urbanization, mean that many of the less palatable aspects of the food system are increasingly kept well out of public view. For example, in the area of animal husbandry, intensive rearing facilities are not normally visible to the public at large, and in the United Kingdom, for example, slaughtering has increasingly been concentrated in large specialized complexes, having been moved out of smaller, more local facilities. The ostensible purposes of such changes are related to efficiency, hygiene, and the facilitation of more stringent inspection standards, but they also have the result of more effectively protecting the food consumer from the likelihood of direct confrontation with scenes that may provoke paradox 3 anxieties.

It is also tempting to suggest that state agencies and various professional groups (physicians, nutritionists, dietitians, health education specialists, etc.) may also be playing a part in the reconstruction of nutritional confidence in relation to paradox 2 (health/disease) anxieties. It could be assumed that professionals working in these areas would see as one of their most important goals the creation of conditions in which consumers can make confident and well-informed choices. However, a degree of caution about how far this can happen in practice is probably called for. In view of the argument advanced earlier concerning the provisional and continually changing nature of scientific insights (and the trans-scientific dimensions of some nutrition-related issues), there is always the possibility that by the time a suitably simplified message has been established in the public domain, scientific opinion will have moved on or controversies will have flared up. These too may enter the public domain, and may reinforce the consumer's skepticism concerning the pronouncements of the experts. Indeed, experts' attempts to bolster the public's nutritional confidence may even produce the opposite effect (Sellerberg 1991:201).

Conclusions

To cast some light upon the ways in which food-related social problems can emerge in modern societies, traditional and contemporary modes of responding to nutritional anxieties and maintaining nutritional confidence have been compared. While such a comparison is essentially a heuristic device aimed at improving our understanding of contemporary cultural processes, once it has been carried through, it does suggest some broader conclusions that are not specifically food related. For example, it may well be that the social construction of social problems in traditional societies is a very different process to that in contemporary societies. In the traditional setting, the response to a whole range of concerns and anxieties might best be characterized, at the cultural level, as a process that involves confronting a deep-seated paradox or conflict and constructing a reasonably coherent set of symbols, rituals, and practices that enables that paradox or conflict to be dealt with, indeed even effectively submerged, as far as the reality of everyday life is concerned. This appears to stand in stark contrast to the dynamics of the contemporary setting, where continuing scrutiny and debate in a whole series of public arenas may mean that a particular issue, far from being submerged, is constantly being reexamined and recycled. While this view is highly speculative, if accepted it does imply that theoretical perspectives on social problems appropriate to modern social systems would not necessarily be transferable to traditional societies, which might well require significantly different approaches.

This chapter has argued that a whole series of far-reaching economic, demographic, and cultural changes have undermined the traditional foodways that can be seen as the foundations of a specific form of nutritional confidence, a confidence that allows the act of eating to maintain its everyday, sometimes mundane, sometimes festive, but always taken-for-granted character. In effect, the cultural devices that produce and sustain this form of confidence appear to have been seriously compromised. The pessimistic view of this situation sees a likelihood of chronic, possibly worsening, states of gastro-anomy and persistent, essentially unresolved conflicts concerning the beliefs, norms, and rules that constitute food ideologies and shape nutritional practices. The more optimistic view is that we may currently be witnessing the short-term tensions and strains involved in the transition to a much more pluralistic nutritional order, which will permit far more flexibility of choice, while at the same time providing novel cultural and institutional supports for the consumer.

It would be foolhardy to attempt to predict with any measure of assurance the likely outcome of what appears to be a contest between two opposed tendencies inherent in the food systems and food ideologies of modern societies. One tendency is essentially in the direction of volatility and instability, and the other in the direction of stabilization and the restoration of at least a provisional form of equilibrium. The forces ranged behind these two tendencies are themselves somewhat equivocal. For example, I have suggested that scientific discourse can have a destabilizing effect, and yet it is perfectly feasible for scientific orthodoxies to become established and to be widely accepted for extended periods of time (although they always remain susceptible to challenge). Conversely, commercial interests may strive to stabilize demands and tastes (in favor of their own products), but may also introduce destabilizing factors (by attempting to generate new wants, by attempting to shift food consumption toward products incorporating higher added value, and so on).

Perhaps the critical question is whether any nutritional culture, in the long run, can tolerate the excessive visibility and obtrusiveness of the kinds of food paradox under examination in this chapter. The answer is that it almost certainly cannot, and that, given the scope of our ingenuity and the breadth of our imagination, there will always be a drive toward the achievement of some accommodation, some protection for the potentially all too delicate sensibilities of the human omnivore.

Note

1. This distinction between sympathetic and contagious magic was originally made by Frazer (1936). See the discussion in Fieldhouse (1986:164–165). For authoritative discussions of the role of magical thought and other related beliefs in traditional societies see, for example, Malinowski (1935) and Evans-Pritchard (1937).

140   Alan Beardsworth

References

Atkinson, P. 1980. "The Symbolic Significance of Health Foods." Pp. 79–89 in *Nutrition and Lifestyles*, edited by M. Turner. London: Applied Science Publishers.

———. 1983. "Eating Virtue." Pp. 9–30 in *The Sociology of Food and Eating*, edited by A. Murcott. Aldershot: Gower.

Beardsworth, A. D. 1990. "Trans-science and Moral Panics: Understanding Food Scares." *British Food Journal* 92(5):11–16.

Beardsworth, A. D., and E. T. Keil. 1992a. "The Vegetarian Option: Varieties, Conversions, Motives and Careers." *The Sociological Review* 40(2):253–293.

———. 1992b. "Foodways in Flux: From Gastro-anomy to Menu Pluralism?" *British Food Journal* 94(7):20–25.

———. 1993. "Contemporary Vegetarianism in the U.K.: Challenge and Incorporation?" *Appetite* 20:229–234.

Burnett, J. 1989. *Plenty and Want: A Social History of Food in England from 1815 to the Present Day*, 3rd ed. London: Routledge.

Cohen, S. 1973. *Folk Devils and Moral Panics: The Creation of the Mods and Rockers*, London: Paladin.

Coon, C. S. 1976. *The Hunting Peoples*. Harmondsworth: Penguin.

Durkheim, E. 1952. *Suicide: A Study in Sociology*. London: Routledge and Kegan Paul.

Elias, N. 1978. *The Civilizing Process Volume I: The History of Manners*. Oxford: Blackwell.

———. 1982. *The Civilizing Process Volume II: State Formation and Civilization*. Oxford: Blackwell.

Evans, G., and J. Durant. 1989. "Understanding of Science in Britain and the USA." Pp. 105–119 in *British Social Attitudes: Special International Report*, edited by R. Jowell, S. Witherspoon, and L. Brook. Aldershot: Gower.

Evans-Pritchard, E. E. 1937. *Witchcraft, Oracles and Magic among the Azande*. Oxford: Clarendon Press.

Farb, P., and G. Armelagos. 1980. *Consuming Passions: The Anthropology of Eating*. Boston: Houghton Mifflin.

Fiddes, N. 1991. *Meat: A Natural Symbol*. London: Routledge.

Fieldhouse, P. 1986. *Food and Nutrition: Customs and Culture*. London: Croom Helm.

Fischler, C. 1980. "Food Habits, Social Change and the Nature/Culture Dilemma." *Social Science Information* 19(6):937–953.

———. 1988. "Food, Self, and Identity." *Social Science Information* 27(2):275–292.

Frazer, G. 1936. *The Golden Bough: A Study in Magic and Religion*. London: Macmillan.

Giddens, A. 1990. *The Consequences of Modernity*. Oxford: Polity Press.

Gluckman, M. 1965. *Custom and Conflict in Africa*. Oxford: Blackwell.

Goffman, E. 1969. *The Presentation of Self in Everyday Life*. Harmondsworth: Penguin.

Gofton, L. 1990. "Food Fears and Time Famines: Some Social Aspects of Choosing and Using Food." *British Nutrition Foundation Bulletin* 15(1):78–95.

Goodman, D., and M. Redclift. 1991. *Refashioning Nature: Food, Ecology and Culture.* London: Routledge.

Grimble, A. 1952. *A Pattern of Islands.* London: John Murray.

Guenther, M. 1988. "Animals in Bushman Thought, Myth and Art." Pp. 192–211 in *Hunters and Gatherers 2: Property, Power and Ideology,* edited by T. Ingold, D. Riches, and J. Woodburn. Oxford: Berg.

Harris, M. 1986. *Good to Eat: Riddles of Food and Culture.* London: Allen and Unwin.

Hilgartner, S., and C. L. Bosk. 1988. "The Rise and Fall of Social Problems: A Public Arenas Model." *American Journal of Sociology* 94(1):53–78.

Kandel, R. F., and G. H. Pelto. 1980. "The Health Food Movement: Social Revitalization or Alternative Health Maintenance System?" Pp. 327–363 in *Nutritional Anthropology: Contemporary Approaches to Diet and Culture,* edited by N. W. Jerome, R. F. Kandel, and G. H. Pelto. New York: Redgrave Publishing Co.

Kent, S. 1989. "Cross-Cultural Perceptions of Farmers as Hunters and the Value of Meat." Pp. 1–17 in *Farmers as Hunters: The Implications of Sedentism,* edited by S. Kent. Cambridge: Cambridge University Press.

Kuhn, T. S. 1970. *The Structure of Scientific Revolutions.* Chicago: University of Chicago Press.

Levenstein, H. 1988. *Revolution at the Table: The Transformation of the American Diet.* New York: Oxford University Press.

Malinowski, B. 1935. *Coral Gardens and Their Magic.* New York: American Book Co.

Manderson, L. 1987. "Hot-Cold Food and Medical Theories: Overview and Introduction." *Social Science and Medicine* 25(4):329–330.

Mennell, S. 1985. *All Manners of Food: Eating and Taste in England and France from the Middle Ages to the Present.* Oxford: Blackwell.

———. 1992. "Indigestion 1800–1950: Aspects of English Taste and Anxiety." Paper presented to the inaugural meeting of the British Sociological Association Sociology of Food Study Group, B.S.A. annual conference, University of Kent.

Messer, E. 1987. "The Hot and Cold in Meso-american Indigenous and Hispanicized Thought." *Social Science and Medicine* 25(4):339–346.

Midgley, M. 1983. *Animals and Why They Matter.* Harmondsworth: Penguin.

Mitchell, V.-W., and M. Greatorex. 1990. "Consumer Perceived Risks in the U.K. Food Market." *British Food Journal* 92(2):16–22.

Paulos, J.A. 1988. *Innumeracy: Mathematical Illiteracy and Its Consequences.* London: Viking.

Pool, R. 1987. "Hot and Cold as an Explanatory Model: The Example of Bharuch District in Gujarat, India." *Social Science and Medicine* 25(4) 389–399.

Regan, T. 1984. *The Case for Animal Rights.* London: Routledge.

Ritzer, G. 1993. *The McDonaldization of Society.* Newbury Park: Pine Forge Press.

Rozin, E., and P. Rozin. 1981. "Some Surprisingly Unique Characteristics of Human Food Preferences." Pp. 243–252 in *Food in Perspective: Proceedings of the Third International Conference on Ethnological Food Research, Cardiff, Wales, 1977,* edited by A. Fenton and T. M. Owen. Edinburgh: John Donald Publishers.

Rozin, P. 1976. "The Selection of Food by Rats, Humans and Other Animals."

Pp. 21–76 in *Advances in the Study of Behaviour, Volume 6*, edited by J. S. Rosenblatt, R. A. Hinde, E. Shaw, and C. Beer. London: Academic Press.

Sellerberg, A.-M. 1991. "In Food We Trust? Vitally Necessary Confidence—and Unfamiliar Ways of Attaining It." Pp. 193–202 in *Palatable Worlds: Sociocultural Food Studies*, edited by E. L. Fürst et al. Oslo: Solum Vorlag.

Sharp, H. S. 1988. "Dry Meat and Gender: the Absence of Chipewyan Ritual for the Regulation of Hunting and Animal Numbers." Pp. 183–191 in *Hunters and Gatherers 2: Property, Power and Ideology*, edited by T. Ingold, D. Riches, and J. Woodburn. Oxford: Berg.

Simoons, F. J. 1961. *Eat Not This Flesh: Food Avoidances in the Old World*. Madison: University of Wisconsin Press.

Singer, P. 1976. *Animal Liberation*. London: Jonathan Cape.

Tracey, M. V. 1977. "Human Nutrition." Pp. 355–360 in *The Encyclopaedia of Ignorance: Everything That You Wanted to Know about the Unknown*, edited by R. Duncan and M. Weston- Smith. Oxford: Pergamon Press.

Turner, B. S. 1982. "The Government of the Body: Medical Regimens and the Rationalization of Diet." *British Journal of Sociology* 33(2):254–269.

Twigg, J. 1979. "Food for Thought: Purity and Vegetarianism." *Religion* 9(Spring):13–35.

Warde, A. 1991. "Guacamole, Stottie Cake and Thick Double Cream: Elements of a Theory of Modern Taste." Paper presented to the British Association for the Advancement of Science Annual Conference, Polytechnic South West.

Weber, M. 1968. *Economy and Society: An Outline of Interpretive Sociology*. New York: Bedminster Press.

Weinberg, A. M. 1972. "Science and Trans-science." *Minerva* 10(2):209–222.

Wilson, C. S. 1981. "Food in a Medical System: Prescriptions and Proscriptions in Health and Illness among Malays." Pp. 391–400 in *Food in Perspective: Proceedings of the Third International Conference on Ethnological Food Research, Cardiff, Wales, 1977*, edited by A. Fenton and T. M. Owen. Edinburgh: John Donald Publishers.

7

Meat as a Social Problem: Rhetorical Strategies in the Contemporary Vegetarian Literature

DONNA MAURER

Introduction

An increasing number of people in the United States—between 8.5 and 12.4 million—call themselves vegetarians (Klemsrud 1975; Krizmanic 1992; Robeznieks 1986).[1] At the same time, meatless diets are gaining scientific legitimacy. The American Dietetic Association officially condones vegetarianism (Havala and Dwyer 1993) and some of its members have formed a Vegetarian Practice Group (Havala 1992). Medical studies support the idea that a healthy diet can be meatless (Chen et al. 1990; Ornish et al. 1990),[2] and President and Mrs. Clinton have recently sought nutritional advice from vegetarian physician Dean Ornish (Apgar 1994). While people generally see cutting down on red meat consumption as a healthy practice, they often compensate by eating more poultry and seafood (Food Marketing Institute 1992:56; U. S. Bureau of the Census 1992), leading the beef and pork industries to launch "healthy meat" campaigns that proclaim beef as "what's for dinner" and pork as "the new white meat." Although the nutritional science community regards vegetarianism as acceptable, current health attitudes seem to be more "antifat" than "antimeat"; meat is still a central component of a typical meal in the United States.

Social movements thrive on the commitment of their members. Where-

143

as most movements demand the adherent's time and money, some movements, like vegetarianism, require personal transformation (Turner 1983: 177). Food habits, as personally embodied and structurally embedded practices, are not easy to change (Bourdieu 1984:467–470; Goldstein 1992:71), yet for vegetarianism to be a viable social movement, advocates must not only convince people to adopt a new ideology, but also persuade them to change their eating routines and cooking practices (Perelman and Olbrechts-Tyteca 1969:26–31). The vegetarian movement hinges not on people *thinking* that meat is bad, but on people acting on that belief; without vegetarians there is no vegetarian movement.

How does a person become convinced that a social condition warrants a change in his or her lifestyle? Although research suggests that most people learn to change their diets through social interaction with already committed vegetarians (Beardsworth and Keil 1992:268; Lustgarden 1993; Maurer 1989), vegetarians seem to learn their "reasons" directly and indirectly through books and magazines produced by claimsmakers within the vegetarian movement. Even new converts who do not read are likely to hear these same arguments rearticulated in social interactions with other vegetarians. In other words, vegetarians learn a "vocabulary of motives" (Mills 1940) that they can then apply to their own experience. Claims regarding the nature of "meat" as a morally ambiguous category structure this vocabulary; in this sense primary claims (Best 1990:87) may become part of the vegetarian's justifications for his or her diet.

Vegetarian books and magazines provide moral reasoning that may inspire potential converts and reinforce dietary change among committed vegetarians. In these primary claims, claimsmakers can fully develop their moral arguments, spelling out detailed reasons and examples. In this chapter, I examine the claims made in 20 vegetarian books and two periodicals (*Vegetarian Times* and *Vegetarian Journal*).[3] I apply Peter Ibarra and John I. Kitsuse's recent rearticulation of social constructionist theory (1993), using their rhetorical idioms of "entitlement" and "endangerment" to address the complex reasoning that underlies the vegetarian discourse.

A Vegetarian Vocabulary of Motives

People who choose vegetarianism have a variety of reasons for doing so, though research suggests that people's motives vary within rather set categories. In a 1991 survey (Scott 1991), for example, *Vegetarian Journal* readers revealed their top four reasons: (1) health (reported by 81%), (2) animal rights (81%), (3) ethics (76%), and (4) environment (75%).[4] Other researchers have found similar categories of reasons, and many vegetarians report more than one motive (Amato and Partridge 1989; Beardsworth and Keil 1992; Dwyer et al. 1973; Krizmanic 1992).[5] What do these categories mean? For example, what is the difference between "animal rights" and "ethics"? What is an "environmental" reason?

Without more qualitative data it is difficult to know how people interpret these categories. Two studies have generated these types of data (Beardsworth and Keil 1992; Maurer 1989). For example, one respondent reported the following environmental motivation:

> The first motivating force for me was a socio-political one, really . . . . Back in 1976, I met a girl who was working at a mental health center with me. And she introduced me to this book—*Diet for a Small Planet*. And what really impressed me was how inhumane it was to eat meat in the face of all the malnourished and impoverished people in the world. And that if you really cared about the planet as well as the people on it, the sensible thing to do was to advocate a food consumption strategy that didn't include meat. (Maurer 1989:79)

A respondent in another study explains his animal rights motivation:

> animals do have rights, I'm sure of that . . . and they have a right not to be exploited by man, the same as people do . . . . I mean, I don't put animals above people . . . but having said all that, I think animals have their life to lead, and why should they be exploited, because they're a lesser being? . . . . So in a way I think we've got a duty, you know, to protect them. (Beardsworth and Keil 1992:269)

Even when we know what the categories "mean" to people, it is not possible to draw concrete causal relationships between the presence of vegetarian texts and people's actual attitudes and behavior without further inquiry (Gardner 1994a:61, 1994b:73; Gronbeck 1981:252). In other words, we cannot predict the likelihood of a person becoming a vegetarian after reading movement literature. Even if it were possible to establish a causal relation between the reading of vegetarian texts and people's articulation of vegetarian motives, it is possible that vegetarian texts "make sense" of previously unarticulated (yet present) attitudes and feelings (Bockman 1991:458). The research I present here, however, suggests that there is at least some correspondence between the reasons vegetarians give for their choices and the prevalent arguments in the vegetarian literature. These vocabularies of motives become a reified set of claims that indicate what the "meat" problem is "about."[6]

Ibarra and Kitsuse's Sociology of Social Problems

In their recent rearticulation of social constructionist theory (see Spector and Kitsuse 1987), Peter Ibarra and John I. Kitsuse (1993) direct sociologists to focus on social problems discourse. They assert that claimsmakers use language as a resource, manipulating words and other symbols to emphasize their positions. Claimsmaking is essentially a rhetorical activity. The use of persuasive language, however, is not limited to overt claims regarding the nature of a particular social condition. Ibarra and Kitsuse use rhetoric in the nonpejorative, nonevaluative sense (Foss et al. 1985:11), so that all communication (even that put forth by social and natural scientists) is defined as rhetorical (see also Aronson 1984; Brown 1992; Gusfield 1992).

The notion that rhetorical and discourse analyses are domains of social constructionist research precedes Ibarra and Kitsuse's admonitions (for example, see Best 1990; Gamson 1988; Gusfield 1981; Hunt 1992; Maynard 1988) and speech communication theorists have long been concerned with role of rhetoric in social movement success and failure (Griffin 1951; Hahn and Gonhar 1971; Simons 1970; Stewart et al. 1989). A distinguishing feature of Ibarra and Kitsuse's approach is the outlining of the various idioms that claimsmakers use in their rhetoric. Rhetorical idioms consist of moral reasoning and vocabularies that reveal what a problem is "about." Claimsmakers use rhetorical idioms both to "evoke the ethos implicit" in a claim and to demonstrate their own moral competence (Ibarra and Kitsuse 1993:32). Ibarra and Kitsuse outline several possible rhetorical idioms: entitlement, endangerment, loss, unreason, and calamity. Claimsmakers may use any of these idioms, but some idioms may be more applicable to certain issues than others.

Rhetorical Idioms of Vegetarian Discourse

People who make claims about meat often (but not always) address such issues as health and food safety, ecology, factory farming, furs, zoos, and animal experimentation. Individuals and organizations that level claims have a variety of interests; they may agree that a particular condition such as meat eating is problematic, but not agree on the reasons *why* it is. Even the claims of people who are on the same side of an issue may vary and conflict.

Vegetarian discourse, as it filters through books and magazines,[7] relies on two key rhetorical idioms: the rhetorics of entitlement and endangerment. Ibarra and Kitsuse characterize the rhetoric of entitlement as "emphasi[zing] the virtue of securing for all persons equal institutional access as well as the unhampered freedom to exercise choice of expression . . . . It is egalitarian in its aversion to forms of discrimination against categories of people" (1993:34). The rhetoric of entitlement emphasizes freedom, choice, and liberation, while it condemns attitudes and actions that are discriminatory and unjust. Claimsmakers who use this idiom "seek to expand the distribution of a good, service, or right," and frame their rhetoric so that any extension of these commodities ultimately benefits all of society (1993:34). Although Ibarra and Kitsuse focus on humans in their definition of this idiom, they note that "entitlement claims have also been extended to animals" and that speciesism may be one form of discrimination that claimsmakers refute (1993:34).

Ibarra and Kitsuse contrast the rhetoric of entitlement with the rhetoric of endangerment. Endangerment centers on "optimal bodily function and health care" (1993:35). Although all rhetorics invoke morality and value judgments, claimsmakers who use this rhetoric emphasize impartiality and scientific judgment: "[M]edical judgment has taken precedence over moral judgment since the understanding of the body that is grounded in scientific knowledge is presumed to be impartial and more factual, hence demonstrably superior to views generated by moral beliefs" (1993:35). Claimsmakers who use the language of objectivity to frame threats to personal health and safety use an "endangerment" idiom. Once claimsmakers appear to be making value judgments regarding other people's health practices, their endangerment claims become less convincing.

Claims in vegetarian discourse follow these two rhetorical idioms. Individual claimsmakers may primarily use one idiom, but they often weave the two idioms together. Claimsmakers who promote vegetarianism on animal rights grounds tend to use an entitlement rhetoric. Often they accomplish this by drawing parallels to other "rights" movements (particularly civil rights and women's rights), sometimes suggesting that the success of these other movements depends on their members becoming vegetarians. Claimsmakers who focus on health reasons primarily use an endangerment idiom. Adopting a more scientific style, these claims focus on the potentially health-damaging effects of meat consumption and on the increased number of people who can be healthily fed when few resources go to animal agriculture. The two idioms overlap when claimsmakers assert that a person gains health benefits by following a morally correct regimen. In this idiomatic combination, a person's physical health depends on the state of his or her spiritual or moral self; a person who acts morally by eliminating meat from his or her diet can expect to reap both spiritual and health benefits.

Meat Eating and Endangerment

Meat poses many threats to health, according to the vegetarian literature: meat consumption damages the health of those who eat it; meat production consumes vital resources, the loss of which harms the environment; and feeding livestock grain endangers the lives of the starving. On at least these three levels, the production and consumption of meat pose a threat to human beings and their social and physical environments. The individual's health, though, seems to take priority. Even authors like Jon Wynne-Tyson (1975), who argue for vegetarianism on moral and ecological grounds, maintain that health arguments must be established first. In other words, although ecology and saving the lives of others are sufficient conditions for the success of this rhetorical idiom, personal health is both necessary and sufficient. People need to be reassured that their health will not suffer if they forsake meat, and that it may be enhanced.

Most vegetarian authors use scientific evidence to back their arguments. For example, according to John Robbins, "Literally thousands of articles published in the last few decades in *The New England Journal of Medicine*, the *American Journal of Clinical Nutrition*, the *Journal of the American Medical Association*, the *British Medical Journal*, *Lancet*, and other publications of similar stature have demonstrated that the less animal fat you take into your body, the healthier you will be" (1992:79). Richard Bargen, author of *The Vegetarian's Self-Defense Manual*, which reviews over 100 nutritional medical studies, states, "Vegetarianism, once it has achieved a solid scientific foundation, will become the 'norm' in Western nations" (1979:31). In *Vegetarian Children*, Sharon Yntema (1987) summarizes 18 studies on the effects of meatless diets on children's health.

Vegetarian authors appear to seek and cultivate scientific legitimacy. This phenomenon points to the intersection of vegetarian discourse with the predominant medical one. Medical and nutritional science provides a "voice of authority" that structures the discourse on what constitutes healthy eating practices (Foucault 1970:50–51). Although the majority of medical professionals may not endorse vegetarianism as preferable to meat eating, vegetarian authors freely cite those who do, such as Dean Ornish, Neal Barnard, and Deepak Chopra. This effort to evoke a sense of scientific legitimacy is especially evident in *Vegetarian Journal* and *Vegetarian Times*. Both magazines review current nutritional and medical research, and both include articles written by and about medical doctors and registered dieticians who advocate vegetarian diets.

The Problem of Protein

Vegetarian authors who seek scientific legitimacy inevitably face the question of protein: Aren't vegetarians endangering themselves by not consuming meat protein? Both nutritional science and popular culture suggest that meat constitutes a superior form of protein as compared with vegetables.[8] Frances Moore Lappé, in the first edition of her book *Diet for a Small Planet* (1971), suggests that vegetarians should "complement" their protein at each meal to ensure that they have consumed all the essential amino acids. Although Lappé's book convinces many people that a vegetarian diet is preferable, her concept of protein complementarity persists [even though she refuted it herself in a later edition of the book (1982)]. Other vegetarian authors seem compelled to erase this idea, especially since it reinforces the popular conception that meat is the best or only protein source. For example, in a *Vegetarian Times* column called "Answering Machine," a reader asks about the relationship between "protein, muscle building, and athletic performance" and his brother's body building regimen (Springen 1993:24–25). Combatting the concept of protein complementarity, the columnist responds:

> And you can reassure your brother that he doesn't need to worry about "complementing" proteins . . . . As nutritional research and knowledge has evolved . . . it's become clear to many (although, alas, not all) nutrition professionals that all of this fussing and combining is not necessary; as long as you're getting enough calories from a healthful diet, plant foods provide all the amino acids you need, all by themselves. So if your brother has oatmeal for breakfast, a bean burrito for lunch, and spaghetti with vegetables for dinner, he'll meet his protein needs without even thinking about it.

Other authors also emphasize that vegetable protein is adequate for a healthy diet. For example, Keith Akers presents a chart of amino acids found in plant foods and argues that potatoes, corn, wheat, and rice are each individually adequate sources of protein (1983:30–31). According to John Robbins, "If we ate nothing but wheat (which is 17% protein), or oatmeal (15%), or even pumpkin (15%), we would easily have more than enough protein" (1987:176). Parham notes that the soybean contains twice as much "complete protein" as meat (1979:35–36).

Vegetarian authors stress the problems associated with the *overconsumption* of protein, and the reduction of risk that follows the elimination of meat from the diet. For example, John Robbins associates the overconsumption of protein with osteoporosis. He quotes two medical doctors from *Lancet*: "They called the connection between meat-based diets and the increasing incidence of osteoporosis an '*inescapable*' conclusion" (1992:60). Keith Akers states that "vegetarians have a greatly reduced risk of suffering from the fatal complications of various cardiovascular diseases" (1983:57). Vegetarian authors cite a variety of other diseases and ailments that are less likely to affect vegetarians than meat eaters, including cancer, kidney disease, gout, arthritis, digestive and elimination problems, hypertension, asthma, anemia, gallstones, ulcers, hypoglycemia, and diabetes.

Although these examples point to the endangering aspects of meat consumption, claimsmakers also emphasize the increased quality of life that the vegetarian experiences. They point to the increased vitality people derive from eating more fruits, vegetables, and whole grains. For example, in "Those Amazing Vegetarian Athletes," Amy Rosenbaum (1993:53) writes, "With magnificent muscles and healthy hearts, the five athletes profiled here are vital, living proof that you don't need to eat meat to excel in your sport." Authors emphasize that the term "vegetarian" does not mean "vegetable eater," but "stems from the Latin *vegetus*, meaning 'whole, sound, fresh, and lively'" (Bargen 1979:4).

Endangerment and Hunger

Many authors also see vegetarianism as a way to end world hunger. These arguments generally stem from Francis Moore Lappé's statement that "for every 16 pounds of grain and soy fed to beef cattle in the United States we only get 1 pound back in meat on our plates" (1982:69). John Robbins claims that although the distribution of grains to hungry people remains problematic, "if Americans reduced their meat consumption by 10 percent, enough grain would be saved to feed sixty million people" (1992:35). At the same time, a reduction in meat consumption saves other natural resources. Akers reports that "[o]ver 90% of all agricultural land . . . is devoted to the production of animal products" (1983:84). Claimsmakers argue that a reduction in meat consumption would save water, forests, and fossil fuel energy, and would reduce soil erosion (Akers 1983:84–85; Boyd 1987:20–21; Lappé 1982:73; Wynne-Tyson 1975:16–29). Meat, then, is seen as endangering both the self and others. Vegetarian authors do not depict meat as having some benefits that are outweighed by the dangers, but as a commodity that has only negative consequences.

Meat Eating and Entitlement

Peter Singer's book, *Animal Liberation: A New Ethic for Our Treatment of Animals* (1975), sparked widespread debate about the moral status of animals. By 1988, over 250,000 copies were in print and "[a]lmost every animal rights activist either owns or has read [it]" (Jasper and Nelkin 1992:17, 90). *Animal Liberation* sets forth the claim that animals' interests deserve equal consideration to those of humans. It states that equality between creatures should not be based on *identity* (the creature's apparent similarity to humans), but on the capacity for suffering. Singer rejects Descartes' view of animals as machines and softens the boundary between humans and animals. He uses the terms "human animals" and "non-human animals" to blur this boundary semantically. In other words, although some of us are "human" and others "non-human," we are *all* animals. Carol Adams (1991:64) also blurs this boundary; she uses gendered pronouns to name animals, substituting "he" or "she" for the conventionally used "it."

Vegetarian rhetoric enjoins humans and animals and opposes them categorically to rocks and other nonsentient objects, which lack the capacity to experience pain, and pleasure. Some sources do not exclude the possibility that plants experience pain but, since it seems less than animal pain, and since humans must eat something to preserve their own lives, it is preferable to consume plants. Also, since more plants are needed to produce meat products than to meet human nutritional needs directly, "[a] vegetarian . . . diet greatly reduces the number of plants killed in order for us to live" (Boyd 1987:32; see also Akers 1983:150; Moran 1985:50; Singer 1975:248–249).

Singer asserts that the capacity for suffering is the baseline characteristic that should determine all our actions. Any other criterion enables potential abuse by people in power who may choose an arbitrary characteristic (such as culturally bound I.Q. test scores) as the determinant of who should be treated "equally." In this way, Singer draws parallels between racism, sexism, and speciesism, which he defines as "a prejudice of attitude of bias toward the interests of members of one's own species and against those members of other species" (1975:7).

Carol Adams (1991) and Marjorie Spiegel (1988) also draw analogies between speciesism and other forms of prejudice.[9] Adams argues that meat is "a symbol and celebration of male dominance" (1991:34) and that "[t]o remove meat is to threaten the structure of the larger patriarchal culture" (1991:37). Men objectify, fragment, and consume both women and animals in the parallel activities of butchering and sexual violence (1991:47–62). For Adams, this is not just an analogy, but a causative relationship; by consuming meat, people reinforce both meat eating and patriarchal values. Therefore, she maintains that all feminists must become vegetarians.

Similarly, Spiegel parallels the experiences of animals and slaves in her book *The Dreaded Comparison: Human and Animal Slavery* (1988). In words and pictures, Spiegel juxtaposes the life experiences of factory-farmed animals and slaves. She asserts, like Singer, that when oppression of any kind is permitted, powerful groups and individuals may make arbitrary distinctions as to who should be dominated: "[A]ny oppression helps to prop up other forms of oppression. This is why it is vital to link oppressions in our minds, to look for the common shared aspects and fight against them as one, rather than prioritizing victims' suffering" (1988:24).

Peter Singer parallels speciesism and racism when he address the hypocrisy of not matching talk and action:

> To protest about bull-fighting in Spain or the slaughter of baby seals in Canada while continuing to eat chickens that have spent their lives crammed in cages, or veal from calves that have been deprived of their mothers, their proper diet, and the freedom to lie down with their legs extended, is like denouncing apartheid in South Africa while asking your neighbors not to sell their homes to blacks. (1975:167)

Singer suggests that the hypocrisy of the racist parallels that of the speciesist and that all forms of oppression are interconnected. These authors claim that if people overlook the oppression of animals, the potential remains for oppressing humans.

Vegetarianism as Boycott

Various motifs that parallel those in other rights movements appear in the vegetarian literature. "Liberation," "oppression," and "suffering" are commonly used words that capture and evoke the moral ethos associated with vegetarianism. Similarly, the term "boycott" expresses the potentially political ramifications of changing one's diet. Authors encourage potential converts that their individual actions have political consequences— and that changing one's diet, compared with other forms of activism, requires little extra energy (for example, Boyd 1987:31; Coats 1989:159– 160; Singer 1975:166–167; Yntema 1987:133). Jay Dinshah encourages the reader to think of the number of animals' lives that can be saved through his or her individual efforts: "Figure your own life expectancy . . . and you can save the life of roughly one sheep, steer, pig, etc., for each year remaining in your lifetime" (1973:45).

Peter Singer argues that, compared with other social problems like "war, racial inequality, inflation, unemployment . . . the reduction of the suffering of non-human animals will be relatively easy" (1975:253). He notes that since "the consequences of speciesism intrude directly into our lives" people should feel compelled to express their commitment in action (1975:167). There is no room for excuses; if a person is truly morally outraged, he or she must move from this outrage to dietary change. Singer notes that anyone can engage in vegetarianism as a form of boycott, since it does not detract from a person's engagement in other social causes because "[i]t takes no more time to be a vegetarian than to eat animal flesh" (1975:233).

An Entitlement Hierarchy

A hierarchy of "interests" emerges through the vegetarian literature; this hierarchy prevails throughout the general population as well (Twigg 1983). The more human-like or human-linked the food source, the more people avoid it (Angyal 1941; Rozin and Fallon 1987; Simoons 1961:106–125). Hence, Americans tend to balk at the idea of eating dog, but find chicken far less objectionable. People more willingly eat the meat of vegetarian animals than carnivorous ones. In line with this hierarchy, vegetarian claimsmakers often encourage people to give up red meat first, followed by poultry, and then seafood (Ballentine 1987; Tracy 1985), and research suggests that people often do eliminate meat products in this order (Maurer 1989).

Dairy products, eggs, and other animal by-products (gelatin, casein, honey, etc.) follow animals and sea creatures in this hierarchy, and plant foods assume the lowest rung. Some vegetarians, called vegans, avoid all animal products and by-products, and some (albeit very, very few) vegans, called fruitarians, limit themselves to those food products that drop effortlessly from a branch or vine, therefore incurring no death— not even to a plant (Kulvinskas 1975:100–109).

Although only about 4% of all vegetarians are vegan (Krizmanic 1992:75),[10] many vegetarian writers claim that the consumption of animal by-products is as damaging as eating meat products directly. Therefore, ovo-lacto vegetarians (those who eat dairy products and eggs) are not entirely morally consistent. For example, Singer writes that living conditions for egg-laying hens are usually worse than those of broilers. Dairy cows routinely have their offspring removed from them; the calves are often either destroyed or raised for veal (Singer 1975:101, 181). According to Keith Akers:

> Animals who provide dairy products and eggs suffer just as much—if not more—than animals raised specifically for slaughter, and most dairy cows and laying hens wind up at the slaughterhouse anyway . . . . Once one admits that what suffering animals experience while they are still alive is an important ethical issue, it is hard to escape the total vegetarian or vegan position. (1983:151)

Although many vegetarian claimsmakers may try to inspire readers to acknowledge the interests of creatures at all levels of the "food hierarchy," they also seem to recognize that although their readers may concur with the *ideology* implicit in the argument, they may have a difficult time matching their behavior with their beliefs.

Practicality and Entitlement

Practicality tempers the rhetoric of entitlement. Ideally, according to most vegetarian authors, a boycott should include avoidance of all animal-derived products and all products tested on animals, but most authors also admit that complete moral congruence is impossible. Some authors urge their readers toward veganism, but they generally recognize that most people, even those motivated to eliminate meat from their diets, have difficulty with the idea of not eating dairy products and eggs. Peter Singer, for example, expresses concern that people could become so overwhelmed "that they end up doing nothing at all . . . and the exploitation of animals will continue as before" (1975:181–182). The vegetarian movement's existence depends upon people giving up meat; if people become slack in their behavior or overwhelmed by dramatic change, then the movement loses momentum. In most social movements, participants donate money and time; these resources enable social movement organizations to grow. While the vegetarian movement needs to nurture these same participant resources, its continuation rests on people participating in the boycott against meat. So, rather than insist that people immediately give up all animal products and by-products (which include many nonfood items such as leather, wool, silk, and goose down), claimsmakers promote the idea of progression: that people should gradually eliminate the products of animal suffering and should strive toward moral consistency.

The concept of progression undermines the "interests" of those animals that produce by-products, and it perpetuates factory farming systems. At the same time, claimsmakers recognize any reduction in the consumption of animal products as a positive move, and since "vegans . . . are ususally vegetarian first . . . [the] expansion of the latter can only aid the former" (Moran 1985:44). The rhetoric of entitlement suggests an ideal to which people might aspire. Rigorous veganism fulfills this ideal, yet claimsmakers encourage people to feel good about whatever changes they make and to not feel guilty if they do not achieve complete moral congruency.

"Meat Is Dead"

A popular bumpersticker reads "Meat is Dead." The oppositional terms "life" and "death" are common to the rhetorics of entitlement and endangerment in the vegetarian discourse. The word "dead" implies both a violation of an animal's right (to live, or at least not to suffer) and a potential endangerment to health. An animal has a "right" to *life*, and externally imposed *death* violates that right. At the same time, plants are *life-giving*, whereas meat presents a *threat to life*, hastening the death of its consumer. The saying "Meat is Dead" connotes both the death of the animal and the deadening quality that the eater assimilates.

The overwhelming majority of vegetarians perceive plant foods as desirable and life-giving (Twigg 1979). By eating food that is more alive, a person becomes healthier, livelier. While animal food is "dead matter," vegetable food lives:

> Take the stem of a spinach plant, cut it into parts. Eat the leaves, but plant the pieces of stem and you will get ten new spinach plants. Can you do that with a lamb? Can you eat its leg and then make the other parts grow into another lamb? No, because it is dead matter. (Satchidananda 1986: 7–8)

> Many plants retain their life-giving energy for many days after they are picked; in fact, they remain still capable of sprouting and growing. Meat, on the other hand, has been in the process of decay for several days. (Parham 1979:57)

Conversely, some authors suggest that by eating meat, one literally "eats death," that one consumes the panic that an animal experiences at slaughter time. This claim follows the homeogenic aphorism, "You are what you eat" to the extreme: one who eats violence becomes violent. Victoria Moran mentions the "phenomenon of 'pain poisoning'" that occurs when an animal is under extreme stress (1985:68; see also Satchidananda 1986:8) and refers to an "indivisibility of violence" in which the violence of slaughter both indicates and inflames violence in other areas of life. Rudolph Ballentine also suggests a connection between meat eating and aggression: meat eating may "create inclinations to inexplicable violence or a pervasive sense of pointless anger and hostility" (1987:72–73).

These vegetarian authors tend to stress the homeogenic consumption and reproduction of *violence* from the animals' slaughter, rather than the consumption and reproduction of the butchered animals' *fear*. This particular emphasis perhaps plays on current concerns about our "violent society"; certainly most people would rank a "violent society" as more problematic than a fearful one (if only because—by definition—a violent society is bound to also be fearful!). John Robbins adds to this motif by suggesting that when we embody the animals' "death fear" (through the digestion process), we react aggressively, "fighting back" as the animals would have had they the opportunity:

When we eat animals who have died violent deaths we literally eat their fear. We take in biochemical agents designed by nature to tell an animal that its life is in the gravest danger, and it must either fight or flee for its life. And then, in our wars and daily lives, we give expression to the panic in which the animals we have eaten died . . . . A nonviolent world has roots in a non-violent [sic] diet. (1987:356)

Robbins and other vegetarian authors emphasize the "fight" component of the "fight or flight" syndrome associated with excessive stress. A nation of people fighting is a more compelling image than a nation of people fleeing.

"Meat is Dead" implies both the problems and solutions as they emerge in vegetarian texts. Although vegetarian authors point to meat as a *social* problem, they portray the solution, at least initially, as a personal one. According to vegetarian discourse, both ethically motivated and health-motivated vegetarians stand to benefit from their avoidance. Jim Mason and Peter Singer write in *Animal Factories*: "The food you consume three or more times daily is your most constant and intimate connection with the environment and the living world around you. If you reflect your concern for them in your food habits, you will be healthier in every way" (1990:188). This promise, which exemplifies the linkage between the rhetorics of endangerment and entitlement, tells the reader that vegetarianism "works" as both an individual health reform and as a boycott against oppression. For the potentially "rights"-motivated vegetarian, added health is a bonus; the "health-conscious" vegetarian gains extra satisfaction in doing "the right thing."

Can a Steak Lover Be Converted?

Vegetarian claims that use entitlement or endangerment rhetoric (or a combination of the two) appear to mirror the articulated motivations of people who become vegetarians, but perhaps these individuals are predisposed to adopt a vegetarian viewpoint before they are ever exposed to these arguments. In other words, the arguments spelled out in the vegetarian literature may "make sense" of people's previously unarticulated feelings and attitudes (Bockman 1991); vegetarian claims give people a convenient language with which to justify and explain their motivations to others (Mills 1940). If this is the primary function of vegetarian claims, how is the vegetarian movement to attract truly "new" members? What sorts of claims are likely to sway the devoted steak lover?

Although some people may experience distress, guilt, or ambiguity over meat (Angyal 1941; Beardsworth this volume; Plous 1993), this does not keep the majority of U. S. citizens from eating it. Cultural mechanisms such as "language surrounding animal use [calling cow meat "beef"], the physical appearance of animal products [wrapped in grocery store cellophane], the remoteness of animal industries, and the way people are socialized to think about animals" enable people to eat meat without focusing on its source (Plous 1993:14–15). Any remaining anthropomorphic tendencies may be overridden by cultural demands and gustatory desires to consume what everyone else is eating and what "tastes good." People generally view meat, like coffee (Troyer and Markle 1984:410–411), as a simple, innocuous, "moral" pleasure.

For most people, abstract ethics are not likely to influence their desires to consume meat. Entitlement claims, which stress an animal's right to pursue its natural interests, do not offer a concrete incentive to the steak lover. Conversely, some people may find claims linking human and animal oppression offensive, asserting that to portray all oppression as equally vile may desensitize people to the necessity of preserving human rights (Jasper and Nelkin 1992:172). At best, adherence to ethical claims may provide a "soft selective incentive" (Fireman and Gamson 1979:20), enhancing a person's self-esteem, or bonding him or her to a circle of friends.

Endangerment claims focusing on the individual's health, on the other hand, promise a more concrete outcome—longer life and more vitality. This endangerment idiom matches prevalent cultural concerns regarding fitness and slimness. Meat (even outside the vegetarian discourse) has a fatty reputation, and many "mainstream" diets, such as Weight Watchers, prescribe minimal amounts of meat. Even though people may treat meat as a "moral pleasure," as suggested above, they may be willing to give it up if they perceive a direct benefit (Belasco 1993:249). Even persuasive endangerment claims, however, may not convince people to give up meat completely—people may instead decrease their consumption without adopting a vegetarian ideology.

Conclusion and Impending Questions

The vegetarian literature provides just one example of how claims-makers use rhetorical idioms in social problems discourse. This analysis is compatible with and extends Ibarra and Kitsuse's original (1993) analysis. First, this analysis suggests that despite the different authors, publication dates, and forms of written material, there is a coherent set of arguments and motives that emerges from the vegetarian literature.

Although many authors combine endangerment and entitlement idioms, the endangerment idiom seems to take priority; authors emphasize that eliminating meat from the diet poses no threat to health. Some authors expand this argument by stressing the vitality that results from eating more vegetables. Claimsmakers using a predominately entitlement idiom stress the unity of human and nonhuman animals, who share a common characteristic of possessing "interests." Adopting a discourse motif of "oppression," claimsmakers link the vegetarian cause with the women's rights and civil rights movements. The two idioms overlap when claimsmakers argue that an "ethical" diet has healthy consequences.

This analysis leaves many unanswered questions: How has the discourse shifted over time? How have the counterrhetorics of meat producers (and consumers) affected the vegetarian rhetoric? How do the authors' interactions (both "in person" and in reading each others' texts) affect the development of discourse? What is the "role of the reader" (Eco 1979; Gamson et al. 1992:388–389) in the interpretation and perpetuation of these idioms? How do vegetarians assimilate the vocabularies of motives implicit in these idioms? How does one learn what the "good" vegetarian books are? Do vegetarian cookbooks also perpetuate these idioms, and if so, how? In view of the evidence that vegetarians are predominantly white, female, and middle-class (Amato and Partridge 1989), to what degree do vegetarian claimsmakers consider their audiences when formulating their claims? How do the discourses of race, class, and gender merge and conflict with the vegetarian one? All of these questions relevant to the vegetarian vocabulary of motives and its rhetorical expression, when generalized as a discourse, point to the complex process of claimsmaking activity.

Acknowledgments

I would like to thank Richard L. Lanigan, Mareena McKinley Wright, Jeffery Sobal, and especially Joel Best for their comments and suggestions on earlier drafts of this chapter. I also want to thank Marilyn D'Antonino and Otto H. Maurer, Jr. for their encouragement and support.

Notes

1.   An accurate count of vegetarians in the United States is elusive because surveys are based on relatively small samples and respondents' self-definition of the category "vegetarian." Keith Akers, a vegetarian activist and author of *A Vegetarian Sourcebook* (1983:13), defines a vegetarian as

one who lives primarily on a plant food diet and abstains from all meat, fish, or fowl; no vegetarian eats any food that *requires* the death of, or injury to, an animal. Some vegetarians, probably the vast majority in the United States, consume dairy products and eggs [ovo-lacto vegetarians]; others abstain from all animal foods and rely entirely on plants [vegans].

However, people's self-definitions may not reflect the "no meat, poultry, or seafood" criteria; apparently, many people who occasionally eat meat consider themselves vegetarians. For example, in one 1973 study, only 64% of the " vegetarian" respondents conformed to this strict definition (Dwyer et al. 1973). To gauge how many people actively practice vegetarianism, the Vegetarian Resource Group recently commissioned a Roper poll in which they asked people specifically if they ever consumed any of the various meat products (Stahler 1994). Using an operationalized definition (a vegetarian is someone who consumes no meat, poultry, or seafood), the Roper poll indicates that between 750,000 and 2,225,000 people in the United States are practicing vegetarians.

2. Also, an International Congress on Vegetarian Nutrition was held in 1992; for the proceedings, see the *American Journal of Clinical Nutrition* (1994).

3. From my own experience as a vegetarian for about 10 years, I selected 20 books published between 1973 and 1993 that represent both the breadth and depth of vegetarian discourse. I examined all 1993 issues of the two periodicals.

4. The other reasons include economics (28%), taste (28%), religion (10%), habit (7%), media articles (8%), friends/family (5%), other (4%), doctor (2%), dietitian (2%). Note that the top four categories reflect the dominant claims in the vegetarian literature.

5. Four primary motivations emerged from Beardsworth and Keil's study of British vegetarians: "moral, health-related, gustatory, and ecological." The authors note that "[i]n the great majority of instances, respondents had no hesitation in identifying their primary motivation in ways which could be classified quite readily under these headings" (1992:269).

6. This is not to say that the discourse of motives simply reproduces itself. Although discourse may become objectivated and hardened, authors can manipulate vocabularies in their texts (Dillon 1986:1–2). Hence, authors may make original contributions to the "language game"; they eventually may alter or even rupture the moral discourse on meat. Although texts may appear to be static phenomena, it is important to remember that the processes of reading and writing are inherently dynamic, interpretive activities (Dillon 1986; Nöth 1990:263). Social constructionists need to conduct more naturalistic research that investigates the authors' reflexivity: how do claimsmakers decide which rhetorical idioms, styles, etc. will be the most persuasive? (Ibarra and Kitsuse 1993:53).

7. As Kress (1985:29) points out, the "genre" of text tends to have a "modal effect which affects the manner in which the text is read. So the expression of a sexist discourse in the genre editorial will carry a different modality from its expression in a short story." Following this, the expression of vegetarian discourse is likely to be expressed (and hence interpreted) differently depending on the avenue of its expression: news broadcast images (secondary claims) structure the discourse differently than books (primary claims). In addition, texts may evoke a number of different (and potentially competing) discourses (Kress 1985:29). For example, *The Sexual Politics of Meat* (Adams 1991) expresses both vegetarian and feminist discourses.

8. Although protein has become a less important concern to nutritional scientists since the 1970s (McLaren 1974) and many nutritional scientists consider

protein complementarity a myth (Young and Pellett 1994), the public still regards meat as a more "strength-producing" food than vegetables (Twigg 1983).

9. Linking vegetarianism to other social movement concerns is not a new phenomenon. In 1851, vegetarian health reformer William Alcott wrote that "[a] vegetable diet lies at the basis of all reform, whether civil, social, moral, or religious" (quoted in Goldstein 1992:26). Vegetarianism (also called "natural diet" and "Pythagoreanism") was an integral part of other reform movements in the Jacksonian period, including temperance, suffrage, women's dress reform, and abolition (Shryock 1931:178).

10. A recent survey of the British population "did not come across a single vegan in a quota sample of 1,997 adults" (Beardsworth and Keil 1992:261).

References

Adams, C. 1991. *The Sexual Politics of Meat: A Feminist-Vegetarian Critical Theory*. New York: Continuum.

Akers, K. 1983. *A Vegetarian Sourcebook: The Nutrition, Ecology, and Ethics of a Natural Foods Diet*. Arlington, VA: Vegetarian Press.

Amato, P., and S. Partridge. 1989. *The New Vegetarians: Promoting Health and Protecting Life*. New York: Plenum.

American Journal of Clinical Nutrition. 1994. Issue on Vegetarian Nutrition 59 (supplement).

Angyal, A. 1941. "Disgust and Related Aversions." *Journal of Abnormal and Social Psychology* 36:393–412.

Apgar, T. 1994. "The White House Wakes Up." *Vegetarian Times* (June):6.

Aronson, N. 1984. "Science as a Claims-making Activity: Implications for Social Problems Research." Pp. 1–30 in *Studies in the Sociology of Social Problems*, edited by J. Schneider and J. I. Kitsuse. Norwood, NJ: Ablex.

Ballentine, R. 1987. *Transition to Vegetarianism: An Evolutionary Step*. Honesdale, PA: Himalayan Press.

Bargen, R. 1979. *The Vegetarian's Self-Defense Manual*. Wheaton, IL: Theosophical Publishing House.

Beardsworth, A., and T. Keil. 1992. "The Vegetarian Option: Varieties, Conversions, Motives, and Careers." *The Sociological Review* 40:253–293.

Belasco, W. J. 1993. *Appetite for Change*. Ithaca, NY: Cornell University Press.

Best, J. 1990. *Threatened Children: Rhetoric and Concern About Child Victims*. Chicago: University of Chicago Press.

Bockman, S. 1991. "Interest, Ideology and Claims-making Activity." *Sociological Inquiry* 61(4):452–470.

Bourdieu, P. 1984. *Distinction: A Social Critique of the Judgement of Taste*. Translated by R. Nice. Cambridge, MA: Harvard University Press.

Boyd, B. R. 1987. *For the Vegetarian in You*. San Francisco: Taterhill Press.

Brown, R. H. 1992. "Poetics, Politics and Truth: An Invitation to Rhetorical Analysis." Pp. 3–8 in *Writing the Social Text: Poetics and Politics in Social Science* Discourse, edited by R. H. Brown. Hawthorne, NY: Aldine de Gruyter.

Chen, J., T. C. Campbell, J. Li, and R. Peto. 1990. *Diet, Life-style and Mortality in China: A Study of the Characteristics of 65 Counties.* London: Oxford University Press.

Coats, C. D. 1989. *Old MacDonald's Factory Farm.* New York: Continuum.

Dillon, G. L. 1986. *Rhetoric as Social Imagination: Explorations in the Interpersonal Function of Language.* Bloomington: Indiana University Press.

Dinshah, J. 1973. "To Tell the Truth." Pp. 43–46 in *Here's Harmlessness,* edited by The American Vegan Society. Malaga, NJ: The American Vegan Society.

Dwyer, J., L. Mayer, R. F. Kandel, and J. Mayer. 1973. "The New Vegetarians: Who Are They?" *Journal of the American Dietetic Association* 62:503–509.

Eco, U. 1979. *The Role of the Reader.* Bloomington: Indiana University Press.

Fireman, B., and W. A. Gamson. 1979. "Utilitarian Logic in the Resource Mobilization Perspective." Pp. 8–44 in *The Dynamics of Social Movements,* edited by M. N. Zald and J. D. McCarthy. Cambridge, MA: Winthrop.

Food Marketing Institute. 1992. *Trends: Consumer Attitudes and the Supermarket.* Washington, D.C.: Food Marketing Institute.

Foss, S., K. Foss and R. Trapp. 1985. *Contemporary Perspectives on Rhetoric.* Prospect Heights, IL: Waveland Press.

Foucault, M. 1970. *The Archaeology of Knowledge.* Translated by A. M. Sheridan Smith. New York: Barnes and Noble.

Gamson, W. 1988. "A Constructionist Approach to Mass Media and Public Opinion." *Symbolic Interaction* 11:161–174.

Gamson, W., D. Croteau, W. Hoynes, and T. Sasson. 1992. "Media Images and the Construction of Reality." *Annual Review of Sociology* 18:373–393.

Gardner, C. B.. 1994a. "The Social Construction of Pregnancy and Fetal Development: Notes on a Nineteenth-Century Rhetoric of Endangerment." Pp. 45–64 in *Constructing the Social,* edited by T. R. Sarbin and J. I. Kitsuse. London: Sage.

———. 1994b. "Little Strangers: Pregnancy Conduct and the Twentieth-Century Rhetoric of Endangerment." Pp. 69–92 in *Troubling Children: Studies of Children and Social Problems,* edited by J. Best. Hawthorne, NY: Aldine de Gruyter.

Goldstein, M. S. 1992. *The Health Movement: Promoting Fitness in America.* New York: Twayne.

Griffin, L. 1951. "The Rhetoric of Historical Movements." *Quarterly Journal of Speech* 38:184–188.

Gronbeck, B. E. 1981. "Qualitative Communication Theory and Rhetorical Studies in the 1980s." *Central States Speech Journal* 32:243–253.

Gusfield, J. 1981. *The Culture of Public Problems: Drinking-Driving and the Symbolic Order.* Chicago: University of Chicago Press.

———. 1992. "Listening for the Silences: The Rhetorics of the Research Field." Pp. 117–134 in *Writing the Social Text: Poetics and Politics in Social Science Discourse,* edited by R. H. Brown. Hawthorne, NY: Aldine de Gruyter.

Hahn, D. F., and R. M. Gonhar. 1971. "Studying Social Movements: Rhetorical Methodology." *Speech Teacher* 20:44–52.

Havala, S. 1992. "Vegetarian Congress Recap." *Vegetarian Journal* 11(6):11–12.

Havala, S., and J. Dwyer. 1993. "Position of the American Dietetic Association: Vegetarian Diets." *Journal of the American Dietetic Association* 93(11):1317–1319.

Hunt, S. 1992. "Critical Dramaturgy and Collective Action Rhetoric: Cognitive and Moral Order in the Communist *Manifesto*. *Perspectives on Social Problems* 3:1–18.

Ibarra, P. R. and J. I. Kitsuse. 1993. "Vernacular Constituents of Moral Discourse: An Interactionist Proposal for the Study of Social Problems." Pp. 21–54 in *Constructionist Controversies: Issues in Social Problems Theory*, edited by G. Miller and J. A. Holstein. Hawthorne, NY: Aldine de Gruyter.

Jasper, J. M., and D. Nelkin. 1992. *The Animal Rights Crusade: The Growth of a Moral Protest*. New York: Free Press.

Klemsrud, J. 1975. "World Vegetarians Meet to Talk—and Fast." *New York Times* August 22:37.

Kress, G. 1985. "Ideological Structures in Discourse." Pp. 27–42 in *Handbook of Discourse Analysis*, Vol. 4, edited by T. van Dijk. New York: Harcourt Brace Jovanovich.

Krizmanic, J. 1992. "Here's Who We Are." *Vegetarian Times* (October):72–80.

Kulvinskas, V. 1975. *Survival into the 21st Century*. Woodstock Valley, CT: 21st Century Publications.

Lappé, F. M. 1971, 1982. *Diet for a Small Planet*. New York: Ballentine.

Lustgarden, S. 1993. "Persuasive Examples." *Vegetarian Times* (October):18.

Mason, J., and P. Singer. 1990. *Animal Factories*. New York: Harmony Books.

Maurer, D. 1989. *Becoming a Vegetarian: Learning a Food Practice and Philosophy*. Unpublished M.A. thesis. Johnson City, TN: East Tennessee State University.

Maynard, D. W. 1988. "Language, Interaction, and Social Problems." *Social Problems* 35(4):311–334.

McLaren, D. S. 1974. "The Great Protein Fiasco." *The Lancet* (July 13):93–96.

Mills, C. W. 1940. "Situated Actions and Vocabularies of Motive." *American Sociological Review* 5:904–913.

Moran, V. 1985. *Compassion: The Ultimate Ethic*. Wellingborough, Northhamptonshire: Thorsons.

Nöth, W. 1990. *Handbook of Semiotics*. Bloomington: Indiana University Press.

Ornish, D., S. Brown, L. Scherwitz, J. Billings, W. Armstrong, T. Ports, S. McLanahan, R. Kirkeeide, R. Brand, and K. L. Gould. 1990. "Can Lifestyle Changes Reverse Coronary Heart Disease?" *The Lancet* 336:129–133.

Parham, B. 1979. *What's Wrong with Eating Meat?* Denver: Ananda Marga Publications.

Perelman, C., and L. Olbrechts-Tyteca. 1969. *The New Rhetoric: A Treatise on Argumentation*. Translated by John Wilkenson and Purcell Weaver. Notre Dame: University of Notre Dame Press.

Plous, S. 1993. "Psychological Mechanisms in the Human Use of Animals." *Journal of Social Issues* 49(1):11–52.

Robbins, J. 1987. *Diet for a New America*. Walpole, MA: Stillpoint.

———. 1992. *May All Be Fed: Diet for a New World*. New York: Avon.

Robeznieks, A. 1986. "How Many Are There?" *Vegetarian Times* (October):16–17.

Rosenbaum, A. 1993. "Those Amazing Vegetarian Athletes." *Vegetarian Times* (March):53–62.

Rozin, P., and A. E. Fallon. 1987. "A Perspective on Disgust." *Psychological Review* 94(1):23–41.

Satchidananda, S. S. 1986. *The Healthy Vegetarian*. Buckingham, VA: Integral Yoga Publications.

Scott, B. 1991. "The Vegetarian Resource Group 1991 Survey Results." *Vegetarian Journal* 10(6):14–17.

Shryock, R. H. 1931. "Sylvester Graham and the Popular Health Movement, 1830–1870." *Mississippi Valley Historical Review* 18:172–183.

Simons, H. W. 1970. "Requirements, Problems, and Strategies: A Theory of Persuasion for Social Movements." *Quarterly Journal of Speech* 56:1–11.

Simoons, F. J. 1961. *Eat Not This Flesh: Food Avoidances in the Old World*. Madison: University of Wisconsin Press.

Singer, P. 1975. *Animal Liberation: A New Ethics for Our Treatment of Animals*. New York: Avon.

Spector, M., and J. I. Kitsuse. 1987. *Constructing Social Problems*. Hawthorne, NY: Aldine de Gruyter.

Spiegel, M. 1988. *The Dreaded Comparison: Human and Animal Slavery*. Philadelphia: New Society Publishers.

Springen, K. 1993. "Pumped Up on Protein?" *Vegetarian Times* (August): 24–28.

Stewart, C. J., C. A. Smith, and R. E. Denton. 1989. *Persuasion and Social Movements*. Prospect Heights, IL: Waveland Press.

Stahler, C. 1994. "How Many Vegetarians Are There?" *Vegetarian Journal* 12(4):6–9.

Tracy, L. 1985. *The Gradual Vegetarian*. New York: Dell.

Troyer, R. J., and G. E. Markle. 1984. "Coffee Drinking: An Emerging Social Problem?" *Social Problems* 31(4):403–416.

Turner, R. 1983. "Figure and Ground in the Analysis of Social Movements." *Symbolic Interaction* 6(2):175–181.

Twigg, J. 1979. "Food for Thought: Purity and Vegetarianism." *Religion* 9:13–35.

———. 1983. "Vegetarianism and the Meanings of Meat." Pp. 18–30 in *The Sociology of Food and Eating*, edited by A. Murcott. Aldershot: Gower.

U. S. Bureau of the Census. 1992. *Statistical Abstract of the United States: 1992*. Washington, D.C.

Wynne-Tyson, J. 1975. *Food For a Future: The Ecological Priority of a Humane Diet*. London: Davis-Poynter.

Yntema, S. K. 1987. *Vegetarian Children: A Supportive Guide for Parents*. Ithaca, NY: McBooks Press.

Young, V. R., and P. L. Pellett. 1994. "Plant Proteins in Relation to Human Protein and Amino Acid Nutrition." *American Journal of Clinical Nutrition* 59:1203S–1212S.

V

Consumer Distrust of Food Processing

8

The Food Information War: Consumer Rights and Industry Prerogatives

CLIFTON ANDERSON

Consumers began to identify themselves as a distinctive interest group in the nineteenth century, and the emergence of the pure food movement in Great Britain and the United States contributed to the consumer awakening. Reformers who fought food adulteration championed the consumer's right to wholesome food. The food industry opposed reform, raising freedom-of-trade arguments that a British reformer dismissed as attempts "to frighten the timid and to throw the public off their guard" (Hassall 1876:871).

Pure food legislation was passed in Great Britain (Collins 1993), and state and municipal governments attempted to deal with food adulteration in the United States (Okun 1986). The need for federal action was recognized, and the Pure Food and Drug Law was enacted in 1906 (Anderson 1958). Since then, consumer advocates and food industry representatives have argued over food policy—primarily disagreeing about how existing regulations should be enforced and what additional regulations may be needed.

Consumer advocates have continued to raise food information issues—questioning the quality and safety of particular foods, inquiring about food fact-finding and regulatory processes in the United States government, and pressing for an expanded flow of public information concerning food, nutrition, and food-related disease. Food industry representatives, apprehensive about the extension of governmental regulations, ordinarily resist requests for disclosure of existing information and development of new food policy-related information. The confrontation between the two sides can aptly be described as a war of words. The rhetoric in the food information war is about many things, but themes concerning science seem especially important. The food information war can profitably be studied as rhetoric that highlights key issues of our time: science's problem-solving potential, citizens' attempts to achieve some degree of control over today's burgeoning technology, and the nation's prospects for improved health conditions in the years ahead.

What people talk about is a valuable clue to the many currents of thought and belief that run through society at all times. What they say they want indicates what people hope to do to shape the future. "Claimsmaking," say Spector and Kitsuse, "is always a form of interaction: a demand made by one party to another that something be done about some putative condition" (1987:78). Claims made in the food information war are evidence of stresses and conflicts that energize our political system.

Food Information and Science

Science is a feature—an enduring component—of the food information frame that claimsmakers are constructing to mobilize support for certain public policies. Members of the public apparently want to have food safety and nutrition policies authenticated by science, and each of the rivals in the food information war claims to have elicited science on "our" side.

Hoping to arouse the public's awareness of the dangers of food adulteration, early-day food reformers publicized researchers' findings concerning the deleterious effects of additives such as alum and lead chromate. However, it soon became evident that the reformers' attempts to sway public opinion with weighty scientific evidence would prompt food industry firms to retain the services of scientists who could offer contradictory evidence.

What science is, what it does, and what it should be doing are recurring themes in the rhetoric of the food information war.

Science as a Resource

Full disclosure of food information is desirable, food reformers have maintained, and they have demonstrated their support of this thesis by encouraging scientists' entry into new areas of research and applied problem solving that could expand society's knowledge base concerning food and nutrition. Food industry leaders have expected to benefit from research aimed at improving their industry's technology, but they have been apprehensive about research that could lead to new restrictions and regulations.

Early in this century, while food information claimsmakers and counterclaimants were involved in rhetoric concerning food additives and adulterants, research in nutrition and dietetics was bringing forth a new issue. That issue, as it has evolved during nearly a century, concerns the individual's need for information about his or her dietary requirements. The nub of the issue: Should the government serve as a resource for public information regarding the foods and the nutritional plans that will help people lead healthier lives?

At first, the question of the government helping with nutrition and dietary planning was not a food information issue. It was a feed information issue, concerning the dietary needs of livestock.

Scientists working at American agricultural colleges conducted much of the pioneering work in nutrition studies. Farmers comprised an important clientele group for these colleges, and farmers were eager to obtain information about livestock feeding programs. In experimental work with livestock, scientists made important breakthroughs in the field of nutrition. They analyzed feedstuffs—determining various feeds' content of protein, fiber, soluble carbohydrates, and ash—and they developed rudimentary guidelines for estimating the dietary needs of cattle, swine, sheep, horses, and poultry.

Later, the planning of livestock rations became more complicated. Scientists discovered vitamins and established their role in nutrition. To be able to feed livestock according to the animals' dietary requirements, farmers needed detailed information on the nutritional values of feeds manufactured by feed mills. They asked state legislatures to mandate informative feed labels, and many states passed feed labeling laws in the early 1900s. Looking back on those days, a representative of the American Feed Manufacturers Association recalled that "the lack of knowledge on the part of the average state legislator led to the inclusion in some of these laws of provisions that were harmful to and interfering with the conduct of the (feed) business" (*Flour and Feed* 1936:7).

Leaders of the milling industry tried to limit the labeling movement. They organized the American Feed Manufacturers Association and sent lobbyists to state capitals. Farmers urged legislators to support comprehensive labeling of feed products. Farmer-owned cooperatives began manufacturing livestock feeds and marketing them under detailed labels. The coops pioneered with "open-formula" labels that disclosed feed formulas the feed industry had always guarded as trade secrets (Knapp 1969:379–382).

After three decades of political maneuvering, farmers achieved the major goals they had sought in the labeling campaign. They persisted through the years because labeling was a vital economic issue for them. They needed information about feeds to plan livestock rations for maximum profitability.

While farmers fought for feed information, American consumer groups set forth proposals for food labeling regulations that would help food shoppers get maximum nutritional value for their money. Consumers Union, established in 1936, has been in the forefront of the campaign for food labeling reform. Gains have been made. In the 1990s, a federal program mandated the use of informative new food labels for almost all processed food products (Barrett 1993; Porter 1993; Wilkening 1993).

Do consumers need informative labels? Critics of feed labeling said farmers would not make use of nutritional information. They were wrong. There are compelling economic reasons for feeding livestock well, and perhaps reformers' arguments for improving human nutrition through education and information lack this bottom-line clarity. Food industry spokesmen have insisted that many consumers will find it difficult to utilize the information on food labels. "It is impossible to make nutritionists out of consumers by legislative fiat or by dictum," a food scientist says (Melnick 1979:210). A food company executive claims most people cannot understand labels that employ "technical language and scientific terminology," and he warns: "The average person is more frightened than helped by language he does not understand" (Belasco 1993:143).

Science and Diet/Health Awareness

The Nutrition Labeling and Education Act of 1990 mandates detailed nutritional information on labels. From a great variety of health-related information categories that might have been included on labels, government experts selected for primary emphasis the amounts of cholesterol, saturated fat, and dietary fiber foods contain. Nutritionists explain: "The intention is to give more attention to nutrients and other food components that have been linked to chronic diseases and less to those associated with particular nutritional deficiencies, which are increasingly rare in the United States" (Senauer et al. 1991:171).

Dietary management of fiber, sugar, fat, and salt is a challenge that health-conscious people now recognize. Awareness of food–health relationships has shown uninterrupted growth since the 1950s when the American Heart Association started to conduct nutrition information programs. The Department of Agriculture, the Department of Health and Human Services, and other federal agencies have developed information programs aimed at encouraging consumers to avoid a high intake of dietary fat. Consumer groups support the campaign to control heart disease through dietary change, and they also cooperate in other food–health awareness efforts.

Despite the public's apparent readiness to consider food–health information, food industry representatives say much of the information is based on theories that have not been adequately tested. Information for consumers should reflect conservative, common-sense views on nutrition, they claim, and consumers should be reassured "about the overall safety of the American food supply" (Tobias and Thompson 1980:123). They are critical of popular books and articles that "exaggerate the hazards of certain dietary factors" and "raise the expectations of the public to unreasonable levels without benefiting either the public or the science of nutrition" (Tobias and Thompson 1980:122–123).

As a practical matter, the food industry has had to accommodate itself to the consumer's heightened awareness of food–health relationships. Products have been redesigned, and merchandising campaigns now feature such terms as low-fat, sugar-free, no cholesterol, and high-fiber. At the same time, the information battle concerning "food faddism" continues. During the long struggle over implementation of the Nutrition Labeling Program, food industry representatives frequently referred to consumer groups as "faddists" and "alarmists." The pejorative labels may reinforce in some minds impressions of food reformers as unrealistic persons not versed in the ways of science. Certainly, scientific knowledge is seen as a key component here. Both food information claimsmakers and food industry counterclaimants apparently feel compelled to set forth their positions as being scientifically defensible.

To be true to science, say the food industry representatives, is to be deliberate, methodical, and unwilling to act prematurely. Instead of proceeding with information programs targeted at modifying the public's dietary habits, they propose to go ahead slowly until the body of scientific evidence is more complete. They are distrustful of decisions concerning dietary goals that result from "emotional reactions, pressures from groups which might profit from the policies, moral and ethical beliefs, and a desire to create the appearance of doing something about a difficult problem that is not understood" (Harper 1981:79–80).

Food information claimsmakers propose to press on with attempts to introduce substantial changes in the public's diet, confident that there is sufficient evidence right now to justify action. "The view that diet modification is impractical or doomed to failure is not justified," says a Canadian physician. "Many people have successfully modified their diets and substantially reduced their blood cholesterol levels" (Graham 1989:ix).

Individual successes in developing healthful dietary practices add up to an impressive record overall. The heart-related death rate of people under 65 has been reduced. In increasing numbers, consumers are interested in learning how to modify their diets to minimize the risk of cardiovascular disease and other serious ailments.

Science, Industry, and the Bureaucracy

When Congress passed the Pure Food and Drug Act of 1906, the United States government took on responsibilities for protecting the safety of the nation's food supply. Regulatory machinery was established, changed, and again revised. Known since 1927 as the Food and Drug Administration (FDA), the regulatory agency has a reputation for working cooperatively with food industry firms. Congratulating the FDA for its "strong, cooperative, practical" approach, a food industry executive once said that the agency has "relied chiefly upon educational processes to bring about reforms and improvements in food production, and on the whole has employed its police powers sparingly" (Thomas 1956:68–69).

Examining the FDA's performance from the consumer's perspective, food information claimsmakers have been critical of the agency's close ties with the food industry firms it regulates. In particular, they have called into question the FDA's reliance on industry sources for data on scientific tests of various products. Critics charge that using the food industry's research data is "like relying on a White Citizens' Council to do research on racism" (Marine and Van Allen 1972:95).

We are concerned here with the rhetoric of the food information war, the exchange of claims and counterclaims. This rhetoric centers time and again on science—the role science should be playing in society versus the actual performance of today's scientific investigators. The performance of the FDA's scientific apparatus has become an important theme in the ongoing rhetoric. Food industry representatives are generally supportive of the FDA's practice of science, while food information claimsmakers find much to criticize.

For instances of "bad science" in the FDA, critics cite reports of various defects in the agency's drug and chemical testing programs. Between 1975 and 1977, two Senate subcommittees heard allegations that G. D. Searle Co. and other pharmaceutical manufacturers had faked safety tests for new drugs, submitting the false data to the FDA. Later, three top officials of Industrial Bio-Test Laboratories, the nation's largest contract testing firm, were convicted of fraud. Their company allegedly faked thousands of tests, and the FDA used some of the bogus data to establish "tolerance levels"—the levels of pesticide residues that are permitted in food products (Schneider 1985:18).

Inside the FDA, according to food information claimsmakers, the agency's scientists have expressed fear that "their laboratory research serves primarily as window-dressing for already arrived at administrative decisions" (Turner 1970:192). The bureaucracy's psychological climate allegedly "tends to filter out and reject evidence that does not support the administrative position already taken and to elevate even the most flimsy information that does support the administrative position" (Turner 1970:193).

While criticizing the FDA's bureaucratic approach to scientific issues, food information claimsmakers stop short of proposing any radical departure from the agency's customary methods for carrying out its research and fact-finding mission. They say there must be improvements— significant changes in the attitudes of government bureaucrats plus increased attention given to the interests of consumers—but they continue to see science as a bulwark, providing the only secure basis on which government food policies can be built. Food industry counterclaimants also accept the centrality of science, but the two sides appear to have conflicting views regarding the functions science should perform.

Inclined to see government as a major patron of science, food information claimsmakers want government to be vigorous and proactive as it attempts to employ science for the common good—first by identifying problematic situations and then by developing problem-solving research and action programs. Food industry supporters, on the other hand, usually prefer a wait-and-see policy concerning problems that may be developing, and they profess to see the possibility for crucial scientific decisions to be made in an environment insulated from political pressures. Viewed from their perspective, a bureaucracy—insofar as it can be shielded from "radicals" and "alarmists"—can be a comfortable environment for decision making to proceed.

Science and the Unknown

Early food reformers wanted consumers to have full information about the dangerous adulterants added to food, and they knew scientific analysis could uncover the information. Today's scientists are being asked to investigate contaminants in food that may cause cancer, mutagenic changes in fetuses, or teratogenic alterations in future generations of people. How vigorously these investigations are pushed may become a key issue in the ongoing food information war.

Speaking for consumers, food information claimsmakers are seeking restrictions on environmental contaminants and increased funding for research. Food industry representatives insist there is little to be concerned about in the "alarmist" misrepresentations regarding hidden dangers supposedly lurking in food. Pesticide residues and other contaminants should not be considered major risks, they say, because natural toxicants in food "present about the same level of risk as environmental contaminants" (Hall 1979:142).

A momentous research task awaits scientists charged with investigating the safety of pesticides and other chemicals. In a lengthy study, the National Academy of Sciences concluded that federal agencies do not have accurate health studies data for most of the 65,000 chemicals presently on the American market. "Of tens of thousands of commercially important chemicals, only a few have been subjected to extensive toxicity testing, and most have scarcely been tested at all," the report stated (Schneider 1985:15).

By filling in the toxicity data gaps, researchers might provide science with a fresh perspective on environmental effects of the widespread use of toxic chemicals. In that case, new research vistas would be open to investigators concerned with health–environment relationships. Of course, there is no guarantee that gap-filling studies will be completed expeditiously. Many food information claimsmakers insist that research into chemical contaminants of food is not being pushed energetically by the FDA. Among the chemicals that enter the food supply, pesticides used in agriculture are said to pose complex problems for investigators (Lefferts 1993).

There are unanswered questions about new strains of disease-causing bacteria that are highly resistant to antibiotics. Has the widespread use of antibiotics by livestock and poultry producers contributed to the emergence of antibiotic-resistant bacteria? What have been the effects on human health of hormones used to promote the growth of poultry and livestock? Ingested over a long period of time, might the milk and meat from cows treated with bovine somatotropin result in health problems for consumers? Again, what are the long-term effects of consuming food preserved by irradiation processes? By asking questions such as these, food information claimsmakers can attempt to alert the public to possible food-related health problems. However, posing questions may not elicit from prospective followers the response leaders of a nascent movement would hope to obtain. A question that is intended to be a call for collective action may arouse some interest—even considerable anxiety—and still not impel people to action. As Sidney Tarrow points out, a collective action frame "is a tool for detaching people from their usual passivity," but the tool is not always employed successfully (1992:191).

Through the years, numerous attempts to stake out new frontiers in environmental science sparked public interest, only to have the interest recede in a short time. A food-related topic that interested both scientists and lay persons during the World War II years was the relationship between soils and nutrition. Russell Lord, an environmentalist, said many people of that era were impressed by a scientist's data showing correlations between the mineral content of soils in various regions and the percentage of military draftees from each region who were rejected for dental deficiencies (Lord 1962:317). These persons knew that in the past high incidence of thyroid disease had been linked to iodine deficiencies in the soil of America's "goiter belt," and it seemed logical to them that other health problems might be associated with the levels of soil nutrients in different regions.

A proposed large-scale research project comparing the nutritional characteristics of foods grown in various regions of the country did not attract support. For the food industry and also for regional business interests, there was no good reason for advancing the idea that the nutritional value of locally grown food will be greater in a region with healthy, well-balanced soils and less in a region with depleted soils. Lord (1962:316) recalls that research in Florida was "first hushed and then halted under chamber of commerce pressures."

The food industry, already troubled by charges that its processing methods cause large losses of nutrients in food products, flatly denied the proposition that health problems occur because mineral-deficient soils produce food of inferior quality. In Congressional hearings regarding regulation of vitamins and health foods, the FDA commissioner supported the food industry's position. He described reports about the depletion of soil fertility as "a lot of nonsense." He continued: "Our soil is naturally rich and the envy of every other nation" (Levenstein 1993:168).

A few research projects have looked at soil–health relationships (Beeson and Matrone 1976; USDA 1980), but the situation that Lord and his colleagues considered to be a social problem has not been a high-priority research topic—and the "soil–health relationship has yet to be even part way explored" (Lord 1962:316). In a similar fashion, any of today's research topics that concern food–health relationships could recede into the background if public support is not forthcoming.

Of course, "grievances are not sufficient to trigger collective action" (Tarrow 1992:177), and food information claimsmakers' calls for expanded scientific research need to have the support of voters who can persuade members of Congress to authorize adequate funding.

Science, Food, and Cancer

Fear of cancer is widespread, and chemicals that may cause cancer share some of the stigma of the dread disease. Since the results of exposure to cancer-causing chemicals may not become apparent for 30 or 40 years, it is impossible for toxicologists to screen the thousands of new chemicals modern technology has created and determine with certainty which are safe and which are not. Through laboratory testing on animals, researchers have determined that certain chemicals are carcinogenic— but they do not know for certain how much exposure to these chemicals humans could tolerate without developing cancer.

Carcinogens that enter the environment as pollutants may contaminate food. The residues of pesticides applied to crops may also represent a carcinogenic threat in food. Food safety reformers ask why carcinogenic pesticides are being used when safer methods of pest control are available. Economic constraints force food producers to cut labor costs by utilizing chemicals, defenders of the food industry reply. Moreover, they add, the risks involved in using agricultural chemicals are minimal.

A comprehensive strategy for eliminating carcinogens from our food supply and general environment should be developed promptly, food safety activists maintain. Sandra Steingraber, a biologist at Columbia College in Chicago, points out:

> Cancer is caused by carcinogens. Astonishingly, you can read entire tracts about cancer published by the ACS (American Cancer Society) and the word *carcinogen* never comes up. These seemingly authoritative agencies have framed the cause of the disease as a problem of *behavior* rather than as one of *exposure* to disease-causing agents. (Paulsen 1993:84)

Since the 1960s, environmentalists have been gaining ground in their efforts to have cancer represented as an intolerable condition that should be prevented and not as just another disease to be treated (Hays and Hays 1987:30–31). In the food information war, claimsmakers concerned about carcinogens in food urge the banning of organochlorines widely used as pesticides. Food industry representatives prefer to speak of carcinogens as "toxicants," and they claim that many toxicants in food are naturally occurring substances that entail little risk to consumers. Oranges, for example, "contain the flavone, tangeretin, which is embryotoxic" (Hall 1980:333). Other common fruits and vegetables contain minute amounts of toxins. Aflatoxin, the most potent carcinogen known, is produced by some strains of mold; residues are found in meat, milk, eggs, and other foods (Alfin-Slater and Aftergood 1981:28).

Toxicants cannot be avoided entirely, food industry spokespersons say, and the role of government regulators should be to make sure that the level of any toxicant in food does not rise above a "negligible risk" level. The government's role should be an aggressive one aimed at controlling the external sources of carcinogens that are entering the food supply, reformers assert. They claim the food industry is trying to "normalize" the presence in food of contaminants that might endanger public health.

Official FDA policy has, in the main, favored the food industry's position. The agency has set tolerance levels for aflatoxin and other hazardous contaminants, taking the position that "zero" tolerance would be impractical and unrealistic. The Delaney Amendment, passed by Congress in 1957, does establish a zero tolerance for carcinogens in additives included in processed food. A long-continued campaign for repeal or modification of the Delaney Amendment is now mounting in intensity, and the rule (never fully enforced) of zero tolerance for carcinogens may soon end.

How can science guide the makers of public policy as they deal with food safety questions? On the question of carcinogens in food, the information claimsmakers ask for an uncomplicated approach. If science reveals the presence of dangerous contaminants in food, they say, then we should get rid of the contaminants. Counterclaimants reflecting the food industry's position say science can establish realistic tolerance levels that will protect human health adequately if imperfectly. Furthermore: "Absolute safety cannot be proven in any aspect of life. Science can only give us a measure of the degree of harmlessness of a particular food or ingredient, which must be measured along with the benefit provided" (Clydesdale 1979:21).

Food Information and Conflict

The food information war is a logomacy, a battle of words. The words have flesh-and-blood targets—designated enemies. Food information claimsmakers are attacking food industry counterclaimants, and vice versa. The combatants aim pejoratives at each other. Beyond the logomacy is a struggle for influence, a contest for the public's support. Each side accentuates the conflictual aspects of their encounters, using conflict as the focus for enlisting new supporters and also for solidifying the loyalties of old supporters.

In this dynamic of conflict, there has come to be a wide circle of involvement—including a variety of groups engaged in transmitting food information. Along with proponents of food reform and representatives of the food industry, the groups involved include academicians, bureaucrats, scientists, and media representatives.

"Impartial" Academicians

When dealing with controversial subjects, educational institutions often strive for impartiality and avoid advocacy. Educators employed by agencies or institutions that are committed to goal-oriented action programs may at times eschew strict impartiality, however. In large institutions, such as the American land-grant universities, some educators may be under constraints of impartiality while others work actively to promote the interests of a particular clientele. Regarding food information, one program at the Connecticut Agricultural Experiment Station should be mentioned as a model of impartiality.

Researchers in Connecticut did not choose to become involved in monitoring food quality in their state. A state law passed before the turn of the century gave the Experiment Station the responsibility for testing samples of food that were suspected of being adulterated. In annual reports, beginning in 1896 and continuing for about 80 years, the Experiment Station listed the results of testing food samples obtained in shops throughout the state. They tested samples because contamination was suspected either by state inspectors or by consumers.

The station's 218-page report of 1973 listed some adverse findings (Hanna 1973). A store in Meriden sold ice cream bars containing small bits of metal. A drugstore in Middletown stocked Metrecal cookies that were insect infested. Blue cheese dressing in a Torrington grocery showed signs of spoilage. Hamburger samples obtained in New Britain had excessive added water, and hamburger in East Norwalk contained a soy flour additive. Most samples had no quality problems, and researchers reported each test result. Essentially, researchers were sharing their test records with the public, without interpretation or elaboration. The information was unbiased, but it was not what the public wanted. Since the mid-1970s, the Connecticut researchers have presented food quality information topically. Believing that consumers want to have detailed information on food products such as tofu, for instance, they have compiled publications comparing characteristics of various brands of products.

Instances of food adulteration abounded in the old Connecticut reports, although authors withheld comment. The reports' authors pointed to situations, but they avoided framing the situations as social problems. Today's educators and researchers cannot respond to the contemporary food issues without focusing on problematic aspects of these issues. Pesticides in food; using food to treat disease, science's competence to set food policy goals, and avoiding *Escherichia coli* contamination are all issues with policy implications.

As educators and researchers consider the issues, they are drawn into the food information war. On the question of *E. coli* contamination, for instance, is the major aspect to be considered the sanitation of the individual food-handler or the clean-up of an extensive industry? Conflicts are shaping up here, and people in academia are becoming involved.

Bureaucracy's Involvement

As noted earlier, the FDA makes use of information supplied by industry while it carries out its regulatory functions. When it makes decisions that serve to define its own functions and powers, the agency can utilize arguments advanced by food information claimsmakers or food industry counterclaimants. The rhetoric of the food information war is available to the FDA as it considers problem areas of food, nutrition, health, and governmental regulation. During its long association with the food industry, the FDA has supported the industry on many issues. For example, officials of the agency have gone on record as favoring abolition of the Delaney Amendment's zero tolerance rule on pesticide residues in food. Inside the agency, according to recent studies and also the Nader Group's study a generation ago, a culture has arisen that is critical of health claims by environmentalists and consumer groups (Lefferts 1993; Turner 1970).

Observers of public bureaucracies report many examples of regulatory agencies being "captured" by the groups they are supposed to regulate. Under the Administrative Procedures Act of 1946, the decision-making processes of the federal regulatory agencies became subject to increased public scrutiny, and public interest groups such as environmental and consumer organizations gained access to information on which regulatory actions were based. Through the years, the public interest groups have publicly criticized actions of the FDA and have questioned the agency's close ties with the food industry. The criticisms of the public interest groups have been noted by the national media, by Congressional committees, and by the FDA. itself. By serving as alert watchdogs, these groups no doubt are altering the behavior of government regulators to some extent. More profound changes may be in prospect at the FDA if important segments of the food industry successfully develop new strategies for dealing with food safety issues. Innovative thinking in the food industry regarding pesticide use could eventually resonate in the FDA.

Food Industry's Resources

In the food information war, the food industry commands impressive resources. Through large-scale advertising, public relations, and lobbying, the industry transmits its views to a variety of publics. Industry representatives, in general, share an aversion to stringent regulation, and they dislike publicity that places their industry and its products in a bad light. The Alar controversy of 1989, which resulted in a huge loss of sales for the apple industry, caused shockwaves in the food industry that persist today.

Alar, a growth regulator, was used on apples to regulate fruit size, coloring, and ripening. When the chemical was depicted on national television as a dangerous carcinogen, millions of consumers refused to buy fresh apples or apple products. The consumer boycott alarmed food processors and producers, and many began to reexamine their use of agricultural chemicals, especially pesticides. In the tomato industry, processors experimented with new nonchemical pest control systems and required producers to reduce their use of chemical pesticides (Lefferts 1993; Wilson 1991).

In other commodity areas, producers took the lead in trying to avoid controversies concerning the safety of their food products. Potato producers organized an effort to prevent farmers who misused pesticides from marketing their potatoes. The livestock industry set up self-policing programs to discourage beef and swine producers from incorrect use of growth promotants and other pharmaceuticals.

Resourceful food producers and processors were trying to avert new food toxicity incidents, and their proactive stance actually caused them to question food production technologies they had previously defended. Certainly, on the pesticide residue issue, consumer groups and food industry advocates were moving closer together. Each side, approaching the issue from a different angle, was framing pesticide residues in food as a problem that required immediate attention.

There are additional signs of change in the food industry. In recent industry-wide meetings, some representatives have continued to oppose the government-imposed nutritional labeling program. Others accept the program and hope to make it operate to the food industry's advantage. One industry leader has predicted that "the day will come when health claims drive the food industry" (Brooks 1993:105). In other words, instead of opposing nutrition labeling and information programs directed at consumers, the industry should be profiting from consumers' awareness of food–health relationships. Here, again, the food industry may be ready to frame an issue along the same lines that food information claimsmakers have drawn in the past.

Possibly, the food industry may yield on peripheral issues while holding firm to its main thesis—that government should not burden the industry with onerous regulations. Industry leaders say "the Alar scare" showed consumers overreacting to inaccurate information about toxicants in food and they are taking steps to avert new toxicity scares. Preplanned public relations and information campaigns will go into operation when a food commodity comes under attack, with the campaigns featuring reassurances from authoritative scientists.

Looking to the future, some industry leaders see food safety and environmental issues being eclipsed by economic concerns. In this view, new international agreements on free trade will prevent the United States from maintaining food safety rules such as the zero tolerance for pesticide residues as set forth in the Delaney Amendment. By requiring food quality and safety regulations to be approved by an international commission, the General Agreement on Trade and Tariffs would move many food policy issues out of the realm of national politics (Truax 1992).

Science as a Province of Politics

Scientists became involved in the food information war early on, not only performing their traditional role of fact-finding but also venturing into the realm of political policy advisors. Through the decades, as science and technology proliferated and became more complex, the number of scientists grew, they came to represent an astonishing variety of specialties, and they also possessed a rich diversity of political and ethical perspectives. Under the circumstances, when scientists express their views regarding food policies or other public issues, they may display more controversy than consensus.

In recent decades, some scientists have become convinced that scientific disputes should be resolved by scientists themselves in their own professional conclaves. Now, if scientists could achieve consensus on questions of concern to their profession, might they also be able to speak with one voice on science-related public policy matters? Along these lines of thinking, the idea of a "Supreme Court of science" has evolved (Cowen 1976; Hays and Hays 1987:361; Kantrowitz 1977). The judges of the proposed court would be scientists who would decide scientific disputes that impinged on work of the FDA or other regulatory agencies. Scientists supposedly would be better qualified than judges to decide scientific disputes. Some representatives of the food industry have indicated they would like to see scientific and technical questions resolved by qualified scientists, but environmentalists and consumer advocates say a science court would likely be elitist and undemocratic. Other observers suggest that "truly impartial scientists could not be found to serve as judges" (Hays and Hays 1987:361).

For good or ill, scientific questions in this nation will often become topics of open political debate. In the food information war, scientists join in rhetoric—and they debate with one another. The idea of science being a place apart, separate from politics, is giving way to a growing realization that, like all other aspects of our lives, science is a province of politics. The ideal of a fair, discerning, contemplative scientific establishment continues to have wide appeal, however, and it recurs frequently in the food information war as a powerful symbol.

Risk Messages in the Media

On Thanksgiving Day 1959, millions of American families had no cranberries with their traditional turkey dinners. After some cranberries were found to have residues of carcinogenic weed killer in excess of the FDA's standard of tolerance, sales of cranberry products plummeted. The media effectively transmitted to consumers an important food–health message: toxic chemicals in food can endanger health. The message was repeated in "the Alar scare" and in other toxicity incidents. Critics of the media charge the media with unbalance, exaggeration, and "fear-mongering." Whatever the information media's excesses may have been, their effectiveness should not be discounted. They impressed on people the danger of toxicants in food. This danger is a theme of the food information war—a message with which consumer advocates have been trying to dent the public's shell of passivity.

Food industry representatives claim the media's reportage is incomplete. News articles deal with toxicity but do not fully explain what benefits pesticides provide to agriculture, or how toxicity risks are assessed. There is drama in danger, however, and a news story can be expected to focus on the dramatic. Indeed, the media's audience will tend to focus on a theme of danger, screening out other messages. During the Alar incident, the initial information about a food risk shocked consumers, and their risk perceptions increased over time as media coverage continued (van Ravenswaay and Hoehn 1991).

Can a food toxicity message backfire? Consumer advocates know that credibility is all-important. Difficult-to-demonstrate claims concerning dangers in food tend to perpetuate the status quo, they say. Before the next food emergency arises, consumer leaders would like to pick the topic, control the timing, and plan the overall claimsmaking strategy. They recognize, however, that the symbol of health risk is available for anyone's use. The media could reveal another food-related health risk at any time. Harvey W. Wiley, the crusader who helped win passage of the Pure Food and Drug Act of 1906, realized that symbols have a life of their own. Pointing to "the old fable of the addition of sand to sugar, of gypsum and terra alba to flour, and of alum to bread," he said many forms of food adulteration continued to be referred to with alarm by speakers and writers even though these practices no longer represented genuine problems (Wiley 1912:595).

Risk messages will continue to recur in the media because they are a major theme in the food information war. Consumer advocates can accentuate the risk theme, possibly giving rise to a new food toxicity emergency, or they can continue to talk about risks without triggering a consumer boycott of some food product. With the best of planning, they still may have to confront the unpredictable situation—the food toxicity crisis that just happens.

Claimsmakers Seek Justice

Early in the food information war, claimsmakers framed their demand for government-conducted information programs as a move to correct an economic injustice. According to claimsmakers, consumers needed information that was being concealed by selfish business interests. The American reformer Harvey Wiley said the sale of adulterated food constituted fraud, since consumers were not getting what they paid for. As the food reform movement progressed, giving increased attention to unhealthful substances used as food additives, the injustice frame was extended to include avoidance of unnecessary health risks. Framing of the food information problem widened further in the post-World War II years when environmental contamination became extensive and people became increasingly concerned about ingesting toxic chemicals with their food. Recently, the injustice frame has been extended again to focus attention on the rights of women to food information and other health-protecting governmental services. The National Breast Cancer Coalition claims women are being treated unjustly, and the group notes the government's reluctance to fund a large research project that would study the effect of diet on breast cancer and also on osteoporosis and heart disease in women (McNutt 1992).

Seeking information on cancer prevention, more and more people who are concerned about cancer may become active and vocal in the food information war. If they do become active, and if they seek implementation of zero-tolerance pesticide residue levels for food, the food information war may heat up to an extreme intensity in the years to come. Claims and counterclaims regarding cancer as social injustice may open a political debate of major proportions. Counterclaimants who defend the agricultural chemical industry are at this moment framing as an injustice the zero-tolerance rule that would take away "the chemical resources which are an important element to an economic and environmental agricultural system" (Richardson 1991).

The Food Information War's Next Phase

Futuristic forecasting must deal with multiple possibilities because the future can develop along an unlimited number of alternative patterns. Forecasters can best stimulate thinking and discussion concerning the emergent future by playing the field—seriously considering the remote long shot as well as the more ordinary and expectable possibilities. The food information war as I have reviewed it involves consumer advocates and other proponents of change, on the one hand, and, on the other, food industry advocates who object to political change that disturbs the economic status quo. The extreme, far-out prediction I offer is a scaling-down of the two sides' rhetoric and, perhaps, the beginning of the end of the food information war.

There are signs, as noted earlier, that some sectors of the food industry are taking a middle-ground position, evidently hoping to avoid toxicity scares and unproductive conflict with consumer and environmental groups. A reconciliation in the food information war conceivably might lead to improvements in the disputes of environmentalists and industrialists concerning pollution and environmental degradation. The scenario of peace and reconciliation is possible but ongoing rhetoric between the claimsmakers does not suggest this outcome will soon occur.

The food information war is likely to continue, and the food industry can be expected to support international trade agreements with provisions that would limit the United States from enforcing certain food safety regulations within its own borders. An interesting phase of the food information war is in prospect, with consumer and environmental groups leading the political fight to modify the powers of the international panels that would resolve trade disputes between GATT trading partners. If they were to lose that fight, they might start campaigning for the establishment of democratic world government!

Cancer risks will in all likelihood be spotlighted as food information claimsmakers tell legislators and the public alarming accounts of carcinogens endangering the nation's food supply. Attempting to involve many people in grassroots demonstrations, organizations concerned with food–cancer relationships will become more active nationwide. If toxicity emergencies occur, extensive educational programs and television specials are likely to be arranged. Using a variety of approaches, the claimsmakers will be framing food-related cancer as a major health problem of the twenty-first century.

It is always possible that the food information war will continue for a time, only to reach a stalemate as people who are "bombarded by nutritional and culinary messages from all sides" become increasingly distrustful of all "pronouncements of experts on food and nutrition" (Levenstein 1993:253). In another possible scenario, members of the public retreat from politics and privatize their concerns about nutrition and health. Political action to extend people's participation in food policy decisions may be impossible to achieve as long as individuals "remain focused on their own arteries and waistlines" (Belasco 1993:249). However, there are other possible outcomes. The food information war need not end in *ennui*. Food information bridging private concerns and social problems may encourage people to continue the struggle for good food, a safe environment, and improved health.

References

Alfin-Slater, R. B., and L. Aftergood. 1981. "Nutrition and Cancer." Pp. 21–33 in *Controversies in Nutrition*, edited by L. Ellenbogen. New York: Churchill Livingstone.

Anderson, O. E. Jr. 1958. *The Health of the Nation*. Chicago: University of Chicago Press.

Barrett, S. 1993. "New Food Labeling Regulations Issued." *Nutrition Forum* 10(3):25–30.

Beeson, K. C., and G. Matrone. 1976. *The Soil Factor in Nutrition: Animal and Human*. New York: Marcel Dekker.

Belasco, W. J. 1993. *Appetite for Change: How the Counterculture Took on the Food Industry*. Ithaca: Cornell University Press.

Brooks, E. 1993. "Marketing Foods for Health Purposes: Realizing the Dream." *Food Technology* 47(9):105.

Clydesdale, F. M. 1979. *Food Science and Nutrition: Current Issues and Answers*, Englewood Cliffs, NJ: Prentice-Hall.

Collins, E. J. T. 1993. "Food Adulteration and Safety in Britain in the 19th and Early 20th Centuries." *Food Policy* 18(April):75–109.

Cowen, R. C. 1976. "Who Decides Between the Experts?" *Ag World* January:11.

Flour & Feed. 1936. "History of American F.M.A." 36(8):7–8, 11.

Graham, A. F. 1989. "Preface" in *The Lighthearted Cookbook*, by A. Lindsay. Toronto: Key Porter Books.

Hall, R. L. 1979. "Food Ingredients and Additives." Pp. 116–150 in *Food Science and Nutrition: Current Issues and Answers*, edited by F. Clydesdale. Englewood Cliffs, NJ: Prentice-Hall.

———. 1980. "Safe at the Plate." Pp. 322–336 in *Issues in Nutrition: An Ecological Perspective*, edited by A. L. Tobias and P. Thompson. Monterey, CA: Wadsworth Health Sciences Division.

Hanna, J. G. 1973. *Food from Connecticut Markets and Farms*. New Haven: Connecticut Agricultural Experiment Station.

Harper, A. E. 1981. "Dietary Goals." Pp. 63–84 in *Controversies in Nutrition*, edited by L. Ellenbogen. New York: Churchill Livingstone.

Hassall, A. H. 1876. *Food: Its Adulterations and the Means for Their Detection.* London: Longmans, Green.

Hays, S. P., and B. P. Hays. 1987. *Beauty, Health and Permanence: Environmental Politics in the United States, 1955–1985.* Cambridge: Cambridge University Press.

Kantrowitz, A. 1977. "The Science Court Experiment." *Bulletin of Atomic Scientists* 33(4):43–50.

Knapp, J. G. 1969. The *Rise of American Cooperative Enterprise: 1620–1920.* Danville, IL: Interstate.

Lefferts, L. Y. 1993. "A Commonsense Approach to Pesticides." *Nutrition Action Health Letter* 20(7):1,5–7.

Levenstein, H. 1993. *Paradox of Plenty: A Social History of Eating in Modern America.* New York: Oxford University Press.

Lord, R. 1962. *The Care of the Earth: A History of Husbandry.* New York: Thomas Nelson.

Marine, G., and J. Van Allen. 1972. *Food Pollution: The Violation of Our Inner Ecology.* New York: Holt, Rinehart & Winston.

McNutt, K. 1992. "Watch Out for Ecofeminism." *Nutrition Today* 27(1):40–42.

Melnick, D. 1979. "Economics in Food and Nutrition Issues." Pp. 178–221 in *Food Science and Nutrition: Current Issues and Answers*, edited by F. Clydesdale. Englewood Cliffs, NJ: Prentice-Hall.

Okun, M. 1986. *Fair Play in the Marketplace: The First Battle for Pure Food and Drugs.* Dekalb, IL: Northern Illinois University Press.

Paulsen, M. 1993. "The Politics of Cancer." *Utne Reader* 60:81–89.

Porter, D. V. 1993. "Food Labeling Reform: The Journey from Science to Policy." *Nutrition Today* 28(5):7–12.

Richardson, L. 1991. "McDecisions." *Agrichemical Age* April: 34.

Schneider, K. 1985. "The Data Gap." *Amicus Journal* 6(3):15–24.

Senauer, B., E. Asp, and J. Kinsey. 1991. *Food Trends and the Changing Consumer.* St. Paul: Eagan.

Spector, M., and J. I. Kitsuse. 1987. *Constructing Social Problems.* Hawthorne, NY: Aldine de Gruyter.

Tarrow, S. 1992. "Mentalities, Political Cultures, and Collective Action Frames: Constructing Meaning through Action." Pp. 156–173 in *Frontiers in Social Movement Theory*, edited by A. D. Morris and C. M. Mueller. New Haven: Yale University Press.

Thomas, G. C. 1956. "The Milling Industry and the Food and Drug Administration." Pp. 68–69 in *The Impact of the Food and Drug Administration on Our Society*, edited by H. Welch and F. Marti-Ibanez. New York: MD Publications.

Tobias, A. L., and P. J. Thompson (eds.). 1980. *Issues in Nutrition for the 1980s: An Ecological Perspective.* Monterey, CA: Wadsworth Health Sciences Division.

Truax, H. 1992. "Coming to Terms with Trade." *Environmental Action* 24(2):31–34.

Turner, J. S. 1970. *The Chemical Feast.* New York: Grossman Publications.

U.S. Department of Agriculture. 1980. "Tracing Elements Through the Food Chain." Pp. 166–175 in *Issues in Nutrition for the 1980s: An Ecological Perspective*, edited by A. L. Tobias and P. J. Thompson. Monterey, CA: Wadsworth Health Sciences Division.

van Ravenswaay, E. O., and J. P, Hoehn. 1991. "The Impact of Health Risk Information on Food Demand: A Case Study of Alar and Apples." Pp. 155–174 in *Economics of Food Safety*, edited by J. A. Caswell. New York: Elsevier.

Wiley, H. W. 1912. *Foods and Their Adulteration*. Philadelphia: P. Blakiston's Son.

Wilkening, V. L. 1993. "FDA's Regulations to Implement NLEA." *Nutrition Today* 28(5):13–20.

Wilson, S. 1991. "IPM Revival." *Agrichemical Age* April:32–33.

9

The Construction of Food Biotechnology as a Social Issue

THOMAS J. HOBAN

Introduction

Since the earliest days of civilization, people have selected and modified plants and animals to increase productivity or enhance desirable qualities. Such qualities include resistance to disease, insects, drought, or other natural pests. Foods have also been processed or modified for centuries to enhance their taste, nutritional content, and handling characteristics. In the past this has generally been a time-consuming and imprecise process.

The last two decades have seen a revolution in biology that has greatly expanded our ability to modify plants and animals at the molecular level. A relatively new set of powerful tools (known collectively as "biotechnology") gives scientists the ability to make precise and rapid changes to any type of living organism. One of the most powerful and controversial techniques is known as genetic engineering, which allows scientists to "cut and paste" hereditary (genetic) material from one type of organism to any other type. Scientists are able to move the desired traits as well. The objectives of food biotechnology are generally the same as previous technologies, but the process is faster and more precise.

During the next decade, the application of biotechnology is expected to have significant impacts on food production and processing. Supporters predict a number of significant economic, social, and environmental benefits. Opponents express concerns about the safety and ethics of biotechnology, including skepticism about the ability of government to adequately control its use. Given the power and wide-ranging implications of biotechnology, a number of important social issues are being raised.

The use of biotechnology in food production is already taking the characteristics of a controversial social issue. Powerful institutions (industry, government, and universities) are staking out their positions in support of biotechnology. Questions are being raised about the potential for negative impacts on the environment. Concerns over the safety of food produced through biotechnology also have arisen, especially from the standpoint of potential food allergens. Some question the ethics of genetic engineering, which some view as an attempt to "play god."

This chapter examines how biotechnology issues are being constructed. Particular attention is paid to the role of the media, government, industry,, and interest groups in defining issues related to biotechnology. I review the contributions of social science theory and research related to the social construction and perception of risk and focus on two of the first applications of food biotechnology (bovine somatotropin and Flavr-Savr^{tm} tomatoes), which have recently been approved for use.

Social Context of Biotechnology

As with any new technology, biotechnology will have a number of important social implications and consequences (Hoban 1989). One of the main issues associated with any technology involves a variety of actual and perceived risks. Recently, a number of groups and organizations have begun to recognize and assess both the risks and benefits of a new technology. This process involves construction of technical and social relationship.

Social Construction of Technical Issues

Social and cultural theories share the idea that perceptions of risk are filtered through perceptual lenses shaped by involvement in social groups (Renn 1992a). People's responses to issues are affected by social influences and communication with friends, family members, and others. A social constructionist approach suggests that risk issues can be understood only in terms of the actors' beliefs and bounded rationalities. This approach views conflicts over risk as a struggle of various groups to have their meanings (i.e., their definitions of risk) imposed on others. The social constructionist perspective on risk does not deny objective reality of hazards and the associated risks. Instead, it draws attention to alternative ways of identifying issues and assessing risks (Short 1992). Conflicts over the risks of all forms of technology have grown more heated and widespread during the last few years.

Hilgartner (1992) develops a system–network perspective on risk. He explains how definitions of risk get built into technology and shape its evolution. Such definitions of risk have at least three conceptual elements: an object that poses the risk, an alleged harm, and a linkage alleging a causal relationship between the object and the harm. Risk objects are linked into complex socially constructed sociotechnical networks. Controversies arise over the construction of risk objects, their harms, and the linkages between them. Definitions and interests change over time; building networks of control around a risk object involves complex struggles among a variety of social actors. For example, social systems develop criteria for prioritizing actions to control serious risks, but deemphasize risks that appear trivial (Renn 1992a). The arenas for constructing risks involve a complex network of facts and machines, policies and regulations, organizations and institutions, research programs, and other interrelated components.

Social Amplification of Risk

The concept of social amplification of risk suggests that events associated with risks interact with psychological, social, institutional, and cultural processes in ways that can heighten or attenuate perceptions of risks and shape risk behavior (Kasperson 1992). These behavioral responses create secondary social consequences that may emerge as economic, environmental, and ethical issues. The secondary consequences, in turn, serve as events that interact with psychological, social, institutional, and cultural processes in ways that can further heighten or attenuate perceptions of risks and shape risk behavior.

Risk amplification occurs when secondary effects trigger demands for additional institutional responses. This is a feedback loop that may lead to overreaction. Risk attenuation occurs when secondary effects place impediments in the path of needed protective reactions. This may lead to some risks being neglected. Amplification stations—individuals, groups, or institutions—collect information about risks, communicate about risks, and undertake behaviors that have social consequences. These stations may either amplify or attenuate reactions to risk.

Individuals process risk information in ways that are shaped by their roles and membership in social groups. Information that is consistent with expectations and beliefs tends to be amplified. Beyond personal role expectations, the general cultural beliefs and values of the larger group to which the individual belongs shape the reaction to risk. Risks have both an objective component and a socially constructed component. The processing of risk information through media and other institutional and cultural filters shapes the social experience of risk. Media coverage stimulates social mobilization and vice versa.

Much of the information people receive about risks comes from the mass media (Sandman 1986; National Research Council 1989). The media collect, interpret, and transmit information about the technical, political, and societal implications of risk. When the media cover a particular story, people assume it is important. Political leaders are more likely to respond to an issue once it is in the media. The media also lend credibility and legitimacy to a particular side in a controversy. By providing a forum for expression, certain groups are able to influence public policies and perceptions through the media. The media have played vital roles in setting the public agenda about biotechnology.

Problems often arise with media communication of complex technical subjects. The media are very selective in terms of the types of stories covered and the information included in a particular story. The media are generally more interested in politics than science, in simplicity than complexity, and in danger than safety (Covello et al. 1988). Media coverage about new technology tends to be sensationalized. They often look for controversy and emphasize opposing views.

Social Arenas of Risk

Social arena theory proposes that various interest groups try to sway public policy in directions that support their own agendas (Renn 1992b). Groups maximize their effect on policy through mobilization of resources. The notion of a "social arena" implies the symbolic location where the struggle for a political solution to a particular issue is played out. There are four major closely related social arenas: administrative, judicial, scientific, and mass media. A variety of groups participate within each arena to influence the outcome on issues associated with technology.

Risk debates within the different arenas tend to focus on two issues:

acceptable level of risk and distribution of risks and benefits across society. Groups whose interests or values are either supported or threatened by a technical development are likely to enter into the arena. Risk issues often serve as symbols of larger distributional conflicts. In other words, the technical risk is often not the motivating factor that pulls a group into the risk arena. Movement into the risk arena may be a way for an interest group to gain notoriety and resources. The groups in the biotechnology arena have a wide range of interests and goals.

Opposing sides are usually formed early in the social arena. Proponents of a technology often have a vested, economic interest in promoting the acceptance of technology. They must assure government agencies, interest groups, and the public that their technology is effective and safe. The companies developing biotechnology products are the most obvious proponents. Other supporters include some government agencies and university researchers.

On the other side, a variety of groups tend to oppose the use of a new technology. Lewis (1990) describes substantial and effective political forces that oppose almost any new technology, based on concern over risks, as well as nostalgia for a simpler life. Opposition to technology has, in fact, become a full-time occupation for some activists. Somewhere between the dedicated proponents and opponents lie the vast majority of people. For the most part, citizens show relatively little interest in or concern for technology until the benefits or risks are somehow brought close to home (such as in food). Given an apathetic majority, the special interests on either side are often left to play the major roles in risk assessment policies and decisions.

Dynamics of Technical Controversy

The construction of biotechnology is taking on the characteristics of a technological controversy (Mazur 1981). Technical controversies are social phenomena that involve three main features. First, the focal point of the controversy is a product or process of science and technology. Second, some or all of the main participants in the controversy are experts in the field. Third, there are experts on opposing sides of the debate who disagree over scientific arguments. Each side tries to build its case through the media and the public policy process. Biotechnology clearly exhibits these three features.

There is often little consensus on technological controversies, because the sides often argue about different aspects of the technology. Supporters of biotechnology tend to stress economic and other benefits, while opponents raise concerns about risk and ethics. Each side states its case so there is little chance for the opposing side to clearly refute what has been claimed. People interpret controversies in line with their position on a particular issue (Mazur 1981). Although ideologies of the two sides may be different, the rhetoric is often similar. Proponents often argue for a technology based on need, effectiveness, and safety. Opponents question technologies on similar grounds. Opponents try to enlist the general public by referring to their groups as "consumer groups" and portraying the establishment as imposing their view on unwilling citizens. The establishment tries to show the challengers as misguided, uninformed, and out to mislead the public. This has already occurred with biotechnology.

Mazur (1981) describes several stages of protest movements to study why certain technologies become controversial and others do not. First, the media carry a warning against a technology that is acknowledged by some of the public. Next, a few activist groups attempt to alter or stop the technology, through such means as protest demonstrations or lobbying. Once the movement becomes widespread it may become incorporated into society at large.

Initial warnings about a technology come to the public's attention through various sources. New technologies often face controversy even within their own promotion circles. In the early 1970s when recombinant DNA (i.e., biotechnology) was first developed, some scientists thought the new life forms could be harmful or uncontrollable if they escaped. They formed a group that cautioned against its use and wrote an article in *Science*. This started a technological controversy that continues today. Warnings appear more readily today because of a large network of environmental and consumer activist groups. They are a strong political force and have access to the mass media.

The next step in the evolution of social protests occurs when a warning is heeded. Groups come together and form national coalitions. Linkages are created to share information and resources. As a technological controversy grows, people on each side emerge as spokespersons and the line becomes more rigidly drawn between the sides. As the activity of protesters increases, the mass media coverage of the controversy increases. As mass media coverage increases, the general public's reaction to the technology becomes evident.

Some technologies are more likely to become controversial than others (Mazur 1981). Technological innovations that are new are more likely to be opposed than are changes in established ones. People are more likely to accept a new technology with little controversy if they can choose to accept it, and if the benefits and risks are balanced in a favorable way. Mazur (1981) concludes that the characteristics of the technology itself are not all that important, relative to the public perception and social construction of the controversy.

Political Context of Biotechnology

Some of the most important and controversial social issues related to biotechnology involve public policies and regulations constructed over the last two decades. Molecular biologists initiated a moratorium on experiments during the early 1970s (Kenny 1989) and regulations have been modified as the technology developed. Meanwhile there has been sporadic media coverage of commercial possibilities and potential risks of biotechnology. Opponents and supporters of biotechnology have tried to shape public policies: litigating through the courts, attempting to influence public opinion, and lobbying government agencies.

Public policies and regulation of food biotechnology have important implications for the types of products developed, as well as the speed with which they reach commercial production (Hatch and Kuchler 1989). Since biotechnology is developing quickly, the political context is in flux. The long-term implications and impacts of biotechnology are not always clear before regulatory decisions have to be reached. In the area of bio-technology regulation, many actors are struggling to meet their private and institutional needs in a battle for position (Kenny 1989).

Several different government agencies are responsible for the regula-tion of food biotechnology. At the federal level, the U. S. Department of Agriculture (USDA), the Food and Drug Administration (FDA), and the Environmental Protection Agency (EPA) have some regulatory respon-sibility for biotechnology. The USDA is responsible for evaluating issues related to the field release of new plants or animals. The FDA is most responsible for the safety and labeling of food products. Both the USDA and FDA have recently tried to clarify their regulations of biotechnology. The EPA is mainly responsible for products of biotechnology that are used as pesticides. Their regulations are still under development.

The potential for either duplication or gaps in the regulatory approach has led to concerns about the overall effectiveness and efficiency of the regulatory process. The tendency has been to regulate biotechnology using existing policies and regulations set up to deal with chemical technologies. The companies and universities developing biotechnology appear satisfied with the current approach and would even like to see the systems streamlined and simplified. On the other hand, activist groups opposing biotechnology argue that the regulations are not strong enough. They feel stronger requirements are needed for testing and public notification (such as through labeling).

The ultimate judge of emerging products of biotechnology will be the consumer. They will appraise the merits of a particular product and determine its success or failure (Stenholm and Waggoner 1992). The

Office of Technology Assessment (OTA 1992) points out that society has become more skeptical of the need for new technologies and that this is a difficult time for a new technology to emerge. Negative experiences with nuclear and chemical industries have made the American public wary of new technologies, and confidence in institutions has eroded. For these and other reasons, biotechnology has been subjected to extensive regulatory oversight, before the products are available.

The government is also taking a more active role in setting the direction for future research and product development related to biotechnology. Al Gore (1991) states that it will be important to invigorate the policy debate to ensure that biotechnology does not just address technological problems in a socioeconomic vacuum, but provides solutions for problems of hunger and disease universally and democratically. He concludes that our society cannot continue to rush forward with this new tool without considering what is at the end of the road.

Our society is involved in a debate about the balance of risks and benefits related to biotechnology (Stenholm and Waggoner 1992). The OTA (1992) explains that for effective policy decisions it is important to clearly distinguish between the technical basis for assessment and regulation of technology-related risks, and what might be done as an extra step to maintain public confidence. Balancing safety and institutional credibility against economic competitiveness represents an important, but difficult, challenge for society and its leaders. The public increasingly expects to play a greater role in such decisions.

The social and political context in which biotechnology is developing may not be very conducive to new scientific or technological innovations. While in the 1950s virtually all Americans believed in "better living through chemistry," people today oppose most chemicals, especially in food (Foreman 1990). In the past, some technologies have been put on the market without adequate examination of the negative consequences of their use. Today, people are much more skeptical about technology. They no longer accept scientific developments without question. Erosion of public confidence in government has also arisen from a decade long legacy of deregulation.

Perceptions of Technologies

One of the outcomes of the social construction of risk and the various political decisions is that actors form perceptions of the risk object. In the case of food products, such as those developed through biotechnology, perceptions will often be strongly held and emotionally driven. It is important to understand perceptions because they are the basis for social actions related to technology and risk. The social construction of a technical issue is based, at least in part, on the perceptions held by various interest groups and the general public.

Perceptions of Risk

Much of the concern expressed about biotechnology is related to the perception that it poses health or environmental risks. Risk has become a major political and social issue, provoking uneasiness about scientific progress. Our society is faced with a difficult dilemma. We are both dependent on technology for enrichment of our lives and suspicious of the associated risks—especially when they are unfamiliar. The public expects government and industry to minimize risks. However, risk management is very complex because of inherent uncertainty, as well as the need to make difficult tradeoffs between the benefits and risks associated with technology (Wilson and Crouch 1987).

Risk perception and management must be considered in its social and cultural context (Heimer 1988; Short 1984). Widespread public concern over technological risks appears to be a relatively recent phenomenon, as are many of the technologies themselves (Lewis 1990). People in affluent societies are preoccupied with safety, while risk is recognized as a normal part of life for the less fortunate. They demand a risk-free world and often resist making any types of tradeoffs, particularly between the economy and the environment (Sandman 1987).

One cause of public controversies over technology is that experts and the public differ in their perceptions of risk (National Research Council 1989). Disagreements between scientists and the public represent problems for each side. Risk assessment professionals and other scientists often become frustrated in their attempts to communicate with the lay public about technical risk assessment and management. Technical experts feel the public misunderstands the "real" nature of different risks. Experts often adopt the counterproductive attitude that they are right and the public is wrong.

Members of the general public often are angered by technical experts who appear cold and impersonal in their use of complex statistical probabilities and bureaucratic jargon (National Research Council 1989). The majority of citizens rely on intuitive risk judgments, typically called risk perceptions. Their information about risk comes largely from indirect sources (i.e., the news media) rather than direct experience. Freudenburg (1988) explains that citizens often reach ill-advised conclusions, but scientists do as well. Although citizen judgments are often based on misinformation, they also reflect a deeper kind of prudence than is commonly realized.

Different, often unrelated, constructions of risk lie at the base of the disagreements between experts and the public (Sandman 1986). Technical experts define risk narrowly to include two main components: the hazard potential (i.e., the likelihood that something will cause harm) and the probability of exposure (i.e., how likely are certain people to be exposed to the hazard). The public defines risk more broadly. They worry about a variety of qualitative and subjective issues (e.g., ethics, control, or the involuntary nature of exposure).

Perceptions of Risks Associated with New Foods

Social construction of general food safety risks sets a context for biotechnology. Food safety has received considerable attention from the mass media, as well as a variety of activist groups. Consumers and scientists disagree over food safety issues (Lee 1989). The FDA and a number of noted scientists have ranked six potential food risks in terms of what people "should" be worried about. They concluded that foodborne pathogens (i.e., microbial contamination) are what really make people sick. The second most serious risk involves nutritional imbalance and malnutrition. The third area of risk involves isolated incidents of environmental contamination (e.g., from lead or mercury). The fourth most serious risk relates to naturally occurring compounds, such as aflatoxin. Risks from pesticide residues are in fifth place. Experts conclude that our least worry should be deliberate food additives (e.g., preservatives and flavor enhancers).

On the other hand, media coverage and public opinion surveys generally reflect the kinds of food safety risks about which the lay public worries. People tend to see a significant risk associated with pesticide residues. They also worry about deliberate food additives (e.g., preservatives). When these are compared to the FDA list it is interesting these two are the least serious risks from a technical perspective. However, these are the food safety issues that get the most attention from the media. People also feel they gain little benefit from these technologies and see them as an involuntary risk.

Lee (1989) provides a detailed discussion of food safety fears, especially as related to new foods, which he terms "food neophobia." The first reason for food safety fears involves the fact that very few people (less than 2%) grow or process their own food. Most consumers have a poor understanding of the food production and processing system. The second cause of food neophobia is that many consumers know very little about chemistry and view new food technology as artificial and risky. Another cause of consumer food fears is the belief that media coverage accurately reflects reality. The mass media play a dominant role in shaping public perception of risks. Consumers often accept news, documentaries, and even entertainment programs, without question. The fourth cause of food safety fears involves the desire for absolute certainty. The driving force behind the desire for zero risk involves the difficulty in understanding very low probability events. Furthermore, in the face of uncertainty people tend to be conservative, especially when the risk involves food. The final cause of food neophobia is the fact that scientists "like to chase zeros." Their ability to detect smaller and smaller quantities is outpacing their ability to explain what the numbers mean. Some of the terms that scientists use in risk assessment (e.g., parts per billion) have no meaning for most people. Extremely small quantities of chemicals cause fear just because they are there.

Many people are especially uneasy about new foods. Unfamiliar foods become familiar through direct exposure (which often happens through childhood), as well as advertising, family influences, peers, and the media (Lyman 1989). The societal context into which a food is introduced is important. If a product is launched amidst controversy or negativity, it creates an unfavorable impression. The idea of novelty about food is a contradictory one. Unfamiliar foods are usually rejected in favor of something known. On the other hand, novelty brings out curiosity and interest in some. As familiarity with new foods increases, their acceptance increases as well.

Socially constructed food meanings and associations are also important for success of new food products. Learned and unlearned associations, images, and other phenomena often create what Lyman (1989) calls "faint copies of other times" (such as nostalgia). Food evokes many images that can be altered by new food technologies. Based on such images, food dislikes may arise even though the food itself has never been tasted. Changing food preferences are a matter of changing attitudes toward foods rather than changing the sensory qualities or taste.

Public concern over food safety has given rise to a variety of alternative food production and marketing approaches (Belasco 1993). During the past two decades people's relationships with food and their frames of reference used to select food have changed. Belasco describes the rise of countercultural cuisine, which involves a tendency to avoid processed food and to shop at coops and natural food stores. Belasco (1993) relates the rise of countercultural cuisine to the environmental movement. During the 1960s, many people began to question human impacts on the environment, including food production. Health food stores offered ecological information, and food became a medium to reach the public with broader ecological messages. Leading simpler, more ecological lives meant rejecting traditional beliefs and seeking different foods. Consumers became less sure if they could trust health claims about food, especially those that came from companies or the government, and the media came to play an important role in the debate over natural foods, including safety concerns.

Perceptions of Biotechnology

Biotechnology is destined to become a major component of our society (Wyse and Krivi 1987). Perceptions of biotechnology will have an important influence on the way that issues are constructed. Biotechnology is developing under intense scrutiny from government and activist groups. Biotechnology could elicit food safety and environmental concerns similar to those expressed about agricultural chemicals. In addition, other dimensions of biotechnology, such as socioeconomic impacts and ethical concerns, will also draw public attention.

During the past few years, four national studies have been conducted to assess public perceptions related to biotechnology (Hoban 1994; Hoban and Kendall 1993; Novo Industri 1987; Office of Technology Assessment 1987). Results seem to be quite consistent over time. Public response to biotechnology will be influenced by the awareness and knowledge people possess. Most studies have found that the majority of people have limited awareness of the term "biotechnology" (Berrier 1987; Hoban and Kendall 1993). However, awareness tends to be higher for specific applications. Higher levels of awareness are associated with more positive attitudes. Most of the information people have about biotechnology comes from the mass media.

Results of all four national surveys show that a majority of people hold positive attitudes about the general use of biotechnology. Results indicate that the public holds fairly high expectations about the potential benefits of biotechnology. People react differently to biotechnology's various applications. Those products that are perceived to have the greatest value and benefit to consumers are more acceptable. People also feel more positive about plant products than they do about animal applications of biotechnology. Consumers will evaluate and respond to new foods in a predictable manner, regardless of whether they are produced through biotechnology.

These studies have also examined the credibility of government agencies regarding their regulation of biotechnology. Credibility has a significant influence on attitudes about biotechnology. People tend to look to government and independent organizations to ensure the safety of food produced through biotechnology. Most people prefer to leave the assessment of food safety to a trusted, independent organization. They also expect the public sector to help shape the research agenda, at least at public universities. Most people also feel that government should pay more attention to what citizens think about biotechnology.

People are clearly interested in receiving more information about biotechnology. The credibility of information sources can also be an important factor in public attitudes toward foods produced through biotechnology. The public is most likely to believe information about biotechnology received from university scientists, public health officials, farmers, and environmental groups. Some sources of information generally receive lower ratings of trust: government agencies, government agencies, food manufacturers, and companies making biotechnology products.

Biotechnology is controversial because scientists are increasingly able to modify and manipulate living organisms. Moral and ethical issues associated with biotechnology will influence public perception of biotechnology (Hoban et al. 1992). Surveys show that people are more likely to object to biotechnology on moral grounds when animals are involved (rather than plants or bacteria). Moral opposition to biotechnology is partly due to religious background, but it also reflects the belief that humans should not extensively modify nature. Moral attitudes have a very significant influence on the social construction of issues associated with biotechnology.

The OTA (1987) concludes that a combination of science interest and media exposure has produced an American public that is aware—if not necessarily sophisticated—about biotechnology. Wyse and Krivi (1987), on the other hand, argue that the public does not understand biotechnology or its potential uses. They believe that most opposition can be traced to scientific illiteracy. Foreman (1990) argues that many scientists and industry officials believe public concerns about biotechnology are based on misperceptions and unjustifiable fears. However, public information and education efforts may not necessarily reduce opposition to biotechnology because the controversy may not be due to lack of information, but may, in fact, reflect basic differences in values and interests.

Case Examples

Two of the first commercial applications of food biotechnology were approved for use in early 1994. One is bovine somatotropin (BST), also known as bovine growth hormone (BgH). The other is a new tomato variety with vine-ripened taste (know as the Flavr-Savr™ tomato). In this section, I will examine how the social issues associated with these two biotechnology applications have been constructed. After a brief description of each application, my comments will include an analysis of the issues, interests, and context for these two technologies. Their current status will be assessed and projections for the future will be provided.

A word about information sources is in order. I have been actively involved with the national level discussions about biotechnology and these specific products for the previous 5 years. My involvement includes a variety of social science data collection activities, as well as consultation with government agencies, nonprofit associations, and private companies. My comments are based on this first hand experience, as well as an ongoing review of mass media accounts and participant observations at a number of meetings, including government hearings and scientific workshops.

Bovine Somatotropin

Bovine somatotropin (BST) is a naturally occurring protein hormone that regulates milk production in dairy cows. Scientists have recognized for decades that supplementing cows with additional BST increases the efficiency of milk production. Using biotechnology, large quantities of BST can now be produced relatively easily and cheaply. Cows receiving supplemental BST produce about 10–20% more milk. During the early 1980s four companies began development and testing of BST. Only one company (Monsanto, based in St. Louis) has been successful in obtaining approval of its version. After a decade of testing, the FDA approved the commercial use of BST in November 1994. Monsanto began selling BST to American dairy farmers in early February 1994.

Significant controversies have been constructed over the use of BST for at least the past few years. It has become a lightening rod for a host of concerns and interest groups. Some of the initial concerns were raised by farm interests and social scientists (rural sociologists and agricultural economists). These early assessments raised questions, not about the safety of BST, but about the potential for socioeconomic impacts on certain groups of farmers. The reasoning was that increasing the supply of milk would depress the prices that dairy farmers received. These interests raised concerns that smaller-scale, "family" dairy farmers would be most affected. Given that milk surpluses represent a chronic problem, this seemed to be an unnecessary technology. This has continued to be an emotional issue.

The government evaluation and approval of BST were based solely on animal and human safety, as well as the efficacy of the product. Social and economic issues were not considered as part of the formal evaluation. The prevailing viewpoint among government and industry interests is that all farmers will be equally able to use BST. Their position is to let the market decide. On the other hand, some activist groups based much of their opposition to BST on concerns over the social and economic impacts. In particular, they generally question the need for BST, given existing high levels of production.

Despite favorable rulings by the USDA, FDA, and others there have been some attempts to amplify the risks and construct a range of animal and human health issues associated with BST. For the most part, the health and safety concerns have been found to be minimal in independent assessment by such groups, as the American Medical Association and the World Health Organization. The basic finding is that milk from cows that receive BST is essentially identical to milk from nonsupplemented cows. Some activist groups have tried to construct and publicize health and safety problems associated with BST, for example, health concerns related to an increased use of antibiotics.

Some interesting coalitions have emerged in the opposition to BST. Small-scale dairy farmers who oppose BST on economic grounds have joined forces with antibiotechnology and animal rights activists. Ironically, these same activists have been very critical of the livestock industry for years. Some try hard to scare consumers away from eating beef. Some opponents have chosen to target their efforts (including ineffectual protests) against food manufacturers and retailers. Grocers are in a particularly difficult position because they have little control over the issue, but have the most contact of any of the actors with consumers.

After approval, the major emphasis shifted to issues associated with milk labeling. The FDA ruled that milk from cows that have received supplemental BST does not need to be labeled since the milk is technically no different from any other milk. No tests are even available to determine if milk comes from cows receiving BST. In addition, the present policy limits any labels from promoting "BST-free milk" because all milk contains the same, small amount of BST. Some companies have begun selling milk or other dairy products they claim comes from cows that have not received any BST. So far, consumers seem unwilling to pay more for milk that is labeled as being from cows that have not received BST. In fact, national milk consumption was not affected by the introduction of BST. Activist groups had hoped that BST would have a significant negative effect on milk consumption.

Right after approval, mass media coverage of BST tended to be strong and relatively balanced (at least in the print media). The television news tended to favor the theatrics of the opponents (dressed up as cows and dumping milk) over the more sedate arguments of government and industry spokespersons. One interesting rhetorical device involves the terms used to describe the product. Opponents always use the term bovine growth hormone to emphasize the emotional term "hormone." Scientists, the government, and industry spokespersons prefer to use the more technical term, "bovine somatotropin." In a related event during the summer of 1994, a movie entitled "I Love Trouble" came out that was loosely based on the whole issue of BST. That and other cultural phenomena help with the social construction of BST issues.

The Flavr-Savr™ Tomato

Another major product of biotechnology received approval from the FDA in May 1994. The product (known as the "Flavr-Savr™" tomato) was developed by Calgene, a biotechnology company based in California. Their goal was to develop better-tasting tomatoes that would be available year-round. In contrast to BST, which results in no difference in product for consumers, the Flavr-Savr™ tomato promised a clear consumer benefit, but at a relatively high price. The product has been available in only a few markets, but demand so far has outpaced supply. It will be available nationally sometime in 1995.

The technical change is relatively simple. Scientists have located and "turned off" the gene that causes tomatoes to spoil after picking. Typically, tomatoes are picked green (about 2 weeks early) so they can be shipped across the country. They are then gassed with ethylene to turn them red. The taste and texture, however, tend to be unacceptable for most consumers. The Flavr-Savr™ tomato can be left on the vine until it is almost ripe, which results in a better taste and texture (even after cross-county shipments).

Some controversies have developed over this product and biotechnology in general during the 2 years since the FDA announced its guidelines for dealing with whole food products, such as the Flavr-Savr™ tomato. Their position is basically not to treat new plant varieties any differently than traditionally bred produce unless there has been a significant change (such as the addition of a known allergen or change in the nutritive value). Industry tends to favor this approach. Activist groups, on the other hand, feel that the policy leaves too much to the discretion of individual companies. They also favor some type of mandatory labeling for all foods produced through biotechnology.

The Flavr-Savr™ tomato was constructed as a test case for the regulation of biotechnology. Calgene decided to submit an optional food additive petition to the FDA to trigger a much more extensive technical review than whole foods ever receive. This decision was in part to build public confidence, as well as to test the FDA policy process. The FDA commissioned a special panel to assess the safety of the tomato, particularly in light of an antibiotic marker gene that had been incorporated into the product for purposes of testing. The FDA panel determined that the tomato was safe and nutritious. The labeling issue is not relevant because the company has chosen to voluntarily label their tomatoes (mainly to differentiate them in the market place).

Opponents of biotechnology concede that the Flavr-Savr^{tm} is likely harmless and that the regulatory process for this product has been extensive enough to ensure environmental and public health. Their main concerns involve the fact that other products of biotechnology will not receive the same level of evaluation. Opponents also want all foods to be labeled as products of biotechnology, just as this tomato will be. Opponents have aimed some of their early protests at the Campbell Soup Company (which is a major user of tomatoes and a supporter of some of Calgene's research). Such efforts have since faded, in part, because processed foods containing the tomato are unlikely in the future (given its high cost). Some activists have also worked to organize chefs in general opposition to biotechnology.

The main problems now facing Calgene and its Flavr-Savr^{tm} tomato involve logistics and competition. They have so far been unable to produce enough of the tomatoes to meet the high demand. They also are attempting to control the whole production and distribution system (bypassing a number of important players in the produce industry). Several other companies have used Calgene's lengthy approval process to develop their own versions of "the better tomato." Regardless of which product ultimately leads the market, the general category of better fruits and vegetables through biotechnology is likely here to stay.

Since the approval of the Flavr-Savr^{tm} tomato, there has been relatively little media coverage (and most of that was quite positive). The early media coverage of the FDA policy and the development of the Flavr-Savr^{tm} tomato was quite interesting. Much of the media coverage was positive about the tomato, but rather negative about biotechnology. Terms such as "Franken-food" sensationalized news stories, and cartoons showed science fiction creations, such as tomatoes with fish-eyes and fins. That particular image was provoked by coverage of an experimental tomato that used genes from an Arctic fish to prevent frost damage. Also, the very popular film "Jurassic Park" contained some strong content related to genetic engineering. These and other cultural artifacts (such as comic books) will influence the construction of societal beliefs and policies relative to biotechnology.

Conclusions and Implications

These two case studies show that the social issues constructed around a new and controversial food technology are multifaceted and complex. These first two products serve as test cases for the extent to which food biotechnology will become constructed as a social problem or just an interesting issue for a number of interest groups and scholars. Based on the early public reaction and the public policy direction, it appears that food biotechnology will not become much of a social problem. Many more products are in the development or approval stage. Most of these will quietly enter the food production system with little fanfare or public attention.

One of the reasons for this prediction is that the support for biotechnology is quite strong (both among organized interest groups and the general public). As with other issues, complex social networks have developed on each side of the biotechnology controversy. The supporting side is strong and well-established, including major international companies, powerful trade associations, prestigious university scientists, and a number of government interests. The opponents appear much less powerful and will likely have a difficult time sustaining any limited momentum they might have gained from their fight against BST. Each side is struggling to have its own meanings legitimized by government agencies and the mass media. The activists have tried to amplify the potential risks through rhetoric and emotional appeals, while the supporters have been willing to let the scientific method and government policy work its course. Consumers appear relatively uninformed and not very concerned about the entire issue.

Biotechnology is being constructed as a complex social issue. Some of the ongoing controversies have a number of important implications for social scientists, public officials, and others. For example, this case allows us to see how important decisions are made about how society balances the benefits and risk of technology in a complex and controversial political environment. The issues address not only health and safety issues, but also ethical and emotional concerns. Philosophical debates are even underway about the fundamental relationship between people and the natural environment. Lessons learned from biotechnology will provide guidance to future research and public policy in related areas.

The public arena for biotechnology could change rapidly in response to a variety of social and technical developments. Activists opposing biotechnology have not had much influence over the regulatory decisions. They are having some impact on broader issues, however. The future of food biotechnology depends on the public reaction to some of the initial products (which so far has been positive). Public reaction will be shaped by the information people receive from the mass media and other sources. Education or communication alone cannot be expected to resolve the value conflicts that inevitably arise over the choice and implementation of new technologies. In fact, risk assessment and communication must be viewed as a political process where power and decision-making are redistributed among various groups.

Society's scarce resources should be focused on the risks that are both serious and important to people. It would be wrong to make policy decisions based only on special interest and public perceptions. It would be equally wrong, however, if such decisions are based solely on technical grounds without any recognition of important public attitudes, concerns, and values. Many different groups have the right and responsibility to become involved in important and difficult societal decisions associated with new technologies.

More social science research is needed that regularly and systematically examines the social construction of biotechnology. Such efforts could further document the strategies and tactics employed by various interests to promote their definition of the situation. Research could also evaluate the relationships among different groups, including the media, government officials, industry, and a variety of interest groups. The social constructionist perspective provides a useful framework for such research.

References

Belasco, W. 1993. *Appetite for Change*. Ithaca, NY: Cornell University Press.

Berrier, R. J. 1987. "Public Perceptions of Biotechnology." Pp. 37–51 in *Public Perceptions of Biotechnology*, edited by L. R. Batra and W. Klassen. Bethesda, MD: Agricultural Research Institute.

Covello, V. T., P. M. Sandman, and P. Slovic. 1988. *Risk Communication, Risk Statistics, and Risk Comparisons: A Manual for Plant Managers*. Washington, D.C.: Chemical Manufacturers Association.

Foreman, C. T. 1990. "Food Safety and Quality for the Consumer: Policies and Communication." Pp. 74–81 in *Agricultural Biotechnology: Food Safety and Nutritional Quality for the Consumer*, edited by J. F. MacDonald. Ithaca, NY: National Agricultural Biotechnology Council.

Freudenburg, W. R. 1988. "Perceived Risk, Real Risk: Social Science and the Art of Probabilistic Risk Assessment." *Science* 242(October 7):44–49.

Gore, A. 1991. "Planning a New Biotechnology Policy." *Harvard Journal of Law and Technology* 5(Fall):19–30.

Hatch, U., and F. Kuchler. 1989. "Regulation of Agricultural Biotechnology: Historical Perspectives." Pp. 51–71 in *Biotechnology and the New Agricultural*

Revolution, edited by J. Molnar and H. Kinnucan. Boulder, CO: Westview Press.

Heimer, C. A. 1988. "Social Structure, Psychology, and the Estimation of Risk." *Annual Review of Sociology* 14:491–519.

Hilgartner, S. 1992. "The Social Construction of Risk Objects: Or, How to Pry Open Networks of Risk." Pp. 39–53 in *Organizations, Uncertainties, and Risks*, edited by J. F. Short and L. Clark. Boulder, CO: Westview Press.

Hoban, T. J. 1989. "Sociology and Biotechnology: Challenges and Opportunities." *Southern Rural Sociology* 6:45–63.

———. 1994. *Consumer Awareness and Acceptance of Bovine Somatotropin (BST)*. Washington, D.C.: Grocery Manufacturers of America.

Hoban, T. J., and P. A. Kendall. 1993. *Consumer Attitudes about Food Biotechnology*. Raleigh, NC: North Carolina Cooperative Extension Service.

Hoban, T. J., E. Woodrum, and R. Czaja. 1992. "Public Opposition to Genetic Engineering" *Rural Sociology* 57(4):476–493.

Kasperson, R. E. 1992. "The Social Amplification of Risk: Progress in Developing an Integrative Framework." Pp. 153–178 in *Social Theories of Risk*, edited by S. Krimsky and D. Golding. Westport, CT: Praeger.

Kenny, M. 1989. "The Debate over the Deliberate Release of Genetically Engineered Organisms: A Study of State Environmental Policy Making." Pp. 73–99 in *Biotechnology and the New Agricultural Revolution*, edited by J. Molnar and H. Kinnucan. Boulder, CO: Westview Press.

Lee, K. 1989. "Food Neophobia: Major Causes and Treatments" *Food Technology* (December): 62–73.

Lewis, H. W. 1990. *Technological Risk*. New York: W.W. Norton.

Lyman, B. 1989. *A Psychology of Food: More Than a Matter of Taste*. New York: Van Nostrand Reinhold

Mazur, A. 1981. *Dynamics of Technical Controversy*. Washington, D.C: Communications Press Inc.

National Research Council (Committee on Risk Perception and Communication). 1989. *Improving Risk Communication*. Washington, D.C.: National Academy Press.

Novo Industri. 1987. *The Novo Report: American Attitudes and Beliefs about Genetic Engineering*. New York: Research and Forecasts, Inc.

Office of Technology Assessment. 1987. *New Directions in Biotechnology— Background Paper: Public Perceptions of Biotechnology*. Washington, D.C.: U. S. Government Printing Office.

———. 1992. *A New Technological Era for American Agriculture*. Washington, D.C.: U. S. Government Printing Office.

Renn, O. 1992a. "Concepts of Risk: A Classification." Pp. 53–79 in *Social Theories of Risk*, edited by S. Krimsky and D. Golding. Westport, CT: Praeger.

———. 1992b. "The Social Arena Concept of Risk Debates." Pp. 170–196 in *Social Theories of Risk*, edited by S. Krimsky and D. Golding. Wesport, CT: Praeger.

Sandman, P. M. 1986. *Explaining Environmental Risk: Some Notes on Environmental Risk Communication*. Washington, D.C.: U.S. Environmental Protection Agency.

———. 1987. "Apathy versus Hysteria: Public Perception of Risk." Pp. 219–231 in *Public Perceptions of Biotechnology,* edited by L. R. Batra and W. Klassen. Bethesda, MD: Agricultural Research Institute.

Short, J. F. 1984. "Toward a Social Transformation of Risk Analysis." *American Sociological Review* 49(6):711–725.

———. 1992. "Defining, Explaining, and Managing Risks." Pp. 3–23 in *Organizations, Uncertainties, and Risks* edited by J. F. Short and L. Clark. Boulder, CO: Westview Press.

Stenholm, C. W., and D. B. Waggoner. 1992. "Public Policy in Animal Biotechnology in the 1990s: Challenges and Opportunities." Pp. 25–35 in *Animal Biotechnology: Opportunities and Challenges,* edited by J. F. MacDonald. Ithaca, NY: National Agricultural Biotechnology Council.

Wilson, R., and E. A. C. Crouch. 1987. "Risk Assessment and Comparisons: An Introduction." *Science* 236(April 17):267–270.

Wyse, R., and G. G. Krivi. 1987. "Strategies for Educating the Public Concerning Biotechnology." Pp. 155–164 in *Public Perceptions of Biotechnology,* edited by L. R. Batra and W. Klassen. Bethesda, MD: Agricultural Research Institute.

VI

Government Food Programs

10

"Do You Teach Them How to Budget?":
Professional Discourse in the Construction
of Nutritional Inequities

KIM D. TRAVERS

Inequalities in health have been defined as "variations in health status among different population groups" (Rootman 1988:2). Historically, inequalities in objective and subjective indicators of nutrition and health status have existed among various groups within society. These inequalities may have biological and/or social determinants. Typically, however, health inequalities among income or class groups "appear to mirror the existence of *inequities* in the distribution of opportunities, resources, services or environmental conditions that are conducive to health" (Rootman 1988:3, emphasis added). Thus, the term nutritional *inequity* implies a social injustice in the construction of inequalities in nutrition and health status.

Professional discourse has historically taken on ideological dimensions that have contributed to the construction of public health problems, including inequities in nutrition and health. I am using the term "ideology" in a Marxian or pejorative sense, as representing the interests of a privileged class (health professionals) while "pretending to be in the interest of the society as a whole" (Nöth 1990:377). Thus, primarily through changing claims regarding responsibility for *inequalities* in nutrition and health, professionals have used ideological discourse in the construction of nutrition and health *inequities*. The purpose of this chapter is to use discourse analysis to examine the changing role of nutrition and health professionals' claimsmaking and other professional activities in constituting nutritional inequities as a social problem.

As a point of introduction, however, it is appropriate to explain the use of the term "discourse." This task of definition is not an easy one as the term is used differently by various disciplines, and thus no single definition proves satisfactory. It is generally accepted that discourse is associated with language, and the term has its roots in linguistics (Bullock et al. 1988:232). However, many social scientists, beginning with Foucault (1971), have expanded the definition to refer to the system of language and conventions that make the knowledge of a particular discipline possible. Philp (1985:69) paraphrased Foucault well: "a discourse can be seen as a system of possibility: it is what allows us to produce statements which be either true or false—it makes possible a field of knowledge." The idea of a system of language and conventions constituting a field of knowledge is the working definition of discourse that will provide meaning within the context of this chapter.

This definition assumes there are multiple discourses. For example, the discourse of sociology is quite different from the discourse of nutrition, which, in turn, is quite different from the discourse of biochemistry. Each field has conventions that help to determine what "counts" as valid knowledge within the discipline and its own language systems (which "outsiders" frequently refer to as "jargon") for interpreting and utilizing that knowledge. As different fields borrow ideas from each other, the discourses inform one another and the fields grow and overlap. So, for example, the field of nutritional sociology will be informed by a discourse that has grown from both sociological and nutritional discourses. The field of nutritional biochemistry will be informed by a discourse that has grown from both nutritional and biochemical discourses. At the same time, however, each subfield develops a more specialized discourse. So, the discourse of nutritional sociology is quite different from that of nutritional biochemistry, and what is valued as knowledge in one may be very different from what is valued as knowledge in the other. Through the failure to recognize the value of knowledge that exists outside of the discourse, discourse can become ideological; some evidence, considered within the field to be irrelevant, can be ignored. Such practice works to construct a partial and misinformed view.

Professional discourses, however, are constructed not only by discourses of specialized academic disciplines, but also by specific sets of rules constituted within the public domain that allow us to judge statements and acts as true or acceptable. Public discourse is usually formed by the dominant culture.[1] As such, public discourse, although reflective of the views of the majority, may serve the interests of only a privileged minority, and thus, may be ideological in nature and function. It is the ideological, and hence seldom questioned, dimension of discourse that contributes to its power in social organization. Some authors (Fraser 1989; Smith 1990) use the terms ideology and discourse almost interchangeably, a practice reflective of that power. In this analysis, I take a similar view.

In this chapter, I map out the ways in which nutritional inequities are embedded within discourse(s). This chapter begins with an historical overview of theories of disease causation in industrialized nations as the basis of the discursive construction of inequities. Noting the pervasiveness of individualistic ideology in professional discourse throughout history and reemerging in the present day, I use a recent ethnographic study of disadvantaged families to illustrate the professional practices and claimsmaking activities that are currently working to construct nutritional inequities. This case study makes clear that the experiences of those living on the disadvantaged side of inequities frequently defy professional discourse. Yet, such discourse remains a powerful influence in a variety of "public arenas," on policy, practice, and public perceptions. As Hilgartner and Bosk (1988:58) proclaim: "statements about social problems thus select a specific interpretation of reality from a plurality of possibilities. Which 'reality' comes to dominate public discourse has profound implications for the future of the social problem, for the interest groups involved, and for policy." The chapter draws to a close by examining the discourse of health promotion and emancipatory nutrition education as possibilities for the reduction of nutritional inequities.

Although some social problems theorists, particularly Spector and Kitsuse (1987), would argue that the conditions themselves (i.e., nutritional inequities) are irrelevant in the study of social problems, I have taken a differing and more critical theoretical stance. I will argue for a change in oppressive discourse toward a reduction in nutritional inequities because, by definition, inequities are a symptom of social injustices and, therefore, cannot *not* be a social problem. I will examine claimsmaking and other professional practices and argue that those activities are constitutive of the social problem of nutritional inequities, yet, I do not suspend judgment on those activities. Whereas it has been argued that one of the weaknesses of the constructionist perspective is that "the sociologist's problem is to avoid participation and, especially, to avoid defending or challenging claims and definitions about putative conditions" (Schneider 1985:224), my thinking follows that of Smith (1987) who claims that it is impossible to study a socially constructed world from outside it. My participation in the discourse is, therefore, intended to be critical with a vision of future social change.

Professional Discourses and Inequities: An Historical Overview

Throughout recent history in western industrialized nations, professional discourse has claimed biology and personal lifestyle behavior as the major determinants of health and disease (Edginton 1989). Scientific and professional discourses appear to assume that improvements in health over the last few centuries have been primarily due to advances in medical technology that can harness the biological cause of disease, or due to voluntary changes in personal behavior that favorably alter risk factors for disease. However, such claims are not grounded in historical evidence. McKeown's (1979) historical analysis of changes in disease and health over the last three centuries reveals that the greatest reductions in mortality have occurred in response to public health measures such as improvements in sanitation and population-wide improvements in access to better nutrition. McKeown argues that greater emphasis should be placed on finding ways to change the environmental and social sources of illness.

But this knowledge of the social and environmental sources of disease is given very little consideration in health discourse. The idea that the social structures within which an individual is embedded are inextricably linked to a person's state of health and perception of that state has only very recently been recognized (at least rhetorically) as "legitimate" within modern western health care. Tesh (1988:3) argues that disease prevention policy is ideological, in that the value dimensions of science and theories of disease causation that form the foundation of such policy are denied. She argues, "not that values be excised from science and from policy but that their inevitable presence be revealed and their worth be publicly discussed." In discussing the historical roles of professional discourse in the social construction of health inequities, it is useful to examine the values and the scientific evidence underlying theories of disease causation. An historical overview of professionals' changing claimsmaking activities can help to illustrate how attention has been diverted from the social and environmental sources of illness despite historical evidence that clearly implicates the social structure in the construction of health and disease.

Inequalities in Health: From an Individual Problem to a Social Problem

According to Tesh, competing theories of infectious disease causation in the nineteenth century bear a striking resemblance to competing theories of chronic disease causation of the twentieth century. She claims that "all [theories] acquired meanings beyond the narrow question of illness, each becoming linked to a different position about the desirability and direction of social change"(1988:4). The similarities between nineteenth and twentieth century theories mirror cyclical changes in professional and scientific discourse reflective of the political ideology of the time.

In the nineteenth century, two competing theories for the cause of infectious diseases were the personal behavior theory and the "miasma" or environmental theory. Discourse consistent with the personal behavior theory suggested that individuals could best decrease their chances of contracting infectious diseases if they adopted certain personal behaviors. Specifically, those who ate well and paid attention to personal cleanliness would provide themselves with the best protection from disease. In fact, there was truth to this theory, as members of privileged classes who had enough money to eat well and to have access to clean water did indeed have some protection. However, this theory had very little relevance for the working class poor, who, for lack of resources, had little chance of changing their nutrition and cleanliness practices. However, the theory of personal behavior advanced the belief in individual freedom and the work ethic that rewards those who work hard and take responsibility for their own health, values consistent with the political ideology of the time. With discourse firmly grounding the cause of disease in individual responsibility, the state was absolved of any responsibility for changing social conditions such as poor sanitation and poverty, which, from an historical perspective, were clearly linked to poor health status (Tesh 1988).

The competing "miasma" or environmental theory removed the source of disease from the individual. Somewhat misguided from a scientific perspective, proponents of this theory believed the source of disease to arise from odors emitted from sewage or decaying organic materials. An 1842 report by Edwin Chadwick entitled *Report of the Sanitary Condition of the Laboring Population of Great Britain* described the appalling living conditions of the Industrial Revolution's working class and recommended improved water supplies and sewage systems to carry wastes and their odors away from people's living quarters. Although the "miasma" theory (implicating odors) was not proven to be scientifically valid in retrospect, the poor sanitary conditions of the time that were endured by the working class were clearly linked to infectious diseases. However, the personal behavior theory was so pervasive that it took years of political struggle by proponents of the miasma theory to implement an environmental approach to disease control with the Public Health Act of 1848. Individualistic discourse diverted attention away from environmental sources of illness and delayed the initiation of public health measures in order to legitimate the freedom of the privileged individual, although the evidence lay elsewhere. Such discursive practices constructed inequities by advancing belief in individual freedom and the work ethic for the advantaged, while failing to provide support for the disadvantaged to initiate personal behavior changes. Inequalities in health status were reduced only when years of political struggle acknowledged environmental links with disease. Public health measures that improved sanitation and nutrition for all were much more effective in improving the public's health. The "sanitary revolution" helped all, not only the rich. Interestingly, the political struggle became effective in initiating social change only when an individualistic discourse was adopted in public campaigns for support. As Tesh (1988:32) argues,

> providing sewerage and clean water was not linked just to disease prevention; it also meant saving money for the taxpayers and assuring a more productive workforce for the industrialists. More important, people saw frugality and efficiency as admirable . . . because these goals expressed values at the heart of nineteenth-century individualism . . . . They meant limited government and social progress.

Although a movement had been made to reduce inequities by shifting from individualistic discourse to a social discourse, the individualistic discourse prevailed in claimsmaking. As such, although inequalities in health status were reduced through providing an environment more supportive of health for all, class-based social inequities remained, leaving open the possibility for health inequities to resurface in the future.

Eliminating Inequities by Reframing a Social Problem as a Technical Problem

With the discovery of microorganisms in the twentieth century, the germ theory of causation began to take precedence over the environmental theory in professional discourse. Professionals claimed that the cause of disease had been isolated in a laboratory, and professional activity led to the advent of vaccines. Although vaccinations helped to eliminate many infectious diseases, the incidence of these diseases had declined dramatically before the development of the technological breakthrough of vaccines, a decline strongly associated with improvements in standards of living (social changes) (McKeown 1979). Tesh (1988) argues that with the cause of disease isolated in a laboratory, health became a technical problem, not a social problem, even though there continued to be a strong relationship between social conditions and the incidence of disease. The responsibility for health was therefore turned over to the technical experts, members of the medical profession, who held the power of cure, the ability to isolate and treat the biological cause of disease. The professionalization of health care ensued, and a discourse of scientific certainty and technical expertise developed (Friedson 1988). Such a discourse constructs health *inequalities* as a result of lack of access to technical treatment. As health and nutrition are removed from the social sphere within such technical discourse, *inequities* are nonexistent. By reframing the problem through professional claimsmaking about biological cause and cure, social inequities in health are eliminated through irrelevance. Technical control of health continues to be a dominant theme in western health care. This is particularly evident in light of recent plans in many nations for health care reform. Plans for reform place emphasis on ensuring equal access to medical (technical) treatment, not on ensuring equal access to resources supportive of health (such as affordable, nutritious food). The situation in Canada, where universal Medicare has been in place for over 25 years but where social inequities in health still exist (D'Arcy 1987), is testimony to the inadequacy of the technical expert approach to resolving health problems with complex social origins.

The Recent Resurgence of Individual Behavior as the Source of Inequalities

More recent ideological positions assert that medical hegemony is no longer acceptable within western society. People are now putting less faith in the ultimate power of physicians and taking responsibility for their own health by changing their lifestyles to decrease their risks of chronic diseases that are leading causes of death and disability. In 1974, the Canadian release of a then revolutionary document, *A New Perspective on the Health of Canadians* (Lalonde 1974), relegitimized the role of personal behavior in health by claiming that individual lifestyle behaviors such as smoking, diet, and exercise were the major factors in the cause of disease. This "new perspective"[2] shifted some of the responsibility for health and disease from the domain of technical health care to the responsibility of individuals, and in doing so, advanced the lifestyle theory of disease causation (Tesh 1988). The Lalonde report served as a model for policy makers in other western countries, such as the United States, who viewed the lifestyle theory as a means to control rising health care costs (Tesh 1988). As Stokes (1979) proclaimed in an editorial for *Science*, "the nation risks losing sight of the fact that one of the cheapest and most effective ways to put a cap on spiraling health care costs is through greater self-care." In 1979, the U.S. Department of Health and Human Services released a similar report entitled *Healthy People: The*

Surgeon General's Report on Health Promotion and Disease Prevention 1979
(Department of Health, Education and Welfare 1979). The discourse continued to be individualistic and grounded in scientific certainty, although
these revered government reports laid a foundation for a shift in professional practice toward prevention of chronic diseases via nutrition and
health education and self-responsibility. The power of these government
reports in advancing the lifestyle theory of disease causation, and ultimately the construction of nutritional inequities, was evident in the chain
of events guiding professional practice that followed.

In Canada, the release of the Lalonde report was followed closely by the
release of nutrition recommendations that formed the basis of professional discourse and practice. Similar recommendations were used throughout the western world, so the Canadian example is simply illustrative. In
1977, Health and Welfare Canada released the first *Nutrition Recommendations for Canadians*, and they became the basis for public education programs. The tone of the recommendations reflected a commitment to
scientific objectivity (witness Recommendation 1: "The consumption of a
nutritionally adequate diet, as outlined in Canada's Food Guide"). The
underlying assumption was that if every member of the population was
made aware of the Recommendations and how to implement them, the
problem of poor nutritional health would be resolved. If inequities were
given any consideration, it was only to imply that they would no longer
exist once the news was out.

With the emphasis on a discourse of objectivity in professional training and in policy documents such as the Nutrition Recommendations, a
commitment to objectivity became the logical choice of standard for
nutrition education practice. Thus, in roles as nutrition experts, educators were to inform, to disseminate scientifically sound nutrition information. To illustrate, the Canadian Dietetic Association's professional
oath pledged "to ensure that our publics are *informed* of the nature of any
nutritional treatment or advice and its possible effects," and "to support
the advancement and *dissemination* of nutritional and related knowledge
and skills" (CDA, no date, emphasis added). Educative practice took the
form of what has been termed by Freire (1970) as the banking concept of
education in which the student (client) is a passive, empty vessel into
which the teacher (nutritionist) deposits knowledge. It is curiously ironic
that the banking concept of education has been named by Sartre (cited in
Freire 1970:63) as the "nutritive" or "digestive" concept of education, in
which knowledge is "fed" by the teacher to students in order to "fill
them out." The goal was to improve people's knowledge of nutritional
facts, assuming the facts would be sufficient to persuade people to
change their "faulty behaviors."

However, claims made by both the Lalonde report and nutrition recommendations reflected an ideological commitment to personal control over health, and the "implicit assumption that the proximal causes of behavior and/or mechanisms for producing behavioral changes lie within the individual, rather than in the social environment" (McLeroy et al. 1988:356). This assumption, however, is inadequate. Causal relationships between behavior and health are quite certain for *populations*, but the relationship between behavior and outcomes are probabilistic, not deterministic, and thus much less certain when applied to *individuals* (McLeroy et al. 1987). In other words, an individual's poor health cannot, with certainty, be attributed to his or her "irresponsible" behavior, nor can a change in behavior be guaranteed to ameliorate the condition. Although individual behavior change may continue to be a cornerstone of preventive nutrition education practice as long as a relationship can be demonstrated between behaviors and disease *risk*, placing *sole* emphasis on individual behavior change pays inadequate attention to the context within which people make their nutrition and lifestyle decisions.

The emphasis on personal control over one's own health reflects acceptance of two pervasive values in a liberal society: individualism and upward mobility. To live a healthy lifestyle represents self-reliance and testifies to membership in affluent classes (Tesh 1988). But are those who do not belong to affluent classes absolved from responsibility for their own health? Are the disadvantaged less healthy because they freely choose to act in "irresponsible" ways that pose risk to their health status or are their choices limited by their social situations? These questions deserve deeper consideration. The distinction between personal lifestyle choices and socioeconomic inequalities in health is not easily made and is subject to heated debate.

Wikler (1987) examined some assumptions that are necessary to place *sole* responsibility for health with the individual. The first suggests that an individual can be held responsible only if he or she knows what to do to stay healthy. At this point in history, there is still a great deal of disagreement among "experts" as to what constitutes healthy behavior. Charles and Kerr (1988) found that many women in their study were reluctant to change their eating practices because they were skeptical of conflicting advice from experts. The other consideration related to the "need to know" argument is, can people be held responsible for inappropriate behavior if scientifically accepted health messages (which they need to know) do not reach them? For example, health professionals and educators frequently rely upon printed materials to disseminate information. Such materials cannot reach segments of the population disadvantaged by limited reading skills. Devault (1991) found that professional counseling is often seen by low income clients as contributing to a sense of inadequacy as there are significant gaps between the advice offered and what can be used with limited resources. These findings suggest that an examination of the discourse and practice of the nutrition profession may be more appropriate than uncritically laying blame on the behavior of individuals.

Wikler's (1987) analysis of the "individualistic ideology" locates a second assumption—that people freely choose their risks. However, inequalities in health may result from an inequitable distribution of choices. For example, a mother may prefer to send her child to school after having fed him or her a nutritious breakfast. But, if that family lives in Nova Scotia and is receiving social assistance, food allowance rates are insufficient to meet nutritional requirements in all but two municipalities (Nova Scotia Nutrition Council 1988). In other words, the "choice" to send a child to school hungry is not freely made and therefore reflects circumstances beyond individual responsibility. The evidence suggests that those who do not participate in healthy lifestyles are not necessarily irresponsible, but may have limited choices, limited knowledge, or insufficient resources to facilitate acting on adequate practical knowledge. Thus, by failing to consider the context within which nutrition and health "choices" are made, individualistic discourse may have contributed to the construction of inequities in nutritional health by diverting attention away from social contributions in claimsmaking about personal lifestyle contributions. By ignoring the possibility that the cause of poor nutritional health could lay in the environment beyond the immediate control of the individual, professional discourse denied the existence of social constraints such as poverty. As such, professional discourse and practice contributed to the reproduction of nutritional inequities.

By focusing on value-free science and objectivity, professional discourse found its power in "truth" and pronounced itself apolitical. However, by accepting the "truth" that arose from claims made in powerful political documents such as the Lalonde and Surgeon General's Reports, professional discourse did not remain neutral, but endorsed the political stance of the time that laid the cause of disease in individual health behaviors. In doing so, professional practice ignored the possibility that the cause of poor nutritional health could lay in the environment beyond the immediate control of the individual. In effect, the existence of constraints such as poverty were denied. By denying poverty's existence, nothing was done to help alleviate it. As Faden and Faden (1978:190) expressed, "To the extent that health educators have ignored or denied the complex social origins of health and disease and inappropriately translated this view into programmatic efforts targeted exclusively toward achieving individual behavior change, they have contributed to social wrongs." Despite professional discourse's claim of objectivity, professional inaction was an unintentional political act that effectively contributed to the construction of nutritional inequities.

The Reappearance of Nutritional Inequities

The early 1980s was a time of economic recession. In 1981, the first Canadian food bank opened its doors to the hungry people of Edmonton (Riches 1989). By the end of the decade they were becoming a Canadian institution. The food bank was but one symbol that indicated no progression toward overcoming nutritional inequities.

As the problem of poverty became hard to ignore, nutrition professionals began to change their claims as to the cause of poor nutritional health. The lifestyle theory that was defensible during the relatively good economic climate during the 1970s became less plausible in view of claims about social inequities arising with the fall of the economy. Instead of locating the problem within the individual, professional discourse located disease causation within the individual's environment. Professional discourse claimed that poverty was the "new" cause of health inequities. People were malnourished for lack of resources.

The immediacy of the problem demanded immediate solutions, and this is where food banks and soup kitchens fit. This time, nutrition educators took a consciously political stance and advocated the charitable process of providing aid to the poor by donating food, money, and time, and by informing the more fortunate members of the public of the extreme need for support. However, politics are not always as they appear. By accepting that poverty was the cause of inequities, and supporting food aid programs such as food banks, a message to "use aid now, and wait for things to get better" (Eide 1982) was sent. Freire (1973:15) calls this type of practice *assistencialism*—"policies of financial or social assistance which attack symptoms, but not causes, of social ills." Professional discourse and practice assumed that, with time, the economic situation would turn around. In the meantime, people were robbed of any responsibility for making a difference by simply being asked to wait. But the economic recession of the early 1980s passed, and the poor did not benefit from economic recovery. The need for food aid grew as the decade progressed. By supporting food banks, professional practice contributed to the illusion that the problem was solved by treating the symptom of hungry poverty. In failing to reflect on the implications of predominantly charitable actions, the underlying social injustices that perpetuated poverty that perpetuated inequities in health, and therefore contributed to the perpetuation of inequities, were ignored.

Then, recognizing the limitations of a practice based upon the charitable model, professional practice emphasized the development of programs that were designed to overcome the stop-gap emergency measures, and to help the impoverished to cope with their misfortunes, on an individual level. With the idea that "nutrition education is the attempt to enable consumers to use available resources optimally to reach valued ends"

(Hornik 1985:21), nutrition counseling and food budgeting workshops to help to ensure that every food dollar was wisely spent became standard practice. When nothing changed, professional discourse blamed the "culture of poverty," the way of life that is inherited through generations of deprivation (Lewis 1970).

A discourse of "helping" people to cope with their environments accepted that they were destined to continue to work with only limited resources. In effect, it endorsed the current distribution of social goods within society. If social change was going to occur, its initiation was going to have to come from the poor. In other words, the "coping" discourse placed all of the responsibility for change on the shoulders of those with the fewest resources and least power to act. By condemning the "culture of poverty" for the perpetuation of inequities, professional practice "blamed the victims" (Ryan 1971) of an unjust social order and sanctioned that social order. Rather than examine continuing victimizing social processes, programs designed to solve social problems were directed at individuals who "had" problems as a result of unusual circumstances. Therefore, programs were developed to teach the victims how to work to make the best of what they had without considering the possibility of social change. Teaching the poor how to budget for food without examining the adequacy of food allowances was an example of such a strategy. Nutrition discourse was political in that it worked to maintain the *status quo*; it was by no means emancipatory. In effect, the "blame the victim" ideology absolved the state of responsibility for transforming the social and environmental problems that made "unhealthy" choices more attractive and accessible (Freudenberg 1978; McLeroy et al. 1987, 1988; Minkler 1989; Wikler 1987). As Freudenberg (1978:374) so aptly put it: "the notion that individual behaviors are the main cause of illness leads to the position that changes in the health care system and the social and economic structure are less essential."

"Do You Teach Them How to Budget?" A Case Study of Professional Discourse and Individualistic Ideology

In the early 1990s, I conducted an institutional ethnography (Smith 1987) of a group of low-income women and their families in a small urban center in Nova Scotia (Travers 1993). For a period of 16 months I observed their nutrition and food-related practices, and conducted 27 group interviews and 15 individual ethnographic interviews with members of a women's group at a local drop-in Parent Center. Analysis revealed the important role of professional discourse and practice in the construction of nutritional inequities.

In some instances, it became apparent that professional discourse, like public discourse, was reflective of individualistic ideology. For example, both public and professional discourses appeared to adhere to the assumption that the poor have sufficient resources, but do not have the knowledge to use them wisely. Lack of budgeting knowledge and skill was assumed to be the source of money problems. To follow this assumption to its logical conclusion, it was their own fault that they ran out of food at the end of the month, or had insufficient funds to pay for a prescription. Research participants were wrongly confronted with accusations of being "out drinking on their welfare check," or having to use the food bank because they did not know how to appropriately budget their food allowances. Yet, analysis also revealed woeful inadequacies of welfare allowances and evidence of advanced budgeting skills among research participants, which should have been sufficient grounds to reject the ideological discourse. But despite this evidence many professionals (and the policy makers who rely upon professional opinion for decision making) continued to blame their clients for their failure to make ends meet. Such a discourse justifies the government practice of providing less than subsistence social assistance allowances (Riches 1986). Individualistic discourse also justifies placing all of the responsibility for breaking free of the welfare system on those living within it, those with the least political power to initiate farther-reaching structural change. Thus, individualistic discourse has a "victim-blaming" ideology (Ryan 1971).

Within discourse generated by individualistic ideology, inequities are not only socially acceptable, but provide a rationale for professionals to continue to practice in a way that attempts to change the "deficiencies" of the individual, while ignoring the social context within which these individuals work. To illustrate, several times throughout the research when I confronted professionals and policy makers with the financial difficulties of the research participants, the immediate and first response was, "Do you teach them how to budget?" Dominique[3] expressed her extreme frustration with this attitude:

> Every time these friggin' people walk in the fuckin' door, that's the first thing that comes out of their mouths is uh . . . that lady, what's her name? [referring to the Minister of Community Services], "Oh, do you have any budgeting programs? Do you teach them how to budget?" You know, and it's like, they give you money but they just don't know how to make it, they don't know to make it last.

I do not dispute the idea that learning to budget effectively is an important skill for anyone to learn, especially for someone with a limited income. In fact, the city's home economist offered budgeting classes at the Parent Center and most of the research participants had taken advantage of them. Because of this opportunity, it is possible that the superior skills the research participants exhibited are not common among other socially and economically disadvantaged citizens. Even members of the women's group recognized such a possibility:

> *Sunny*: But that is true sometimes too, . . . I mean like you get a young girl who first goes on social services with her baby and you give her this big giant check and you tell her to go pay rent, go pay her phone bill, go pay her lights, go get her groceries, clothe her baby and clothe herself, and she doesn't know how to do it.

This blanket assumption suggests that learning to budget will in some way erase the inadequacies of welfare allowances. Again, the onus is on the victims of the system to change within it; the system remains unquestioned. Unfortunately, such professional discourse contributes to inequities through systematic discrimination against their clients by professionals.

Looking specifically at the specialized discourse of nutrition professionals, analysis revealed the penetration of professional nutrition discourse into the research participants' daily work of feeding their families. Contrary to commonly held professional opinion that still appears to be informed by Lewis' (1970) "culture of poverty" hypothesis, the data revealed that these women were not simply adhering to a "live for today" mentality, but were planning for long-term food security, receiving the messages that professionals believe they should hear, and acting upon them when their resources permit, *if* they had relevance/practical application for their families. It is appropriate, then, to explore in more depth how nutritional discourse was received and acted upon by the research participants.

Current nutrition recommendations encourage Canadians to limit their salt and fat intakes, and to optimize consumption of foods rich in essential nutrients, such as vitamins and iron (Health and Welfare Canada 1989). The following quotes are but a few examples that illustrate that research participants were aware of such recommendations, and were attempting to plan their eating practices accordingly:

> *Janice*: I don't usually put salt in anything I'm cooking. . . . I guess basically because I don't care for salt and I figure there's enough salt in the food already when you buy it.
>
> *Tina*: Well, I guess its um, trying to get enough, or trying to get more foods with iron. Whenever I've got my hemoglobin checked its always low, its always been low since I was a teenager.
>
> *April*: That's the other reason I'd like to go to 2% [milk] for both the kids and him. I don't think he needs as much fat as he's getting.

In all of the families studied intensively, there was evidence of attention to and application of nutritional discourse in meal planning, preparation, and eating.

As regular patrons of the Parent Center and its services, all of the research participants had access to nutrition education through the Center's home economist, and through regularly scheduled seminars by the city's nutritionist. Therefore, the penetration of professional discourse into their daily practices was not surprising. It is also possible that such a penetration may not be characteristic of the entire population of socially and economically disadvantaged persons, although other ethnographic research revealed that even the homeless were paying attention to nutritional discourse when scavenging for food (Hill and Stamey 1990).

Curious about the source of the discourse, I asked most participants where they received their nutritional messages. The sources were varied. As expected, some participants cited the Parent Center as a predominant source of general information. Some remembered learning nutrition in home economics in school. Others heard messages through the media, although most messages heard via media channels were tied to commercial interests that took nutrition information out of context to promote a product. For most, however, health professionals and hospitals were cited as sources, particularly when referring to specialized information regarding a specific nutritional concern. For the women, pregnancy and childbirth were cited most as events that stimulated nutrition discussions between themselves and health professionals, as Janice's quote indicates:

> You get all kinds of stuff in the hospital when you have babies. *Was that stuff useful to you?* Yea, it was, yea, especially when I had Ian. *The first one you always . . .* Yes, read. Yes, my sister, she started, she's due in September and I think she's read every book that was possible already. Every time I see her, it's, "Look at this book, look at this, look at this."

Contrary to commonly held professional opinion, these women were interested in learning whatever they could to facilitate a healthy pregnancy outcome and a healthy infancy. Motivation to learn, during pregnancy and at other times of their lives, was not usually the limiting factor leading to suboptimal nutritional intake.

However, implementing the nutritional recommendations received was not always straightforward. The type of information given or the "education" process used by the professionals was not always relevant or useful to the women. During the research, I had the opportunity to observe education sessions given by the city's nutritionist, and to question the women regarding their impressions and ideas after the session. The following discussion took place after the nutritionist facilitated a working session on healthy lunches for children:

Sunny: I did not realize that you are supposed to use all the food groups for each meal. I always thought that it was something that had, as long as you had all the food groups within the run of a day, then you were doing OK. But I didn't realize that you needed that balance at every single meal. [There is group agreement on this point, and I confirm that her impressions are correct.]

Lana: I don't go by that I just, . . . figure out what I'm having for dinner and do that but I don't go by . . . *You don't go by food groups?* No. *Most people don't go by food groups?* No. But if I sit down and try, if I sit down and watch it, I do, I am giving her all from it but I don't sit down and say you know, this is from this, and this is from this . . . *No, it just sorta comes together.* Like when you're grocery shopping you don't wanna have a double list.

Dominique: Like when we have supper we have, you know, like we have ham steaks or whatever you have, we always have baked potato or rice and I always make sure there's a vegetable right? You know. And it all straightens out.

Although the nutritionist had avoided lecturing and was successful in attaining the women's participation, the message received by the majority of those in attendance was to follow Canada's Food Guide in planning each meal, a useful message but one they had all heard before. In fact, most of the women were already acting on the message, even though their work was routinized as opposed to thought through carefully at each meal. However, by suggesting that the women plan to choose foods from all four food groups at each meal rather than throughout the day (which is acceptable), the message contributed to feelings of inadequacy and guilt for not doing as well as they might.

As long as professional practice continues to place primary emphasis on changing individuals without consideration of the context within which they work, the potential remains high for victim blaming on the part of professionals, and guilt on the part of the individual who is unable to live up to expectations. For these research participants, guilt for failing to adhere to recommendations they knew were best for their families was ever present. The following passage from a discussion with Tina over what she fed her toddler when he was suffering from a cold is illustrative of guilt:

Tina: I had some of that chicken noodle soup in there, . . . I remember I gave Josh some of the noodles, it has a lot of salt in it but, I gave him some of the noodles out of the can anyway.

Kim: *Do you worry about, a couple of times you mentioned to me you know there's a lot of salt in something, do you worry about too much salt in food?*

> *Tina*: Yea I guess I do. I don't know where I got it from but yea, I guess it's those books . . . that you get at the hospital, from Birth to Year One Feeding Baby? [This is a Department of Health publication, the actual title of which is *Year One: Food for Baby*] . . . . They just mention that canned, canned stuff like vegetables and soups, they always say they're not a good choice because they have a lot of salt.

Tina's son was sick and had a poor appetite. Wanting to feed him something, she resorted to a can of chicken noodle soup she had received from the food bank. Yet, she felt pangs of guilt for feeding her son something that was not consistent with a nutrition message she had received. Dogmatic nutrition messages do not assist the disadvantaged in making reasonable and moderate choices among available alternatives, which the chicken soup decision could have been, but foster a sense of inadequacy and guilt for failing to live up to the standard set by them. These findings are similar to those of Devault (1991) who reported mothers' feelings of inadequacy when they found themselves unable to implement recommendations following nutrition education designed specifically for low-income women. Considering that economically disadvantaged citizens are becoming reliant upon food banks, which often provide less than optimal nutritional choices, professional discourse is becoming even more damning as options are limited.

At times, however, unnecessary guilt generated by unrealistic expectations was not as big an issue as was the sheer impracticality of following nutrition recommendations. The following discussion between Tina and me illustrates an example of the impracticality of implementing nutritional recommendations:

> *Kim*: When you went to visit [the nutritionist] in her office, . . . what kind of advice did she give you on diet and . . . ?
>
> *Tina*: She gave me a few pamphlets and that, um, and there was, she asked me if I was taking my prenatal vitamins. . . . I remember we were talking about iron . . . and I told her, I said every time I have my iron taken, it's usually down around 10 or 11, a little below normal, so she suggested that I, she gave me a list of different foods, but I already knew them . . . to try to eat more iron . . . to try to eat more of those. I do try to eat more but, you know, I don't think I eat enough to make a difference, you know?. . . . I can't eat too much of that . . . so I can eat a little but not enough things to make a difference, so I keep taking iron pills I guess, those prenatal vitamins. . . . The other pamphlets were just about, one was about breast feeding, one was about nutrition during pregnancy. . . . I had already read them.

Since this was not Tina's first pregnancy, she had already heard the

usual lecture on nutrition and pregnancy, and had read the more common pamphlets. She was sufficiently literate (Grade Eight) to read and
understand the pamphlets, and motivated to review them. She was also
aware of her greatest nutritional problem in iron-deficiency anemia. Yet,
despite her knowledge and motivation, her nutritionist was unable to
assist her in improving her food choices. The standard list of iron-rich
foods that the nutritionist provided were foods either unfamiliar, objectionable, or too expensive for Tina to consume in sufficient quantities to
make a difference. The advice she received was not practical information
that would assist her in incorporating unfamiliar and inexpensive foods
into her diet in acceptable ways, but merely a list of foods. The nutritionist did disseminate nutrition information, but did not educate. In addition, the information may not have even been received if it were not for
Tina's literacy and motivation.

For Tina, and many of the other research participants, the nutritional
quality of her diet was improved more by structural and policy initiatives than by dissemination of irrelevant and impractical nutrition information. Tina was relatively advantaged as her prenatal vitamins were
paid for by municipal social assistance; for others, prenatal supplements
were an unaffordable luxury. As well, all pregnant women on social
assistance in the municipality studied were eligible to receive an additional food allowance or vouchers toward the purchase of milk and
orange juice to help meet their increased nutritional requirements during pregnancy. For the women I studied, the nutritional counseling that
accompanied these programs was less helpful.

April's situation can be used to illustrate the possibilities after welfare.
Within the context of making nutritional recommendations accessible
and realistic, April's situation illustrates how a structural change, in this
case the availability of resources, can make an impact on one's abilities to
implement nutritional change.

> April: I find the more you know about food, the healthier you are. I find
> when my children were babies, things I ate then and what I eat
> now, I do see a difference. . . . I really watch what the children eat
> and make sure that they are getting everything from the food
> groups. I feel the more education you get, then the more, and just
> talking to other Moms to get ideas.

For April, who had more resources than other research participants,
nutrition information was more relevant and pragmatic.

The above quote not only illustrates April's ability to implement recommendations to the extent that she can meet the standards set by professionals and thus remain guilt-free, but also brings to light the role of

differences between clients and professionals in constructing nutritional inequities. Most professional nutrition educators would argue that they are better able to provide more relevant and practical advice to "clients" most like themselves. Part of this could be lack of understanding of the context within which the socially and economically disadvantaged make their nutrition decisions. April was, at the time of the research, joining the ranks of helping professionals. She therefore identified more with the professional nutritionists she dealt with, and they with her. In addition, however, April's example reveals a skill in obtaining relevant information from a professional. April seemed to understand how to get the information she needed; she once told me "I'm the type of person that wouldn't settle for pamphlets either." She learned to press further, to challenge the nutritionist to provide more than pamphlets. Yet, identifying with professionals has its pitfalls, as a great deal of valuable learning from nonprofessionals can be undervalued. Although April's quote reveals she has also learned a lot from "just talking to other Moms to get ideas," this sort of learning was not equal in value to professional nutrition education in her assessment. Although April was able to measure her nutritional knowledge against the standard of professional nutritional discourse, one wonders if her outstanding abilities to feed her family on a less than optimal income are related to her knowledge of the academic subject matter (gained from professionals) or to her practical knowledge (gained from experience and talking with other Moms) of implementing what she felt was best.

I was able to explore the idea that professionals do not have sufficient understanding of the context within which the socially and economically disadvantaged make their nutrition decisions more deeply with John, a research participant training to become a health professional. John was living in a low-income situation, and I therefore expected him to be more understanding of the context and less tied to professional discourse. As the following conversation between John and his wife Bessie illustrates, I was mistaken:

> *John*: And nutritionally it's not, it's not so much a situation where people can't afford the food, it's that they're in such a position financially, emotionally, so much stress in low income areas, just with the fact that you have a low income and so on, that lower income people smoke more on the average, they eat more, but it's generally not nutritious food, especially the adults.
>
> *Bessie*: But that's not, I don't think that's always the case. I mean we're low income.
>
> *John*: It's not always the case but it's more prevalent in a low income society than it is in a higher income . . . .

> *Bessie:* But anybody who has any brain at all knows that you need fruit, vegetables, meats and breads.
>
> *John:* No I'm sorry, I beg to differ with you there, because one of the high functions of a nurse is to ensure proper nutrition in their patients. And so much focus is put on it because lower income groups especially, are not generally getting the nutrition they need. And it's more an education situation than it is . . . .

John seems to think his family is the exception in planning nutritious meals. His nursing training has taught him that people living in low-income situations have more health problems and poorer health habits, which is extensively documented in professional literature. Yet, he does not seem to fully appreciate the possibility of structural "barriers" to healthy living (although the commercialization of food does enter into his analysis). Instead, he attributes poor health habits to "stress," believing the answer to lie in individual education. The valuing of individual health education reflects the dominant individualistic ideology subscribed to by health professional schools. John has dismissed his own personal experience of living in poverty as exceptional, and has placed more value on his newly attained theoretical knowledge, which does not locate the health problems and habits of the poor into social context. His practices suggested an internalization of the oppressive, individualistic discourse. By viewing his antistereotypical situations as exceptional, he reinforced public discourse and participated in the reproduction of nutritional inequities. John's adoption of the professional discourse reinforces popular discourse confirming his ability to rise above the problems of poverty as a result of his own knowledge and hard work. Because he feels his family is the exception, his potential to appreciate the context within which health decisions are made is tempered. John is not unique. An American study comparing indigenous paraprofessionals' and professionals' perceptions of EFNEP (Expanded Food and Nutrition Education Program) clients' beliefs and practices revealed that indigenous paraprofessionals and professionals consistently underestimated the abilities of their low-income clients, and attributed their problems more to "deficiencies" of the poor rather than structural issues (Bremner et al. 1994). So, like many other health professionals, John's professional practice will likely work to modify the habits and beliefs of the individuals within the current social order, rather than to critique the social structure as a potential source of inequities.

As the examples presented in this case study attest, professional discourse is powerful. It penetrates the everyday practice of eating directly through conveying nutritional messages to individuals, it intersects with the commercial sector when it is coopted to sell a product, and it permeates policy by informing decision makers. Because of its consistency with individualistic ideology, professional discourse can accentuate inequalities in nutritional health by failing to examine the fabric of society as a source of inequities, and laying blame upon the disadvantaged individuals who, despite their best efforts, are unable to live up to expectations set by professionals. Taken even further, discourse is dangerous when it is used to exert the power of the state over individuals who are struggling to work within an inequitable system. The following quote illustrates the potential for state intervention in the lives of these women based on nutritional discourse, which places sole responsibility for change upon the individual:

> *Lana:* I'm going through a custody case right now, and I've got a grandmother who's trying to take my daughter from me, between her and her father. And they had all this mumbo jumbo that I wasn't feedin' her the right food and that and I wasn't cookin' her home-cooked meals, it was precooked food. I don't know where they got all that anyway, they said uh, I shouldn't be givin' her hamburger and French fries and Kraft dinner and all that. I said, "Why cook somethin' the child is not gonna eat, when you know the child is gonna eat the Kraft dinner and stuff, why can't you cook it?" So, . . . the judge just looks at them when he was reading through this, the list they had wrote, and he said, "Well it's certainly economical for . . . " 'cause where I was on welfare at the time, and he just laughed in their faces.

Thankfully, the judge in this situation was appreciative of the struggles Lana faces to feed her family, and did not place blame on her for failing to conform with idealistic nutritional discourse. Dominique, however, was quick to point out one of the structural sources of inequities that Lana faced, one that the judge did not acknowledge: "You know what he should've done, he should've turned around to them and he shoulda said, 'well I think we better up that child's support another $100 a month or $50 a month so that child can eat better'." Lana's ex-husband was ordered to pay only $50 per month in child support, yet she was expected to feed her child as if she drew upon unlimited resources, and risked being deemed an "unfit" parent incapable of custody. When abused to justify decisions beyond the scope of professional practice, discourse can be dangerous indeed.

In sum, if one were to examine the eating practices of the socially disadvantaged population in isolation, and to impose nutritional discourse from the perspective of the professional, it may be easy to come to the conclusion that the poor do not pay attention to our messages and that their "unwise" food choices, such as expensive convenience foods, are made as a result of living in a "culture of poverty." However, by analyzing practices from the perspective of the participant, and by tracing how eating is embedded within social constructs, it becomes more readily apparent that nutritional messages are attended to and acted upon if resources permit, and that purchasing convenience foods is logical if basic ingredients are not available at reasonable prices locally, or if food preparation facilities are less than ideal. Nutrition educators need to be cognizant of the potential to too easily "blame the victim." As part of a move toward a reduction in nutritional inequities, the discourse must be changed.

The Discourse of Health Promotion: Future Possibilities for Reducing Inequities?

In 1986, Canada hosted the first International Conference on Health Promotion, and the *Ottawa Charter for Health Promotion* (WHO, HWC, CPHA 1986) was released. With the release of this landmark document, professional discourse became more politicized, explicitly recognizing the inextricable relationships between people's health, their individual behaviors, and their social environment. The *Charter* was grounded in the philosophy of health promotion, "the process of enabling people to increase control over, and to improve, their health" (WHO, HWC, CPHA 1986:426), and called for a reduction in inequities through the strengthening of community action and public participation in creating healthy public policy. The *Charter* put health on the agenda of policy makers, recognizing that public policy has the power to deny or grant opportunities for health. Although professional practice lags behind, the possibilities for a health promotion perspective in the reduction of nutritional inequities are of interest.

One component of a health promotion perspective is a reconceptualization of nutrition and health education from information dissemination to a social change or emancipatory focus. Nutrition education for social change is not a totally novel concept. Paulo Freire (1970) conceived of empowerment education in response to his experiences with hungry Brazilians who were illiterate, unable to participate in democratic processes, and oppressed by powerful land owners. Freire appeared to recognize that hunger was not caused by poverty per se, but arose from imbalances in power. In a way, his "pedagogy of the oppressed" was a form of politicized nutrition education as its aim was to empower the hungry to improve their social conditions, and ultimately, to improve their health and well-being. This was long before nutrition educators, such as Eide (1982), began to name conflict of interest as the cause for inequitable access to food within nations.

Perhaps it is not coincidental that Freirian philosophies of education have been given recent attention in nutrition education literature. Eide recommends the use of Freirian strategies in changing "the nutrition educator's role in access to food from individual orientation to social orientation" (1982:14).

Reports describe adaptation of Paulo Freire's empowerment education as a model for nutrition programs (Kent 1988; Rody 1988). As Kent (1988:194) so eloquently stated, "Nutritional literacy means more than knowing the technical aspects of nutrition . . . teaching of nutrition should include examination of the world which generates nutrition problems." Kent describes the purpose of these programs as "to support people in making their own analyses so that they themselves can decide what is good for them" (1988:193). However, participants' analyses are not simply a regurgitation of the nutrition educator's analysis. Instead, the educator poses problems to the participants, and the participants draw from their own experiences and practical knowledge to try to make sense of their situation on their own terms. They are free to challenge the educator's (and each other's) interpretations. The emphasis is on creating a dialogue among group members, and from the sharing of experiences and interpretations emerges a collective knowledge that helps people to uncover the "root causes of their place in society" (Wallerstein and Bernstein 1988:382). As "consciousness-raising" progresses, participants begin to see ways of actively making changes in their situation. People become empowered to transform their reality.

Health movements, such as the women's health movement and the ecology movement, have used Freirian-like strategies such as consciousness-raising groups to stimulate changes in health services and to initiate political action for health-promoting legislative changes. Such political changes evolve following intense public pressure arising from long-term, cumulative effects of changing public opinion and cultural values (Faden 1987). In effect, democratic deliberations have played a large role in shaping healthy public policy; this is health education for social change. "Health education for social change identifies the health-damaging elements in our society. Its goal is to involve people in collective action to create health-promoting environments and life-styles" (Freudenberg 1978:375). Such "politicizing" of health education has had a major impact on all members of society. The benefits are not limited to only those who participated in the movements (Freudenberg 1978).

But nutrition education for social change need not be limited to Freirian consciousness-raising. As the community is composed of power structures that control issues to be placed on the public agenda, entire communities can be potential sites for enlightenment. The problem of inequities is best addressed at this level, as

> those with the most severe health problems within a community are often
> those with the least access to community power . . . such groups are often
> left out of the process of defining problems and developing programmatic
> solutions . . . . An essential component of community health promotion,
> then, is increasing access by the disadvantaged to larger community politi-
> cal and power structures. (McLeroy et al. 1988:364–365)

It is important at this point to caution against accepting any community intervention as emancipatory. The rather general language used in
documents such as the *Charter* make it possible for agencies or programs
to continue to proceed with business as usual, while couching it in the
language of health promotion (Hexel and Wintersberger 1986). McLeroy
et al. (1987:101) are worth quoting at length on this point:

> One of the most critical issues in health promotion is the accusation that it
> is largely targeted to, and addresses the needs of middle and upper socio-
> economic groups. As such, it is directed at the most advantaged segments
> of society and ignores the needs of the poor, the elderly, and minorities. To
> the extent that health promotion ignores social, economic, and cultural
> realities, this is a legitimate criticism. Moreover, by targeting health pro-
> motion at those who can afford to pay, we reinforce the idea that health is
> a commodity.

Without active participation of the disadvantaged, even community interventions can continue to perpetuate inequities by creating a more
healthy environment for those already predisposed to healthy lifestyles,
while ignoring the impact (or lack of impact) on those who need environmental change the most. For example, Glanz and Mullis' (1988) review of
environmental interventions to promote healthy eating reveals that
most programs have focused on point of choice nutrition education in
restaurants and supermarkets. Unfortunately, these programs have little
impact on those who cannot afford to eat in restaurants or those whose
food choices in grocery stores are necessarily motivated by price, not
nutrition. Although this critique is not meant to begrudge the more
fortunate of useful community interventions, it *is* meant to highlight the
potential injustices created if community interventions ignore the needs
of the less powerful to meet the needs of those already in a position to
implement change.

Although professional practice lags behind and health promotion discourse risks cooption, a shift in professional discourse from an individualistic perspective to a more politicized discourse that recognizes the
inextricable relationships between people's health, their individual behaviors, and their social environment opens up possibilities for a reduction in nutritional inequities.

Summary and Conclusions

With a deliberately critical theoretical stance and a vision of future social change, this chapter has examined the discursive construction of inequities in nutrition and health in industrialized nations. Historically, ideological theories of disease causation have formed the basis of professional discourse and practice. Although historical and recent ethnographic evidence reveals that objective social conditions frequently defy discourse, the discourse remains a powerful influence in a variety of public arenas, on policy, practice, and public perceptions. In particular, the pervasiveness of individualistic ideology in professional discourse throughout history and reemerging in the present day draws to light the power of discourse in diverting attention away from underlying structural causes of inequities. Such a perspective justifies a practice that decontextualizes individual behaviors and accepts the social conditions that give rise to these behaviors as given. The chapter draws to a close with an argument for a change in oppressive discourse toward a reduction in nutritional inequities. The discourse of health promotion and emancipatory nutrition education are examined as possibilities for the reduction of nutritional inequities.

Notes

1.　This is not meant to imply that specific subgroups will not have their own public discourses, but simply that only certain discourses will become popular and acceptable within the public domain. Just as small bits of the discourse of nutritional biochemistry will become prevalent in popular discourse (the word "cholesterol" for example), so will pieces of discourse from various subcultures. By and large, however, the discourse of the dominant culture is most likely to pervade mainstream thinking.

2.　"New" is really a misnomer. The Lalonde report represented a return to the nineteenth century's personal behavior theory described previously.

3.　All names of respondents are pseudonyms. Italicized text refers to the interviewer's comments and questions.

References

Bremner, B., C. C. Campbell, and J. Sobal. 1994. "Comparison of the Beliefs and Practices of EFNEP Clients with Staff Perceptions of Clients." *Journal of Nutrition Education* 26:123–130.

Bullock, A., O. Stallybrass, and S. Trombley (eds.). 1988. *The Fontana Dictionary of Modern Thought*, 2nd ed. London: Fontana Press.

Canadian Dietetic Association. no date. *Code of Ethics*.

Charles, N., and M. Kerr. 1988. *Women, Food and Families*. Manchester: Manchester University Press.

D'Arcy, C. 1987. *Reducing Inequities in Health: A Review of the Literature* (Cat. No. HSPB 88-16). Health Services and Promotion Branch Working Paper. Ottawa: Health and Welfare Canada.

Department of Health, Education and Welfare. 1979. *Healthy People: The Surgeon General's Report on Health Promotion and Disease Prevention 1979* (No. 79-55071). Washington, D.C.: Public Health Services Publication.

Devault, M. L. 1991. *Feeding the Family: The Social Organization of Caring as Gendered Work*. Chicago: University of Chicago Press.

Edginton, B. 1989. *Health, Disease and Medicine in Canada: A Sociological Perspective*. Toronto: Butterworths.

Eide, W. B. 1982. "The Nutrition Educator's Role in Access to Food—From Individual Orientation to Social Orientation." *Journal of Nutrition Education* 14:14–17.

Faden, R. R. 1987. "Ethical Issues in Government Sponsored Public Health Campaigns." *Health Education Quarterly* 14:27–37.

Faden, R. R., and A. I. Faden. 1978. "The Ethics of Health Education as Public Health Policy." *Health Education Monographs* 6:180–197.

Foucault, M. 1971. *The Order of Things: An Archaeology of the Human Sciences*. New York: Random House.

Fraser, N. 1989. *Unruly Practices: Power, Discourse and Gender in Contemporary Social Theory*. Minneapolis: University of Minnesota Press.

Freire, P. 1970. *Pedagogy of the Oppressed*. New York: Continuum.

———. 1973. *Education for Critical Consciousness*. New York: Continuum.

Freudenberg, N. 1978. "Shaping the Future of Health Education: From Behavior Change to Social Change." *Health Education Monographs* 6:372–377.

Friedson, E. 1988. *Profession of Medicine: A Study of the Sociology of Applied Knowledge*, 2nd ed. Chicago: University of Chicago Press.

Glanz, K., and R. M. Mullis. 1988. "Environmental Interventions to Promote Healthy Eating: A Review of Models, Programs, and Evidence. *Health Education Quarterly* 15:395–415.

Health and Welfare Canada. 1977. *Nutrition Recommendations for Canadians*. Ottawa: Health Promotion Directorate.

Health and Welfare Canada. 1989. *Nutrition Recommendations . . . A Call for Action*. Catalogue No. H39-162/1990E. Ottawa: Minister of Supply and Services.

Hexel, P. C., and H. Wintersberger. 1986. "Inequalities in Health: Strategies." *Social Science and Medicine* 22:151–160.

Hilgartner, S., and C. L. Bosk. 1988. "The Rise and Fall of Social Problems: A Public Arenas Model." *American Journal of Sociology* 94(1):53–78.

Hill, R. P., and M. Stamey. 1990. "The Homeless in America: An Examination of Possessions and Consumption Behaviors. *Journal of Consumer Research* 17:303–321.

Hornik, R. C. 1985. *Nutrition Education: A State-of-the-Art Review*. Rome: United Nations Administrative Committee on Coordination, Nutrition Policy Paper No. 1.

Kent, G. 1988. "Nutrition Education as an Instrument of Empowerment." *Journal of Nutrition Education* 20:193–195.

Lalonde, M. 1974. *A New Perspective on the Health of Canadians.* Ottawa: Health & Welfare Canada.

Lewis, O. 1970. "The Culture of Poverty." Pp. 67–89 in *Anthropological Essays.* New York: Random House.

McKeown, T. 1979. *The Role of Medicine: Dream, Mirage or Nemesis?* London: Nuffield Provincial Hospitals Trust.

McLeroy, K. R., N. H. Gottlieb, and J. N. Burdine. 1987. "The Business of Health Promotion: Ethical Issues and Professional Responsibilities." *Health Education Quarterly* 14:91–109.

McLeroy, K. R., D. Bibeau, A. Steckler, and K. Glanz. 1988. "An Ecological Perspective on Health Promotion Programs." *Health Education Quarterly* 15:351–377.

Minkler, M. 1989. "Health Education, Health Promotion and the Open Society: An Historical Perspective." *Health Education Quarterly* 16:17–30.

Nöth, W. 1990. *Handbook of Semiotics.* Bloomington: Indiana University Press.

Nova Scotia Nutrition Council. 1988. *How Do the Poor Afford to Eat? An Examination of Social Assistance Food Rates in Nova Scotia.* Halifax, NS: Unpublished NSNC.

Philp, M. 1985. "Michel Foucault." Pp. 65–81 in *The Return of Grand Theory in the Human Sciences,* edited by Q. Skinner. Cambridge: Cambridge University Press.

Riches, G. 1986. *Food Banks and the Welfare Crisis.* Ottawa: Canadian Council on Social Development.

———. 1989. "Responding to Hunger in a Wealthy Society: Issues and Options." *Journal of the Canadian Dietetic Association* 50:150–154.

Rody, N. 1988. "Empowerment as Organizational Policy in Nutrition Intervention Programs: A Case Study from the Pacific Islands." *Journal of Nutrition Education* 20:133–141.

Rootman, I. 1988. "Inequities in Health: Sources and Solutions." *Health Promotion* Winter: 2–8.

Ryan, W. 1971. *Blaming the Victim.* New York: Vintage Press.

Schneider, J. W. 1985. "Social Problems Theory: The Constructionist View." *Annual Review of Sociology* 11:209–229.

Smith, D. E. 1987. *The Everyday World as Problematic. A Feminist Sociology.* Toronto: University of Toronto Press.

———. 1990. *The Conceptual Practices of Power. A Feminist Sociology of Knowledge.* Toronto: University of Toronto Press.

Spector, M., and J. I. Kitsuse. 1987. *Constructing Social Problems.* Hawthorne, NY: Aldine de Gruyter.

Stokes, B. 1979. "Self Care: A Nation's Best Health Insurance." *Science* 205:64–71.

Tesh, S. N. 1988. *Hidden Arguments: Political Ideology and Disease Prevention Policy.* New Brunswick, NJ: Rutgers University Press.

Travers, K. D. R. 1993. *Critical Nutrition Education for Social Change: Toward Reducing Inequities through Participatory Research and Community Organization.*

Unpublished Ph.D. Dissertation, Dalhousie University, Halifax, Nova Scotia.

Wallerstein, N., and E. Bernstein. 1988. "Empowerment Education: Freire's Ideas Adapted to Health Education." *Health Education Quarterly* 15:379–394.

Wikler, D. 1987. "Who Should Be Blamed for Being Sick?" *Health Education Quarterly* 14:11–25.

World Health Organization, Health & Welfare Canada and Canadian Public Health Association. 1986. "Ottawa Charter for Health Promotion." *Canadian Journal of Public Health* 77:425–427.

11

The Food Stamp Program and Hunger: Constructing Three Different Claims

MARK R. RANK and THOMAS A. HIRSCHL

Hunger in the United States is a frequently constructed social problem. The image of children and adults going hungry in a prosperous and wealthy nation is a disturbing picture. For example, a recent *Newsweek* article (Shapiro 1994) featured a large photograph of a child standing in a soup kitchen line, with the title underneath, "How Hungry is America?"

In this chapter, we examine a major social welfare program—the Food Stamp program—whose stated purpose is to reduce hunger in America. To what extent does the Food Stamp program meet this objective? Further, what are the perceived problems associated with the program in reaching this goal?

Consistent with the overall theme of this book, we rely upon a constructionist perspective to shed insight into this examination (e.g., Best 1989; Miller and Holstein 1993; Spector and Kitsuse 1977). We explore the claims of the following groups: (1) the recipients of food stamps, (2) the research policy analysts of the Food Stamp program, and (3) the general public. These groups constitute three sets of key players in that they represent the consumers of the program, the analysts of the program, and the taxpayers of the program. Furthermore, the first author has had extensive experience interacting with all three groups of claimants. We conclude with a discussion that juxtaposes the various claims made regarding food stamps and hunger.

Background

The Food Stamp program constitutes a major welfare program in the United States. As Ohls and Beebout note, "It offers the only form of assistance available nationwide to all households on the basis only of financial need, irrespective of family type, age, or disability" (1993:1). Recipients are given food coupons, which come in various denominations and may be exchanged for food products in grocery stores and supermarkets that choose to participate in the program. The program was established in 1964, and modified in 1977 (for a historical background and description of the program, see Berry 1984; DeVault and Pitts 1984; MacDonald 1977; Ohls and Beebout 1993; as well as Poppendieck in this collection).

The Food Stamp program is federally funded and administered by the Department of Agriculture; consequently, benefits do not vary across states. Income, assets, and family size determine eligibility and benefit levels. Families must be below approximately 130% of the poverty line to qualify.

In 1993 the average monthly food stamp benefit was $68.00 per person (Committee on Ways and Means 1994). Between 20 and 30 million people generally receive food stamps in the United States, or approximately 1 of every 10 individuals. Like all public assistance programs, the specific number of recipients varies from month to month and year to year, depending on a range of factors, such as the strength of the economy.

One of the major purposes of the Food Stamp program is to reduce hunger and malnutrition in the United States by providing low-income households with the ability to purchase an adequate diet. As stated in the House Committee on Ways and Means' *Green Book: Overview of Entitlement Programs*, "Food Stamps are designed primarily to increase the food purchasing power of eligible low-income households to a point where they can buy a nutritionally adequate low-cost diet" (1994:757).

To what extent does the Food Stamp program meet this objective? Further, what are the problems associated with the program in reaching this goal? We examine the perspectives and claims made by three different groups.

Three Differing Claims

The Recipient's View

We begin with the viewpoint of those closest to the Food Stamp program—the food stamp recipient. We rely upon a series of in-depth interviews that Mark Rank conducted with a wide range of welfare recipients. These interviews captured several of the predominant attitudes and claims of recipients toward the Food Stamp program (for further detail, see Rank 1994a, 1994b).

From the perspective of the food stamp recipient, two overriding themes emerge: (1) food stamps generally do not provide enough assistance to avoid serious shortages of food during a typical month; and (2) there are significant psychological difficulties in using food stamps as a result of the overall stigma attached to the program. These two themes are discussed below.

Shortage of Food Assistance. Perhaps most apparent when one listens to welfare recipients describe their daily lives and routines is the constant economic struggle that they face. This includes not having enough food, difficulties in paying monthly bills, worrying about health care costs, and so on. The amount of food assistance and income received each month is simply insufficient to cover all of these necessary expenses. For those on public assistance, life is reported as an ongoing struggle to survive economically.

Carol Richardson was asked to describe what her day-to-day problems were (all respondents' names have been changed to protect their confidentiality). Having lived in poverty for most of her 45 years, she could be considered an expert on the subject:

> Making ends meet. Period. Coming up with the rent on time. Coming up with the telephone bill on time. Having food in the house. It looks like we've got enough now. I got food stamps last month. Otherwise we would be down and out by now. It's just keepin' goin' from day to day. Carfare, busfare, gas money . . . .

The recipients' economic struggles become even more difficult toward the end of each month; Food Stamp and Aid to Families with Dependent Children (AFDC) benefits are received monthly. These benefits are usually not enough to provide adequately throughout a particular month (e.g., Brown and Pizer 1987; Cohen et al. 1993; Food Research and Action Center 1991; Simpson 1990). For example, many recipients find that their food stamps routinely run out by the end of the third week. Even with the budgeting and stretching of resources that recipients try to do, there is simply not enough left at the end of each month. Tammy and Jack Collins, a married couple in their mid-30s with six children, describe the process:

> *Tammy:* Mainly it's towards the end of the month, and you run out of food stamps and gotta pay rent. Tryin' to find enough money to buy groceries. It's the main one.

> *Question*: When that comes up, do you turn to somebody to borrow money, or do you just try to stretch what you've got?
>
> *Tammy*: I try to stretch. And sometimes his Ma will pay him for doin' things on the weekend for her, which will help out. She knows we need the money.
>
> *Jack*: We collect aluminum cans and we got a crusher in the basement and we sell them.
>
> *Q.*: What happens when you run out of food?
>
> *Tammy*: That's when his Ma helps us.

Recipients often rely on some kind of emergency assistance such as food pantries or family and friends to help them through. Such networks provide an important source of support. Of the food pantries Rank visited, all reported that the numbers of individuals coming in for emergency food supplies increased dramatically during the last 10 days of each month (Rank 1994a). The reason for this is that welfare benefits simply run out a week or so before the month is over.

Carol Richardson was asked if she ran out of food, particularly at the end of the month:

> *Carol*: Yeah. All the time.
>
> *Q.*: How do you manage?
>
> *Carol*: We've got a food pantry up here that they allow you to go to two times a month. They give you a little card. And in between those times, we find other food pantries that we can get to. We've gone to different churches and asked for help all the time. And we get commodities at the end of the month. Cheese and butter. And then we usually get one item [food commodity] out of it, which helps an awful lot.

In short, the end of the month represents a time when the recipients' economic struggles become even more magnified. It is a period when even the basic necessities may be hard to come by. It is seldom a question of improperly budgeting one's finances. Rather, it is a question of not having enough money to begin with to cover the monthly expenses. Among the poverty stricken, this is a major reoccurring problem. Public assistance programs may help, but they simply do not provide enough. Households are forced to routinely make hard choices among necessities.

One particularly hard choice facing some households in the wintertime is choosing between heat or food. This has been referred to by social workers as the "heat-or-eat" dilemma. Lacking enough money to cover the basic needs, does one choose to have heat in one's house but therefore go hungry, or not to go hungry but therefore freeze? A 3 year study done by the Boston City Hospital showed that the number of emergency room visits by underweight children increased by 30% after the coldest months of the year. In explaining the results, Debrorah Frank, who led the study team noted, "Parents well know that children freeze before they starve and in winter some families have to divert their already inadequate food budget to buy fuel to keep the children warm" (*New York Times* 1992). As a result, the ability of an underweight child to fight infection and disease becomes even more impaired when that child is also malnourished.

Hunger is thus a real consequence of surviving on food stamps. Many of the families Rank talked to admitted that there were times when they and their children were forced to go hungry and/or significantly alter their diet. An example of altering one's diet during the latter part of the month is the case of Edith Mathews. A widow in her 60s, Edith lives in a working class, elderly neighborhood. Although she has been receiving 45 dollars a month worth of food stamps, it is not enough to provide for an adequate diet. Edith suffers from several serious health problems, including diabetes and high blood pressure. The fact that she cannot afford a balanced diet compounds her health problems. She explains:

> Toward the end of the month, we just live on toast and stuff. Toast and eggs or something like that. I'm supposed to eat green vegetables. I'm supposed to be on a special diet because I'm a diabetic. But there's a lotta things that I'm supposed to eat that I can't afford. Because the fruit and vegetables are terribly high in the store. It's ridiculous! I was out to Ceder's grocery, they're charging 59 cents for one grapefruit. I'm supposed to eat grapefruit, but who's gonna pay 59 cents for one grapefruit when you don't have much money? But my doctor says that that's one thing that's important, is to eat the right foods when you're a diabetic. But I eat what I can afford. And if I can't afford it, I can't eat it. So that's why my blood sugar's high because lots of times I should have certain things to eat and I just can't pay. I can't afford it.

Nancy Jordon was asked about not having enough food for her three children. In her mid 30s and working as a cosmetologist, Nancy has been receiving public assistance for 2 months. Her income from work is simply too low to survive on as a single parent. She explains that not having enough money for food has had physical consequences not only upon her children, but upon her as well:

> *Nancy:* Well as long as I got money. If not, I have to resort to other measures. It's a sad thing but a woman should never be broke because if she's got a mind, and knows how to use it, you can go out in the streets. Which is the ultimate LAST resort is to go to the streets. But at a point in a woman's life, if she cares anything about her children, if she cares anything about their lifestyle,

> they'll go. Matter of fact, some would go to the streets before they
> would go to aid.
>
> Q.:   Have you had to do that, in the past, to feed your kids?
> *Nancy*:   A couple of times yes.

In short, the first claim often made by those who rely on food stamps
is that the assistance is not nearly enough to avoid serious shortages of
food during a typical month. Living in poverty and on public assistance
is both harsh and difficult. It is marked by an ongoing economic struggle
that becomes more acute by the end of the month. This ongoing struggle
is manifested in the reported constant companion of the Food Stamp
program—hunger.

The Stigma of Using Food Stamps.   A second claim typically made by
those receiving welfare in general, and food stamps specifically, is the
degree of perceived stigma in using these programs. Slightly over two-
thirds of the people that Rank interviewed reported specific instances of
feeling that they were treated differently by the general public when it
became known that they were receiving public assistance (Rank 1994a,
1994b). These occurrences ranged from blatant antagonism to more subtle forms of disapproval. The most frequently cited cases occurred with
the use of food stamps.

Several examples are illustrative. Janice Winslow, a 37-year-old separated mother of three, discusses the difficulties in using food stamps:

> You really do have to be a strong person to be able to use food stamps and
> not get intimidated by how people treat you when you use them. And
> even then it's still hard. You feel people's vibes, you know, in the line. And
> the checkout people are almost without exception rude, unless you really
> get to know them. And I always feel like, "God, I'll be glad when I don't
> have to use these." They never ever leave any change in there. So every
> time you check out, they always have to go up to the office to get change,
> so you got all these people waitin' in line—it's like, you know, "These food
> stamp people."
>
> Once about six weeks ago I turned to the woman behind me and said, "I
> don't know, I have not once come up here and bought something with
> food stamps where they didn't have to go and get change for, like a five or
> something, that they had in the drawer." She says, "Well, I guess it's just
> one of those ways that they're not making it easy for you."

A second example comes from a married couple who were asked if
they had noticed any difference in the grocery store when they used
food stamps:

> It's absolutely blatant in the stores. They'll smile and be chatting with you,

and then they see you pull out the food stamps—they just freeze up. And they scrutinize the food. I mean, I get really hyped. If it's a birthday or something, and I'm buying steak so that we can have a birthday dinner at home—ohh, the looks they get on their faces. Once I had a clerk tell me, "You buy really good food with your food stamps" (laughter). Jeez. Yeah, there is a difference.

Recipients may develop several strategies for dealing with the stigma of having to use food stamps. Some shop at off times or go to checkers whom they know personally. For example:

When I go to buy with food stamps, I try to go at night so not too many people get behind me. Especially when the employees ask about the I.D. And then they want to see one more I.D. And it's very, very uncomfortable. I guess I cannot be like other people that just carry their food stamps in their hands like money. I just . . . can't do that.

Similarly, Jody Edwards, a 23-year-old single parent, explains:

I try really hard to hit a day that nobody's gonna be at the store because I just get all flustered. I have a terrible time using my food stamps. Just hate it! Just hate it.

Others may go to stores where the use of food stamps is fairly common. For example, one rural woman often goes into the metropolitan area to shop instead of going to her rural neighborhood grocery store:

Well, when I went grocery shopping, I usually went to Ceders [a supermarket]. Because I figured a lot of people go in there and use 'em, you know, so I wouldn't feel out of place. Otherwise, it would look bad, and I still felt stupid.

Alternatively, recipients may send someone else to use their food stamps, or perhaps dress differently:

I feel like I have to be dressed really nice and look nice to use 'em. I don't wanna look all dumpy and look like I fit it [the image of a welfare recipient].

The use of food stamps is particularly hard for many individuals because it constitutes a stigma symbol—it identifies the user as a member of a stigmatized group (see Goffman 1963). Likewise, living in subsidized housing, the use of a Medicaid card, and so on, function as stigma symbols and hence cause various degrees of anxiety among welfare recipients.

If the strategy of concealment is impossible (as with the case of food stamps), then an attempt may be made to either minimize contact with the general public (when having to reveal one's welfare status), or to physically dissociate oneself from the image of a "typical" welfare recipient (by dressing according to middle class standards, watching what one buys in the supermarket, and so on). Consequently, a second overriding claim made by those who rely upon the food stamp program is the considerable degree of discomfort when using food stamps.

In summary, the ability of food stamps to combat hunger, from the recipient's point of view, is weakened by the fact that the assistance is not enough to purchase an adequate diet throughout the month. A second claim made by food stamp recipients is that when they do use the stamps, there is a psychological penalty to be paid as a result of the stigmatization surrounding the program. Not surprisingly, these claims are often reiterated by advocacy groups and agencies who work directly with the poor. The credibility and legitimacy of these claims rest upon the firsthand knowledge and direct experiences of recipients.

The Policy Analyst's View

From the perspective of the research policy analyst, statistical analysis has been the tool that has shaped and informed the discussion regarding the Food Stamp program. This research has relied heavily on large scale, demographic surveys involving low-income households and food stamp recipients. Such policy analysts are found primarily within federal government agencies or universities. They tend to have advanced degrees in economics, sociology, or public policy.

Although research policy analysts have explore several lines of inquiry (e.g., administrative costs, targeting accuracy, work incentives), a major issue that has largely framed the policy discussion has been that of participation or nonparticipation in the program. Much of this research has been sponsored by the United States Department of Agriculture (USDA), which oversees the Food Stamp program. For example, Carole Trippe and Pat Doyle begin their report's executive summary, which was prepared for the USDA's Food and Nutrition Service, with the following: "Policymakers are concerned about the extent to which the Food Stamp Program (FSP) serves its target population, as well as about which subgroups of the target population are more or less likely to participate in the program" (1992:vii). Likewise, the Food and Nutrition Service begins a report dealing with food stamp participation rates with the following: "The Food and Nutrition Service (FNS) has a keen interest in the extent to which Food Stamp Program (FSP) benefits reach those who are eligible for them. The participation rate—the ratio of the number of participants to the number of eligibles—provides a picture of a program's success in reaching this target population" (Trippe et al. 1992:ix).

One of the concerns from the policy analyst's perspective is that approximately 40 to 50% of the food stamp eligible population fail to participate in the program (see Committee on Ways and Means 1994). The impact of food stamps on combatting hunger is therefore substantially reduced, in that nearly one-half of low-income eligible households are not participating.

Rank and Hirschl have examined in detail this process of nonparticipation in the Food Stamp program (Hirschl and Rank 1991; Rank and Hirschl 1988, 1993). They argue that within the eligible population, participation in food stamps depends primarily on three factors. First, an individual must be aware that a program exists. Without such knowledge, participation is highly unlikely. Second, the individual must believe that he or she can qualify for the program; persons who know about a specific program but believe they are ineligible probably would not apply. Third, the individual must have the desire and ability to apply for public assistance. Consequently, even though individuals may be aware of a particular program and believe they are eligible, they may decide not to participate if they hold negative attitudes about the use of food stamps.

Rank and Hirschl then apply this model to explain why eligible households in rural areas are much less likely to participate than their counterparts in urban areas. They argue that the above three factors vary according to the degree of urbanity. The first two depend strongly on access to and exchange of accurate eligibility information. Welfare programs are not advertised; rather, most individuals learn about such programs through word of mouth or by other informal means. Such interactions are more likely to occur in densely populated areas, particularly because these areas often are segregated on the basis of class and race. Low-income households in urban areas are more likely than their rural counterparts to encounter other low-income households who have firsthand knowledge about the welfare system. Such interactions can make eligible persons more aware of the existence of welfare programs and can provide a rough gauge of the eligibility criteria.

In addition, increased interaction among low-income households resulting from population density can reduce some of the stigma and the adverse attitudes surrounding the use of public assistance. Proximity to other low-income individuals who receive welfare can reduce one's own disapproval through the firsthand knowledge that there are others who also need assistance. Indeed, although social stigma is attached to public assistance in both rural and urban areas, such disapproval has been shown in prior research to be greater in areas of lower population density. Rural residents are more likely to view those who accept public assistance as lazy and dishonest.

Rank and Hirschl's empirical tests confirm these hypotheses. Their statistical analyses lend strong support to the fact that households in rural areas use the Food Stamp program significantly less than households in urban areas. As hypothesized, the underlying mechanism behind this relationship is that individuals in rural areas hold less accurate eligibility information and more adverse attitudes toward the program. Both of these factors result in reduced use of the Food Stamp program.

Based upon these findings, and based upon the fact that poverty tends to be higher and more extreme in rural areas, Rank and Hirschl make the following claim:

> Consequently, where the need for welfare provision is greatest, the use of such programs is smallest. Our analysis has shown that participation in food stamps is not equal across geographic regions of the United States. This finding leads us to ask whether access is also unequal across different regions. We believe that equality of access should be a guiding principle of programs directed to low-income individuals. The stated purpose of such programs is to assist the needy; that need is felt in all regions of the country, but particularly in rural America. The irony is that where the need for food stamps is strong, so too is the inability to participate in the program. (1993:619)

Other policy analysts have analyzed additional population groups that have been underserved by the Food Stamp program. These have included the elderly (Cohen et al. 1993) and the homeless (Burt and Cohen 1988). The claims made by these researchers mirror the claims made by Rank and Hirschl. For example, Hollonbeck and Ohls (1984) summarize their findings in the following way:

> It is estimated that approximately half of the elderly persons who are eligible for food stamps fail to take advantage of the benefits to which they are entitled. The most important reason for their non-participation appears to be their uncertainty or lack of knowledge about program eligibility, suggesting that professionals who work with the elderly should encourage them to take the steps necessary to determine their possible eligibility. Perceived stigma and transportation barriers are also factors leading to non-participation for some elderly persons. (1984:616)

From this perspective, the ability of food stamps to reduce hunger is compromised by the fact that the program fails to reach 40 to 50% of the target population. Furthermore, various policy analysts point out that particular groups, such as those in rural areas, the elderly, or the home-less, face considerably more constraints and barriers in using the program than do other subgroups. Consequently, researchers such as Rank and Hirschl introduce into the policy discussion the claims of underutilization and unequal access to the Food Stamp program, limiting its effectiveness in reducing hunger for specific demographic groups in America. These policy analysts rely upon the rubric of "objective scientific" research to persuade their audiences that such claims are credible.

The General Public's View

A third key group involved in the Food Stamp program are those who ultimately pay the bill—the taxpaying general public. The public's view of welfare programs in general, and the Food Stamp program in particular, is predominately negative. Survey results during the past two decades indicate that the general public is quite hostile toward individuals and households relying on public assistance programs. Those receiving welfare are perceived as lacking in morality and ability, abusing the system, and so on (e.g., Feagin 1975; Kluegel and Smith 1986). For example, Kluegel and Smith's analysis of the general public's attitudes toward welfare recipients found "70–80% of respondents endorsing the common stereotypes that they are lazy and are dishonest about their need" (1986:152). Likewise, a recent *Times Mirror* poll on the subject found the following attitudes by the general public regarding welfare:

> A striking finding is that welfare is considered odious by every demographic subgroup in the survey. Fully 75% of respondents said the current welfare system changes things for the worse by making the recipient dependent on the government. Only 12% said it creates change for the better by helping those unable to support themselves, a figure that is less than the percentage of those who are now or were recipients of welfare. (1994:26)

What these survey results indicate is that a considerable amount of stigma and disgrace is attached to the use of public assistance programs (Camasso and Moore 1985; Horan and Austin 1974; Keith 1980; Moffitt 1983; Waxman 1983; Williamson 1974). One reason for this stigma is that the use of welfare tends to jar against the value of independence in which most Americans take pride (Gans 1988). Consequently, those who rely on government assistance for financial support (rather than on their own efforts) are perceived as failures. An example of this comes from a 1978 study by Coleman et al. In interviews conducted in Boston and Kansas City, respondents were asked who they felt constituted the lowest class in society.

The word used most often by our sample members to characterize the life
style and income source of people at the bottom was welfare . . . .The
principle enunciated . . . was that the welfare class and people at the
bottom are nearly synonymous terms, that any American for who welfare
has become a way of life is thereby to be accounted among the nation's
lowest-class citizens. (1978:195)

In addition, as Rank (1994a) argues, welfare recipients stand in sharp
contrast to the widely held American value of self-reliance and the
dream that the United States is a land where opportunities exist for all
who are willing to work for them. Rank writes:

In pointed contrast stand those who do not support themselves economically. Those who depend upon the government for their survival. Those
who are no longer self-reliant. In short, those whom we call welfare recipients. Because their predicaments are in sharp contradiction with the
American dream, we often look at them with disdain, blaming the individual for the problem. (1994a:201)

One of the frequently made claims by the general public regarding the
Food Stamp program is that its recipients abuse the system. This is
illustrated in the commonly told story of the welfare recipient who
drives up to the grocery store in a brand new Cadillac, proceeds to use
their food stamps to buy extravagant items like sirloin steak, and then
purchases alcohol or cigarettes with the leftover change.

As an illustration of this, the first author has had substantial experience with various talk radio programs around the country. He is occasionally asked to discuss the myths and realities of the welfare system
and its participants. The above claim and accompanying story are frequently recounted by those who call in to voice their opinions. As Joel
Best writes, "Claims often begin with dramatic examples . . . . Particular
cases often shape our sense of social problems, and claims-makers draw
attention to examples that seem to justify their claims" (1989:1, xx–xxi).

For instance, the following individual telephoned a syndicated radio
program in New Orleans as the first author and host were discussing the
welfare system. The caller came on the air and first made the claim that
welfare recipients were routinely abusing the system, and then illustrated it with a dramatic example:

You know, I've got a classic example. I've called before. I was at the tax
collector's office, or the assessor's office, tryin' to find out why my real
estate taxes are 350 dollars a month. I'm driving my four year old vehicle
with a six digit income, and across the street somebody's pullin' up to get
their food stamps in a brand new 1994 vehicle. Got a package of cigarettes
in their pocket. The store owners let 'em take these food stamps—they
buy a carton of milk—get cash for the rest of the money, go back and get

cigarettes, beer, whatever the heck they want. And they got kids that are starvin'. (Crescent City Connection 1994)

Obviously those who participate in talk radio do not represent a random sampling of the population, yet they do voice many of the same claims found in randomly conducted surveys. In addition, such claims and accompanying examples are occasionally expressed by those in political power. For example, when asked about the 1983 budget deficit, President Reagan responded with "a story about an unnamed young man in an unidentified grocery who used Food Stamps to pay for a single orange, then bought a bottle of vodka with the change" (Morganthau et al. 1982).

From the perspective of the general public, one of the major problems with welfare programs overall, and the Food Stamp program in particular, is that they work too well. They are viewed as providing attractive benefits that encourage people not to work as hard as they might, and to become increasingly dependent upon the government. Charles Murray has written positively about this "common sense" perspective:

> This popular wisdom, which is as prevalent today as it was then, is just that—the views to be heard in most discussions in most blue-collar bars or country-club lounges in most parts of the United States. It is the inarticulate constellation of worries and suspicions that helped account for Ronald Reagan's victory in 1980 . . . . The popular wisdom is characterized by hostility toward welfare (it makes people lazy). (1984:146)

Consequently, the claims often made by the general public regarding welfare overall and food stamps in particular have little to do with addressing specific needs such as hunger. Rather, they have to do with the perceived disincentives and abuses associated with the programs. These claimsmakers routinely use the example of the neighbor down the street who is abusing the system to validate their claims. These claims are also made by a variety of conservative politicians and think tanks, arguing that they are reflecting the public sentiment. The credibility and legitimacy of these claims rest upon the popular common sense appeal that welfare programs encourage laziness.

Discussion

The constructionist perspective suggests that social problems are shaped and defined by various groups making claims about them. Furthermore,

> Claims-makers inevitably hope to persuade. Typically, they want to con-

vince others that X is a problem, that Y offers a solution to that problem, or that a policy of Z should be adopted to bring that solution to bear. While the success of claims-making may well depend, in part, on the constellation of interests and resources held by various constituencies in the process, the way claims are articulated also affects whether they persuade and move the audiences to which they are addressed. (Best 1987:102)

In this chapter we have examined the claims of three different groups regarding the Food Stamp program and hunger—the recipients of the program, the analysts of the program, and the taxpayers of the program. Each group views the Food Stamp program and its goal of reducing hunger in a different light.

From the recipient's point of view, the program is lacking because it fails to provide an adequate amount of assistance to avert serious food shortages throughout the month. Furthermore, substantial psychological costs (in the form of perceived stigma) hinder the use of the program. First-hand knowledge provides the grounds on which these statements are based.

From the research policy analyst's perspective, the program's objective of reducing hunger is compromised by the fact that it statistically fails to reach approximately 40 to 50% of the eligible population. Likewise, particular groups in need, such as rural residents or the elderly, are even less likely to participate in the program, due to a lack of information and/or stigma surrounding the program. The claim of inequality of access is subsequently raised. Statistical research provides the grounds on which this argument is based.

From the general public's view, the Food Stamp program is regarded as severely flawed because it is perceived as violating several important American values, and it is believed to encourage abuse and dependence. It is thus looked upon with disdain. The problem is not with hunger, but with the program itself. By scaling back such "give away" programs, these claimmakers argue that people would work harder and avoid hunger all together. Appeals to common sense provide the grounds on which these statements are based.

Consequently, depending upon the group making the claim, the Food Stamp program provides too little assistance, too much assistance, or assists too few people. These three claims are routinely reported in the media. And it is in the media where the debate regarding legitimacy often takes place. As Schneider notes, "Social problems participants usually hope the news media will help them publicize claims and thus enhance their legitimacy" (1985:221).

An example illustrating all three claims can be found in a recent *Newsweek* story, "How Hungry is America?" mentioned at the beginning of this chapter (Shapiro 1994). The article centers around a study of hunger in America, conducted by Second Harvest (a nationwide network of food banks). They report the surprising finding that 1 of every 10 Americans make use of food pantries, soup kitchens, and other emergency food-distribution programs. The article begins with the story of Eileen, who recently lost her job and apartment.

> She and her 13-year-old daughter went on welfare and moved into public housing. In January, Eileen signed up for food stamps. "It's very humiliating," she says. Each month she gets $130 in food coupons, but now there are two weeks to go until the next allotment, and no food in the house. (58)

The article goes on to quote several individuals in agencies dealing directly with the poor. They support the claim that food stamps are not enough to survive on, thereby forcing people to turn to emergency assistance. Their first-hand knowledge is used for credibility—"people at the front lines of hunger relief say that the study confirms what they see daily" (58).

Midway, the story takes a different slant. It introduces the general public's claim of abuse in the welfare system. The author describes Theresa:

> At 30, she's been on welfare much of her life and feeds her four kids by faking residence in several Massachusetts towns, so that she can use their emergency food programs . . . . Often Theresa and her children take home so much food they end up feeding leftovers to the birds. Even the family's pet iguana is provided for: It gets shredded carrots and escarole. (59)

This claim is then given credence by quoting from a member of the Heritage Foundation (a conservative think tank), who provides the popular, common sense wisdom.

> "You could never spend your way out of this problem," says Robert Rector . . . who is a strong critic of federal antihunger programs. He maintains there is no evidence for widespread hunger or undernutrition in America, and dismisses the results of the Second Harvest study as a "pseudodefinition" of hunger. "The more programs you have that hand out food for free, the more people will use them," he says. (59)

Finally, the above quote is immediately followed by the policy analyst's claim that the problem lies in food stamps not reaching enough people.

> "There is some welfare fraud," agrees J. Larry Brown, director of the

Center on Hunger, Poverty and Nutrition Policy at Tufts University in Medford, Mass. But he believes it's the economy that prompts most people's visits to food programs, not their desire for free red gelatin. "We could end hunger in a matter of six or eight months," he says, by expanding the food-stamp program and increasing funding for such targeted programs as WIC (Special Supplemental Food Program for Women, Infants and Children). Research backs up Brown's view. (59)

The *Newsweek* story represents in a microcosm the three claims detailed earlier in this chapter regarding the Food Stamp program—that it provides too little assistance, too much assistance, or assists too few people. As Best writes, "many contemporary claimsmakers use the mass media to reach their audiences. If the press can be convinced that their claims are newsworthy, the media will spread their message" (1989:1). In this case, the message and accompanying grounds are quite different depending upon the group making the claim.

Yet there is one theme connecting all three claims—the importance of stigma. The general public attaches considerable stigma to welfare overall, to food stamps specifically, and to those who rely on the assistance. This is experienced first-hand by individuals using food stamps. Likewise, policy analysts report the importance of stigma in understanding why more eligible people do not use the program. In this sense, it would appear to be the general public that has successfully defined the parameters and boundaries of the debate.

References

Berry, J. M. 1984. *Feeding Hungry People: Rulemaking in the Food Stamps Program.* New Brunswick, NJ: Rutgers University Press.

Best, J. 1987. "Rhetoric in Claims-Making: Constructing the Missing Children Problem." *Social Problems* 34:101–121.

———. (ed.). 1989. *Images of Issues: Typifying Contemporary Social Problems.* Hawthorne, NY: Aldine de Gruyter.

Brown, J. L., and H. F. Pizer. 1987. *Living Hungry in America.* New York: New American Library.

Burt, M. R., and B. E. Cohen. 1988. "Feeding the Homeless: Does the Prepared Meals Provision Help?" Prepared for the U. S. Department of Agriculture, Food and Nutrition Service, October.

Camasso, M. J., and D. E. Moore. 1985. "Rurality and the Residualist Social Welfare Response." *Rural Sociology* 50:397–408.

Cohen, B. E., M. R. Burt, and M. M. Schulte. 1993. "Hunger and Food Insecurity Among the Elderly." Project Report. Washington, D. C.: The Urban Institute.

Coleman, R., L. Rainwater, and K. McClelland. 1987. *Social Standing in America: New Dimensions of Class.* New York: Basic Books.

Committee on Ways and Means, House of Representatives, U. S. Congress. 1994. *1994 Green Book.* Washington, D. C.: U. S. Government Printing Office.

Crescent City Connection. 1994. WWL Radio Station, New Orleans. June 9.

DeVault, M. L., and J. P. Pitts. 1984. "Surplus and Scarcity: Hunger and the Origins of the Food Stamp Program." *Social Problems* 31:545–557.

Feagin, J. R. 1975. *Subordinating the Poor: Welfare and American Beliefs.* Englewood Cliffs, NJ: Prentice-Hall.

Food Research and Action Center. 1991. *Community Childhood Hunger Identification Project: A Survey of Childhood Hunger in the United States.* Washington, D.C.: Food Research and Action Center.

Gans, H. 1988. *Middle American Individualism: The Future of Liberal Democracy.* New York: The Free Press.

Goffman, E. 1963. *Stigma: Notes on the Management of Spoiled Identity.* Englewood Cliffs, NJ: Prentice-Hall.

Hirschl, T. A., and M. R. Rank. 1991. "The Effect of Population Density on Welfare Participation." *Social Forces* 70:225–235.

Hollonbeck, D., and J. C. Ohls. 1984. "Participation Among the Elderly in the Food Stamp Program." *The Gerontologist* 24:616–621.

Horan, P., and P. Austin. 1974. "The Social Bases of Welfare Stigma." *Social Problems* 21:648–657.

Keith, P. M. 1980. "Demographic and Attitudinal Factors Associated with Perceptions of Social Welfare." *Sociology and Social Welfare* 7:561–570.

Kluegel, J. R., and E. R. Smith. 1986. *Beliefs about Inequality: Americans' Views of What Is and What Ought to Be.* Hawthorne, NY: Aldine de Gruyter.

MacDonald, M. 1977. "Food Stamps: An Analytical History." *Social Service Review* 51:642–658.

Miller, G., and J. A. Holstein (eds.). 1993. *Constructionist Controversies: Issues in Social Constructionist Theory.* Hawthorne, NY: Aldine de Gruyter.

Moffitt, R. 1983. "An Economic Model of Welfare Stigma." *American Economic Review* 73:1023–1035.

Morganthau, T., J. Buckley, D. Weathers, M. Achiron, and P. Abramson. 1982. "Reagan's Polarized America." *Newsweek* (April 5):17–19.

Murray, C. 1984. *Losing Ground: American Social Policy 1950–1980.* New York: Basic Books.

New York Times. 1992. "Study Hints of Hard Choice for Poor: Heat or Food." September 9:C20.

Ohls, J. C., and H. Beebout. 1993. *The Food Stamp Program: Design Tradeoffs, Policy, and Impacts.* Washington, D.C.: The Urban Institute Press.

Rank, M. R. 1994a. *Living on the Edge: The Realities of Welfare in America.* New York: Columbia University Press.

———. 1994b. "A View from the Inside Out: Recipients' Perceptions of Welfare." *Journal of Sociology and Social Welfare* 21:27–47.

———. 1988. "A Rural-Urban Comparison of Welfare Exits: The Importance of Population Density." *Rural Sociology* 53:190–206.

Rank, M. R., and T. A. Hirschl. 1993. "The Link between Population Density and Welfare Participation." *Demography* 30:607–622.

Schneider, J. W. 1985. "Social Problems Theory: The Constructionist View." *Annual Review of Sociology* 11:209–229.

Shapiro, L. 1994. "How Hungry is America?" *Newsweek* (March 14):58–59.

Simpson, P. 1990. "Living in Poverty: Coping on the Welfare Grant." Community Service Society Working Paper Series, Poverty Perspectives.

Spector, M., and J. I. Kitsuse. 1977. *Constructing Social Problems*. Menlo Park, CA: Cummings Publishing Company.

Times Mirror Center for the People and the Press. 1994. "Economic Recovery Has Little Impact on American Mood." News Release, April 6.

Trippe, C., and P. Doyle. 1992. "Food Stamp Program Participation Rates: January 1989." United States Department of Agriculture–Food and Nutrition Service.

Trippe, C., P. Doyle, and A. Asher. 1992. "Trends in Food Stamp Program Participation Rates: 1976 to 1990." United States Department of Agriculture–Food and Nutrition Service.

Waxman, C. I. 1983. *The Stigma of Poverty: A Critique of Poverty Theories and Policies*. New York: Pergamon Press.

Williamson, J. 1974. "The Stigma of Public Dependency: A Comparison of Alternative Forms of Public Aid to the Poor." *Social Problems* 22:213–228.

VII

Government Food Policies

12

Political Struggle over Scientific Definitions: Nutrition as a Social Problem in Interwar Norwegian Nutrition Policy

UNNI KJÆRNES

Introduction

What is nutrition policy all about? This has long been a matter of debate. This chapter will take the view that different definitions of nutrition as a social problem are expressed through specific positions in nutritional science. Moreover, it will argue that these positions are related to certain issues and conflict alignments on the political agenda. Most Western countries have established nutrition policies, but their form and extent are highly variable. The chapter deals with Norwegian nutrition policy in a historical perspective, focusing on the interwar period. It was during this period that nutrition emerged as a political issue in Norway. This period is also interesting in view of the development of the welfare state as well as agricultural policy and market regulation. Furthermore, it marks a shift in the history of nutritional science, accompanied by substantial changes in the understanding of nutritional problems. Therefore, this empirical case may provide a basis for discussing various ways of formulating nutritional problems as well as diverging policy strategies.

Inadequate nutrition is in the first place experienced as a problem for the individual, within the private sphere. When nutritional problems enter the political agenda it is because some actors also regard them as social problems that affect either all of society collectively or certain groups. They find this situation unacceptable and want some kind of action, most often in the form of state involvement.

In different policies, various actors have brought the issue to the political agenda: politicians and political parties, interest organizations, grassroots movements, etc. Nutrition scientists have a dominant role in the formulation of nutritional problems and nutrition policy. Conflicts in nutrition policy have often been expressed or made visible within a scientific context, in terms of conflicts between groups of experts. Therefore, the following questions will be discussed in this chapter: What were the most important ways in which scientific findings in nutrition were translated into social problems in the interwar period? How was science applied in policy making in Norway? What were the relationships between scientific and political conflict, and the consequences for policy formulation?

Defining Social Problems

Social Problems and Political Agenda Setting

It is important to recognize the subjective nature of social problems: "social problems are what people view as social problems" (Best 1989:xvi). This means a process in which people designate certain social conditions as social problems (Schneider and Kitsuse 1984:viii). The constructionist tradition has defined social problems as "the activities of individuals or groups making assertions of grievances and claims with respect to some putative conditions" (Spector and Kitsuse 1977:75).

Political scientists have dealt with agendas and political agenda setting in a rather parallel manner to social problems work by sociologists.[1] An agenda may be defined as "the list of subjects or problems to which governmental officials, and people outside government closely associated with those officials, are paying some serious attention at any given time" (Kingdon 1984:3). Policy making may be regarded as essentially a "definitional activity" in which policy actors select a particular definition of a problem as well as its solution from an array of alternatives (Zebich 1979:19). Identification and definition activities will usually involve conflicts between actors who want to "possess" the problem, to define the problem and the policy. "The definition of the alternatives is the supreme instrument of power" (Schattschneider 1975:66). According to Schattschneider (1975), the success of any given item on the agenda will be influenced by the powers, positions, and resources held by the various actors. The conflicts involving the most powerful actors, adhering to existing basic alignments and with many people drawn into the conflict, will most likely end up on the agenda and get the most attention.

This means that problems and conflicts emerging from less established alignments and less influential actors will have greater difficulty in becoming a part of the political agenda. To obtain support for policies aimed at common interests, it is necessary to establish alliances and to arouse public attention. When public attention is drawn to a conflict, the result is highly dependent upon reactions of the *"third parties,"* often the public or the state. Their response will provide the conflict with a public arena and give publicity to the issue, as well as protect the weaker part. Furthermore, measures can be taken to solve the problems. From this perspective it is easier to understand why issues are brought onto the public agenda—or rather why some actors try to do so.

However, only a small number of social problems are successful in receiving public attention. Therefore, there will always be competition (Hilgartner and Bosk 1988). Actors are involved in a continuous struggle over the agenda, to have their specific issues defined as the most important, their problems as the largest crisis. It is a "conflict over conflicts" (Schattschneider 1975). Second, within each substantive area, there is competition over definitions, between alternative ways of framing the problem. While the ability to choose reflects power, the choice of conflict and definitions also distributes power. New definitions of alternatives may change conflict alignments completely. On the other hand, in the process of expansion through public attention and alliances, *the scope* will inevitably change. "A change of scope makes possible a new pattern of competition, a new balance of forces and a new result . . . but it also makes impossible a lot of other things" (Schattschneider 1975:17). The agenda may gain attention and acceptance, but a number of solutions to the problems may become impossible or irrelevant.

Science and Social Problems

Scientists may be viewed as political actors competing over how to define a social problem. Aronson has discussed science as an arena for the construction of social problems, which seems useful also in a policy formulation context (Aronson 1984a). Aronson starts with internal relations, the interaction among scientists. She terms claims about findings to other members of the research community *cognitive claims*. In external relations, the interaction of scientists with nonscientists, science serves as an ongoing arena for the social construction of social problems. Scientists' claims to outsiders refer to the broader implications of research findings for the particular concerns of the nonspecialist audience. These,

Aronson terms *interpretative claims*. Two types of interpretative claims could be distinguished within this context. One type is expert advice, where claims are made in the light of administratively defined objectives and contingencies. A second form asserts the existence of a social problem that a particular scientific specialty is uniquely equipped to solve.[2] The cognitive claims of scientists give rise to specific social problem interpretative claims. In a study of leukemia research Aronson finds several major approaches (Aronson 1984b). Scientists representing each approach to leukemia made competing cognitive and interpretative claims, each represented by a different type of expertise. On the basis of its own definition of biological cause (cognitive claim), each group made a different recommendation (social problem interpretative claim) for government intervention to solve what was seen as the "social problem" of leukemia. Such differences are readily understandable. Within a whole range of interdependent factors influencing the problem, each specialized group of scientists will interpret evidence in terms of its own narrow concerns. These concerns include their own ability to influence the situation. In other words, the alternatives seen by the scientist will be influenced by professional interests as well as by the setting in which interpretative claims are made.

Nutrition Science and Problem Formulation

Different ways of formulating nutrition as a social problem, a problem that should attract attention, have distinct consequences for the policy outcome. One aim of this chapter is to identify such differing approaches in nutrition research. In turn, I want to discuss links between these differences, items on the political agenda, and the resulting policy formulation.

However, I will first discuss how science per se has had various implications for how food is conceived as a social problem, for food policies, and social policies in the interwar period. Scientific arguments implied that people—or politicians—could not decide by themselves what is adequate nutrition: experts had become central. One had to *know* the contents and properties of the food (Levenstein 1988). Second, the importance of dietary composition has made it relevant to assess and become involved in individual behavior and private life in a detailed manner. In the Scandinavian countries, this involvement on behalf of the common interest fits into a pattern in which society and expertise have sought to change family life so as to create "the good life" through elaborate systems of public policy (policies of family, nutrition, welfare, education, etc.) (Hirdman 1990; Kjærnes and Jensen 1994).

A scientific understanding of nutritional problems has also had other consequences. Developing norms (recommendations) on nutrient intakes and proper diets has been a central aim of studies of the linkage between dietary habits and health. For most application purposes, this knowledge has to be translated into dietary advice (Botten and Kjærnes 1987). Such recommendations state that some foods are more healthy than others—resulting in a priority list, with immediate consequences for the market (Levenstein 1988). In this way, translating scientific findings into recommendations and policy goals becomes an important part of the process of policy formulation in which not only scientists, but also market actors, are involved. The formulation of interpretative claims becomes an arena in which conflicts between different economic interests unfold, as well as between suppliers and consumers. By extending the conflict with new actors and new arguments, the scope of the issue must be expected to change. The final outcome may not necessarily be in accordance with the original ambitions of those who first brought up the issue.

Problem Definitions and Policy Changes: The Case of Norway

Prewar Nutrition Research in Norway

Ever since nutrition was recognized as a research subject just before the turn of the century, nutrition scientists and nutrition research institutions in Norway have generally been an integral part of the international scientific community. The start took place gradually within established medical research institutions, unlike, for example, early nutrition research in the United States, where it was developed as a new branch of applied agricultural research (Aronson 1982; Levenstein 1988). From the 1890s, there was some scientific debate on nutritional topics, but high visibility and intense debate emerged only during World War I.

During the initial phase of nutrition research, most questions (cognitive claims) concerned the adequacy of food and the need for protein.[3] Studies concentrated on experimental balance studies (i.e., analyses of nutrient intake vs. excretion and body weight changes) and chemical analyses. Health consequences were discussed primarily in terms of working capacity (measured as oxygen uptake). A second phase of nutrition research started when biochemists detected essential micronutrients just before World War I. The concept of "vitamin," first introduced in 1912, led to a completely new understanding of nutrition. Whereas nutrition formerly had been regarded as a quantitative question, the new perspective underlined the qualitative aspects of diet: dietary composition (Levenstein 1988;

Rustung 1940). It was now recognized that a quantitatively adequate diet could have poor nutritional quality, perceived as low vitamin content. Increasingly, scientists came to understand health consequences as specific deficiency diseases. Moreover, growth and the more general effects in relation to resistance to infections were given greater emphasis. Accordingly, recommendations were now to relate to "optimal" needs that could promote good health, rather than to "minimum" needs for survival as previously had been the case.

Nutrition research was first taken up in Norway by physiologists and hygienists (Falkum and Larsen 1981; Reichborn-Kjennerud et al. 1936). The Department of Physiology at the University of Oslo was a major contributor to basic research in nutrition related to needs of energy-providing nutrients, metabolism, etc. (called "nutrition physiology").[4] Here the main approach was laboratory and clinical studies. Hygienists in Norway were also concerned with diet and nutrition as part of living conditions. Their contributions were partly in the form of dietary and anthropometric surveys, and partly through their role as health reformers (Falkum and Larsen 1981:180).

Physiologists worked within the framework of minimum needs investigated through balance studies of individuals: what is needed to survive? Hygienists, on the other hand, concentrated on better knowledge of normal body processes, especially growth, something that required large samples and data that were collected and evaluated in a standardized manner. A general call was to improve the "quality of the population."[5] This new orientation became especially evident after the end of World War I (Erichsen 1993).

How to define nutritional needs and dietary recommendations was a matter of major controversy among nutrition scientists, which illustrates the association between cognitive and interpretative claims. In Norway, this resulted in highly differing perceptions of nutrition as a social problem. Scurvy was traditionally a common ailment among Norwegian sailors. Physiologists and hygienists had diverging views on its cause (Reichborn-Kjennerud et al. 1936:226). Sofus Torup, a professor of physiology, believed that the cause was a monotonous diet and a chronic low-grade poisoning from inadequately preserved foods. His proof was that scurvy had not occurred during Fritjof Nansen's polar expeditions, where Torup had planned the food provisions. Axel Holst, professor of hygiene, and Theodor Frœlich, a pediatrician, on the other hand, had performed studies of what they called "ship beri-beri," which indicated a specific dietary deficiency. Their results were presented in 1907, and the studies later contributed to the identification of vitamin C. Torup eventually had to revise his views. However, these differences in recognition of the role of vitamins persisted for several decades (Langfeldt 1933). Later in the

1930s, however, scientific controversies were to become far more moderate. Evaluations and statements then seem to refer to a shared basis of scientific knowledge (Evang and Hansen 1937; Statens Kostholdsnemd 1940). That this shift must be understood within a political context will be the topic of the following section.

Nutrition as a Social Problem

Three major types of perspectives related to nutritional science may be pointed out concerning social problem claims. The first is that malnutrition is not a major problem. The second is that malnutrition is a problem of great significance, linked to structural features in society, and that measures should aim at relieving poverty. The third perspective involves acknowledging problems of nutrition, but regarding them as a question of individual lack of knowledge and motivation. Whereas the first position was clearly associated with claims of minimum needs, the other positions emerged from the recognition of nutritional quality and optimal needs.

In the 1920s and 1930s, an attitude common among physiologists seems to have been that nutrition was important as a scientific topic, and that scientific knowledge could be applied, for example, in product development and planning of diets (for war provisioning, institutions, ship provisions, etc.). As these scientists saw minimal physiological needs, the general diet was sufficient. They did not consider the extent and types of nutritional problems to be sufficiently acute to call for public action (Statens Kostholdsnemd 1940:62). Nutrition was *not seen as a social problem*. Nutritional well-being was primarily an individual responsibility in which the government should be involved only to ensure that subsistence needs were met. To the extent that problems other than lack of scientific documentation did exist, these concerned the lack of knowledge and motivation and poor morale on the part of the general population. While these views of very limited and strict social policy measures reflected ideas of the nineteenth century, they were greeted with renewed interest during the economic recession of the early 1930s (Seip 1987).

The opposite position, highly visible in the political debate on nutrition in the 1930s, held nutritional problems to be central, linked to widespread poverty and unemployment; malnutrition was regarded as a *problem of welfare*. The causes of nutritional problems were seen as inadequate economic or practical opportunities. This in turn would indicate a need for redistribution measures, in the form of social security or public services. This perspective could be found first in Norway's social-democratic Labor Party and in other groups on the political left. Presumably it was the welfare aspects that made nutrition interesting as a political issue. Scientific arguments were also important, and socialist physicians, with Karl Evang as a leading figure, were central to the process (Jensen 1991). Karl Evang and his associates performed a study of the diet among unemployed and other low-income groups that concluded that nutritional quality was closely linked to income, and that for many it was scarcely possible to obtain a nutritionally adequate diet according to (British) nutritional recommendations (Evang and Hansen 1937).[6] This problem was most severe in families with many children. Here per capita income was lower, while children had greater need for the more expensive protective foods. Evang mounted an attack on public authorities and the level of poor relief.

Another group of experts also presented social problem claims linked to the welfare perspective. Since the 1880s, economists and statisticians had been undertaking studies of household income, consumption, and expenditure in Norway. The problem in focus was primarily poverty, but for a long time nutrition was not used as a yardstick. In the 1930s, the orientation of economists changed radically from Liberal to Keynesian theory. Economists also took an interest in income inequality as evaluated by nutritional norms, applying a concept of "standard of living" in which food constituted a major part. A "nutritional standard" was developed, with nutritional needs (according to optimal norms) forming the basis. These standards (including housing, clothing, etc.) were in turn incorporated into a huge macroeconomic planning model that embraced production as well (Wold 1941). However, while left-wing physicians and politicians focused on economic redistribution measures, economists were more open to other measures, such as relief in kind and food as part of public services. They saw these measures as more direct and therefore more effective (Wold 1938).

The third perspective, regarding nutrition as *a problem of knowledge and behavior*, views the main problem as the lack of sufficient knowledge and motivation to buy, prepare, and serve food that is healthy. Often this perspective has been linked to the household task of planning an acceptable diet with limited financial means. Contrary to the welfare-oriented understanding, nutrition and diet are here individual responsibilities. A focus on housewives and their knowledge of nutrition was common to all groups of experts, who moreover agreed on the element of lack of motivation. Hygienists relied mainly on this approach. Unlike their British and U.S. colleagues, many Norwegian hygienists did somewhat agree that nutrition was a welfare problem by acknowledging income as an important reason for inadequate nutrition among the poor (Falkum and Larsen 1981). Their own epidemiological surveys revealed such connections. But they did not make any social problem claims on this. Instead, they relied on measures under their own control, such as education (Kjærnes 1989).

In contrast to Britain, Norway had no centralized health administration supervising the health situation and health services in this period (Erichsen 1993). Measures such as school medical examinations and school meals[7] emerged piecemeal on the local level. Hygienists developed their ideas with a close association between scientific ideas and practical reforms. Their role in nutrition was hardly visible in the political debate. Socialist physicians, on the other hand, believed in a centralized administrative system in which health, together with other concerns, was to be incorporated into large planning models and coordinated strategies.

All these perspectives concern nutrition and well-being in relation to food consumption patterns. Soon other aspects were to become significant. The interwar years saw a severe economic crisis, especially in agriculture. A common call, agreed on by most parties and groups, was to "buy Norwegian." This was also the attitude of all expert groups referred to above. Norwegian products should be preferred by housewives as well as by public authorities (for meals in institutions, poor relief in kind, etc.). From mid-1930s, the combination of health demands and production demands was to be developed into a more coordinated approach.

Food supply is generally a question of meeting market demands, without considering nutritional needs. But nutrition may also be regarded as a *problem of supply*. Nutritional problems may be understood as the outcome of a food market that does not satisfy the needs of the population. Deficiency can be explained by too low or wrong production in relation to calculated "needs" for specific food items, or because of other conditions that influence supply and demand. The challenge thus became to introduce market regulations that could stimulate production and distribution of the foods needed. Scarcely surprising is the fact that market actors were in favor of this approach. Its strongest advocates, however, were experts who had already been concerned with structural perspectives related to nutrition: leftist physicians and planning-oriented economists.

Subsistence *versus* Optimal Health

So far, various social problem definitions have been treated separately. The political agenda and the emergence of nutrition policy were, however, strongly influenced by the positions of the claimsmakers, the involvement of other actors, and general political events. A highly visible controversy in 1935 came to represent a schism, a change of domination over the political agenda—from minimalist-oriented physiologists and status quo defending civil servants, to the advocates of a broad policy of welfare and redistribution. This conflict was expressed as a scientific controversy, but had clear political overtones and consequences (Kjærnes 1990). A similar debate was underway in Britain (Webster 1982), and both sides in Norway referred to British expertise to support their views.

Since World War I, the Department of Physiology at the University of Oslo acted as advisors for public authorities in nutritional matters. In 1932 the Ministry of Justice (under the then Agrarian Party government) tasked the Department to develop food lists to be used as a basis for distribution of poor relief in municipalities that had gone bankrupt and depended on governmental support. The aim of poor relief was to ensure subsistence, at the same time keeping costs as low as possible. This led to intense and open conflict with other experts and with the political left—on scientific conclusions concerning needs, on the existence of nutrition problems, on food requirements of the poor, and on the responsibility to be taken by public authorities. The Department disregarded any claims related to dietary diversity or enjoyment; even the extra needs of children were regarded with distrust (Medicinsk Selskap 1935).

Karl Evang and his associates took a different position. First, minimum needs were not acceptable as a frame of reference. The unemployed could not be expected to "lead a life completely at rest" (Medicinsk Selskap 1935: 138). And, furthermore, "we know that such a dietary reduction will lead to considerable lowering of working capacity, and that it is not compatible with a normal physical development of children. Such a low standard would therefore be unjustifiable as a measure of the needs of those depending on relief in this country" (Medicinsk Selskap 1935:144). This view was supported by hygienists like Carl Schiœtz. The socialist physicians went further, stressing that food was a basic source of pleasure and well-being: "Nutrition is surely a very important factor among other measures which should be undertaken in order to maintain the joy of life" (Medicinsk Selskap 1935:196).

Politically this meant a departure from the principle of mere subsistence, which had implied that the responsibility of society and public authorities was limited to preventing starvation. The new idea was to ensure optimal health. The critique aroused considerable attention in the media and in political circles (Nordby 1989). With some modification, the left wing perspective won the battle, while the minimalist approach lost most of its legitimacy (Kjærnes 1990).

Dietary surveys, debate, and inspiration from countries such as Sweden and England were soon to expand the issue.[8] By using "objec-

tive standards" as a basis for evaluating consumption, nutrition problems were linked to poverty as such. This extension was made explicit
by Evang and Hansen (1937:133). In Norway as well as in international
fora (ILO League of Nations) nutrition thus became linked to demands
for improved living conditions for the working class and for the unemployed (ILO 1936). Nutrition as a welfare demand implied a considerable
expansion of the understanding of needs, including the possibility of
maintaining a traditional or socially acceptable diet, sensory quality, etc.
Moreover, the welfare perspective involved concern for distribution and
social inequality, as well as a departure from degrading or stigmatizing
measures. Nutrition as a welfare demand thus implies that the use of
scientific knowledge is turned upside down, as arguments for expanding,
rather than limiting, wage demands and public social security. This was in
contrast both to the practice of Norwegian Poor Laws and to the approach
of nutritional expertise. On the other hand, the debate strengthened the
widespread belief in science as a basis for designing the good life through
some kind of "rational diet" (Kjærnes and Jensen 1994).

Nutrition on the Political Agenda: A Change of Scope

Nutrition emerged on the political agenda as a question of welfare and
social distribution, linked to central economic demands in social democracy and the labor movement. This redefinition of nutrition as a social
problem took place in a period when the general attitude in society was
positive to science and scientifically based progress (Seip 1989). "Scientific eating" was in the interwar years a matter of both great optimism—
a solution to social problems—and deep conflict, an issue of intense
controversy. But there was more to it than merely a scientific reorienta-
tion. New aspects were soon added, and the focus changed. The relationship between nutrition and food production became increasingly
evident when the need for special foods could be documented. Milk, for
example, was "needed" for its vitamin content (Kjærnes 1993). The political breakthrough for a nutrition policy came when welfare perspectives
became linked to production.

This implied a new and active role for the state. Planning was a central
instrument, emerging as a trademark of Norway's social democracy
(Østerud 1975). Nutrition proved a very useful instrument in this planning policy. Its scientific, calculable basis could easily be included in the
"standard of living" concept so central in the early development of social
democratic welfare policy. Nutrition could also provide direct links to
production (Wold 1941). Improved welfare could be obtained while at
the same time supporting a crisis-ridden industry. A focus on rural

poverty[9] could also improve the electoral basis of the Labor Party in these groups.

According to the new ideas, different interests were to join hands in common efforts toward a more rational use of production resources, while at the same time improving the general welfare of the population. In this period, agriculture experienced severe problems of surplus, falling prices, and debt crisis. Farmers traditionally had a firm basis in Norwegian politics through a political party and strong interest organizations, and this position was further strengthened in the interwar period. Nutrition became a useful argument for increased state support to agriculture and regulated prices on agricultural produce. This was given further support when economists claimed that through public policy, agricultural surplus could be used to satisfy needs beyond the existing market demand (Frisch 1941). Here dairy products were at the center of attention (Kjærnes 1993). There was hunger in the midst of surplus. Calculations of total "needs" according to the new norms showed that production should be increased.

Toward the end of the 1930s a strong and highly understandable alliance was established between nutrition and agriculture. However, in this process of establishing a nutrition policy, which—notably—took place just before and immediately after World War II, problem definitions in nutrition policy also changed, from welfare to food supply. Poverty problems almost vanished from the agenda. This can be explained only partly by increased incomes and established social measures. It was in this context that ideologically it was no longer considered appropriate to discuss social inequality, injustice, etc. After World War II the welfare perspective disappeared among experts as well as in nutrition policy. Several measures were no longer regarded as relevant, were deemphasized (such as school meals), or were delinked from nutrition policy, such as consumer subsidies. The supply perspective did, however, prevail: nutrition was defined mainly as a problem of planning supplies; production was insufficient for certain foods, especially dairy products. Karl Evang, now Director General of Health, was a particular exponent of this shift of emphasis. The "nutrition physiology" community, on the other hand, remained skeptical to this close alliance with "the milk lobby."

Institutionalization

The selection of strategies and political alliances has consequences for the structure and organization of a policy. A nutrition policy concentrating on services, such as school meals and other measures of public food distribution, would probably lead to an administrative apparatus for implementing a special law and developing a team of specialists. No such policy was established, however. Instead welfare was to be ensured through general programs of economic redistribution. A policy focused on knowledge would need a body to formulate and communicate information at the central, and possibly also the local level. Such a system was in fact established, as part of home economics and consumer education (Kjærnes 1989). But this was not what was regarded as a nutrition policy body.

Norwegian nutrition policy was formulated and institutionalized within the setting of seeking nutritional goals through cooperation and planning (Kjærnes 1990). Its structure clearly set out the relationship between the actors, involving all "concerned parties": various producer interests, nutrition scientists, and, in the beginning, economists (Lien 1990). Consumers, however, were not regarded as a "concerned party," so they were not included in the organization that was established. A first proposal for a coordinating body came up in 1938.[10] A National Nutrition Council organized according to these principles was established in 1946. Its role was mainly to provide advice in administrative and political questions related to agriculture, planning of production, etc. This type of policy did not require a large administration, special measures, or the development of a nutrition profession. The Council provided a forum for the presentation of food production figures, an exchange of information, and last, but not least, negotiations over policy views and strategies. The supply orientation and the structure made the policy an integrated part of the vast agricultural corporative system of committees and councils.[11]

The organization of nutrition policy was highly divergent from other parts of the health and social sector. Other programs of health prevention— medical examinations, individual counseling and dietary (or medical) treatment—have not been part of, or even associated with, nutrition policy in Norway, although this type of nutrition-related work had already been established, for example, in the form of mother and child centers.

Discussion

The consequences of the interwar economic depression on nutrition are contested.[12] The topic was a matter of intense controversy in contemporary academic and political debate. In focus were cognitive claims made by various groups of scientists related to the understanding of nutritional needs. Together with the distinction between different types of interpretative claims, these concepts have helped to characterize the differences between groups of scientists concerning nutrition as a social problem.

However, problem definition is a dynamic process, including several actors who influence each other. The academic debate, the differences in cognitive claims, was at that time between the traditional physiological approach and the newer biochemical and epidemiological approaches of the hygienists. Neither of these groups, however, had any urgent need to attract attention and claims for governmental intervention concerning nutrition as a social problem. Whereas the physiologists remained loyal to the government, the hygienists had a very different arena for promoting their cause, the municipal health care system. Actors other than those directly related to the nutritional science community were decisive in bringing nutrition to the political agenda. These other actors, socialist physicians in particular, also actively made reference to science in their claimsmaking. However, these new actors used science to show that nutrition was a social problem of large proportions. Drama was added to the conflict (Hilgartner and Bosk 1988). An intense conflict over poor relief developed. According to Schattschneider (1975) the conflict was socialized, becoming known and visible and attracting new groups.

In seeking support for state involvement, new alliances were made. The political situation linked nutrition to yet another major conflict: the economic crisis in agriculture. Nutrition thus became a major issue involving many actors, one that was linked to an important contemporary conflict alignment. With new actors and alliances, the scope changed, and with them the framing of the problem of nutrition. Nutritional inadequacy was turned into a problem of supplies and marketing. Prominence was accorded new arguments of support to national food production (to solve the farmers' problems of sale, thereby improving their living conditions), while the question of public responsibility for the poor and unemployed receded into the background. New conflict alignments formed a new scope, and former arguments and former conflicts became irrelevant.

The legitimacy and confidence of established nutritional science are considerable, and nutrition experts have an evident and strong position in nutrition policy. While the relationship between science, expertise, and public policy has been studied in a number of fields (see, for example, Fischer 1990; Jasanoff 1990), little attention has been paid to the field of nutrition—although social consequences of different policy goals and strategies are considerable. Moreover, most studies have been performed in a North American setting. Scandinavia offers an opportunity for studies of similar issues in very different types of societies. Although goals in the form of health and well-being may be similar, the role and structure of public policy are quite different.

The conflict over nutrition in relation to poverty and public responsibility is classical in societies where basic needs are not met. One question is related to responsibility: whether poor nutrition is a matter of individual motivation and morale or whether people are victims of larger social processes that should be regulated through public policy. However, a central question found here was not whether malnutrition was related to social inequality—that was self-evident—but rather the norms and criteria to be used to evaluate the nutritional situation among the poor. Recommendations aiming at optimal nutrition led to a conclusion of malnutrition as a large and pressing social problem, while those based on a minimum for survival did not. The level of recommendations became an important issue of scientific, as well as political, conflict, dominating the question of cause. The cleavages had a clear relationship to a political left–right dimension. While the first question showed a continuity from social policy controversies in the late nineteenth century, the latter question of norms was closely related to the emergence of modern nutritional expertise, and it came up somewhat later in Norway than in, for example, the United Kingdom or the United States. While the point of departure, the size and causes of nutrition as a poverty problem, was similar to conflicts over nutrition in other countries, the following development was closely related to the specific Norwegian debate and the positions of the different actors.

The harmony that developed on the issue of nutrition may explain the (seemingly) new agreement on nutritional recommendations. The introduction of new powerful actors was followed by a change of scope and a redefinition of nutrition as a social problem. The new relationship between groups of scientists and the changing attitudes toward nutritional recommendations showed that this had consequences for the scientific community and cognitive claimsmaking. From 1935, different scientific views tended to merge into a common agreement on scientifically developed "optimal" standards for nutrition, linked with the firm belief that science could solve social problems—"above" politics and conflicts of interest. Accordingly, topics related to social class inequality were deemphasized. The belief in coordinated, harmony based solutions, that all Norwegians should join in common efforts to build a welfare society, was further strengthened when the National Nutrition Council was established soon after the end of World War II. In the postwar period, the setting obstructed a redefinition that turned the problems upside-down, questioning excessive intakes of certain nutrients (fats) as well as the close alliance with agriculture.

Notes

1.   An agenda may be defined as "the list of subjects or problems to which governmental officials, and people outside government closely associated with those officials, are paying some serious attention at any given time" (Kingdon 1984:3).

2. A third form highlights the importance of science as a general cultural resource, seeking ideological support for all of science as an end in itself. These claims generally seek to justify both expenditures of science and the autonomy of science.

3. There is no written history of nutrition research in Norway. Several books and articles deal with the topic in other countries (for example, Aronson 1982, 1989; Hirdman 1983; Jones 1986; Levenstein 1988; McCollum et al. 1939).

4. A professorship in nutrition ("nutrition physiology") was established as a result of a donation from the industrialist Johan Throne Holst early in the 1930s. A decade later he formed a foundation that led to the establishment of a Department of Nutrition at the University (Rudeng 1989:345).

5. In Norway, professor of hygiene Carl Schiøetz was a central proponent for this tradition, performing large-scale anthropometric studies of children.

6. Evang made explicit reference to recent British studies, especially that of Sir John Boyd Orr Evang et al. (1937:9).

7. Schiøetz was a well-known reformer of the school meals system.

8. There were close links between Norwegian and other European nutrition scientists—through scientific journals and conventions, personal contacts, and, eventually, also through representation in international advisory bodies.

9. Inadequate diets were found to be especially frequent among agricultural laborers and cottagers (Evang and Hansen 1937).

10. An ad hoc body tasked with adjusting food consumption, so that nutritional needs could be met in times of war, was established in 1939. Its plans were probably important for the relatively good nutrition situation maintained in occupied Norway during World War II (Statens Kostholdsnemd 1940; Strøm 1948).

11. Other alternative forms of organization have also been presented. The first National Nutrition Council established in 1937 was an expert body, aimed at advising public authorities on these matters. The representative council that eventually was established kept this function in a special subcommittee for nutrition (Kjærnes 1990).

12. See, for example, Webster (1982).

References

Aronson, N. 1982. "Nutrition as a Social Problem: A Case Study of Entrepreneurial Strategy in Science." *Social Problems* 29:474–487.

————. 1984a. "Science as a Claims-making Activity: Implications for Social Problems Research." Pp. 1–30 in *Studies in the Sociology of Social Problems*, edited by J. W. Schneider and J. I. Kitsuse. Norwood, NJ: Ablex.

————. 1984b. "Comment on Bryan Turner's 'The Government of the Body: Medical Regimens and the Rationalization of Diet'." *British Journal of Sociology* 35:62–65.

————. 1989. "Why Weren't Vitamins Discovered Earlier?" *Knowledge and Society* 8:87–105.

Best, J. (ed.). 1989. *Images of Issues: Typifying Contemporary Social Problems*. Hawthorne, NY: Aldine de Gruyter.

Botten, G., and U. Kjærnes. 1987. "Behov for Mat og ¢nske om Matvarer." *Scandinavian Journal of Nutrition* 4:116–120.

Erichsen, V. 1993. "The Health of the School Child? An Historical Comparison of Inspection Schemes in Britain and Norway." *Dynamis Acta Hispanica ad Medicinae Scientiarumque Historiam Illustrandam* 13:29–53.

Evang, K., and O. G. Hansen. 1937. *Norsk Kosthold i Små Hjem.* Oslo: Tiden.

Falkum, E., and Ø. Larsen. 1981. *Helseomsorgens Vilkår: Linjer i Medisinsk Sosialhistorie.* Oslo-Bergen-Troms¢: Universitetsforlaget.

Fischer, F. 1990. *Technocracy and the Politics of Expertise.* Newbury Park, CA: Sage.

Frisch, R. 1941. "Sosial¢konomiske Problemer ved Kostholdet." Pp. 1–23 in *Kosthold og Levestandard. En ¢konomisk Unders¢kelse,* edited by K. G. Wold. Oslo: Fabritius & S¢nners Forlag.

Hilgartner, S., and C. L. Bosk. 1988. "The Rise and Fall of Social Problems: A Public Arenas Model." *American Journal of Sociology* 94:53–78.

Hirdman, Y. 1983. *Magfrågan: Mat Som Mål och Medel Stockholm 1870–1920.* Stockholm: Rabén & Sjögren.

_____. 1990. *Att Lägga Livet Till Rätta - Studier i Svensk Folkhemspolitik.* Stockholm: Carlsson Bokförlag.

ILO. 1936. *Workers' Nutrition and Social Policy.* International Labour Office, Studies and Reports, Series B (Social and Economic Conditions) No. 23. London: P. S. King & Son, Ltd.

Jasanoff, S. 1990. *The Fifth Branch: Science Advisers as Policymakers.* Cambridge: Harvard University Press.

Jensen, T. ø. 1991. *The Political History of Norwegian Nutrition Policy.* Presented at the 2nd Biennial Conference, International Commission for Research into European Food History: The Origins and Development of Food Policy in Europe. Brunel University, Uxbridge.

Jones, G. 1986. *Social Hygiene in Twentieth Century Britain.* London: Croom Helm.

Kingdon, J. W. 1984. *Agendas, Alternatives, and Public Policies.* Boston: Little, Brown.

Kjærnes, U., 1989. "Ernæring, Næring og Forbrukerne." Pp. 36–45 in *Forbruksforskning. I Går - i Dag og i Morgen,* edited by E. Bergan, T. Bergh, B. N. Fjeldheim, et al. Lysaker, Norway: National Institute for Consumer Research.

_____. 1990. *Velferdskrav og Landbrukspolitikk: Om Framveksten av Norsk ernæringspolitikk.* SIFO Report No. 7. Oslo: National Institute for Consumer Research.

_____. 1993. "A Sacred Cow: The Case of Milk in Norwegian Nutrition Policy." Pp. 91–106 in *Regulating Markets–Regulating People: On Food and Nutrition Policy,* edited by U. Kjærnes, L. Holm, M. Ekström, et al. Oslo: Novus Forlag.

Kjærnes, U., and T. Ø. Jensen. 1995. "Political Dilemmas of Designing the Good Life—the Case of Nutrition and Social Democracy." In *Constructing the New Consumer Society,* edited by J. Holmwood, H. Radner, G. Schulze, and P. Sullivan. New York: MacMillan.

Langfeldt, E. 1933. "Plan for Kostholdet i Norge Bygget På Landets Egen Produksjon." *Stats¢konomisk Tidsskrift* 47:77–94.

Levenstein, H. A. 1988. *Revolution at the Table. The Transformation of the American Diet*. New York: Oxford University Press.

Lien, M. 1990. *Kunsten å Gjøre Alle til Lags: Statens Ernæringsråd i Norsk Ernæringspolitikk*. SIFO Report No. 5. Oslo: National Institute for Consumer Research.

McCollum, E. V., E. Orent-Keiles, and H. G. Day. 1939. *The Newer Knowledge of Nutrition*, 5th ed. New York: Macmillan.

Medicinsk Selskap. 1935. *Forhandlinger i Det Norske Medicinske Selskab*. Oslo.

Nordby, T. 1989. *Karl Evang: En Biografi*. Oslo: Aschehoug.

Østerud, Ø. 1975. *Samfunnsplanlegging og Politisk System. En Analyse av Offentlig Planlegging som Politikk og Ideologi*, 2nd ed. Oslo: Gyldendal Norsk Forlag.

Reichborn-Kjennerud, I., F. Grøn, and I. Kobro. 1936. *Medisinens Historie i Norge*. Oslo: Grøndahl & Søns Forlag.

Rudeng, E. 1989. *Sjokoladekongen*. Oslo: Universitetsforlaget.

Rustung, E. 1940. *Kostholdsstudier*. Oslo: Johan Grundt Tanum.

Schattschneider, E. E. 1975. *The Semisovereign People: A Realist's View of Democracy in America*. Hinsdale, IL: The Dryden Press.

Schneider, J. W., and J. I. Kitsuse (eds.). 1984. *Studies in the Sociology of Social Problems*. Norwood, NJ: Ablex.

Seip, A. L. 1987. "Fattiglov og Fattigvesen i Mellomkrigstiden - et Forsørgelsessystem Under Krise." *Historisk Tidsskrift* 66(3):276–300.

―――. 1989. *The Influence of Science on Social Policy in Norway in the 1930s*. Paper presented at the "Welfare State in Transition" conference, University of Bergen.

Spector, M., and J. I. Kitsuse. 1977. *Constructing Social Problems*. Menlo Park, CA: Cummings.

Statens Kostholdsnemd. 1940. *Aktuelle Kostholdspørsmål i Norge*. Oslo.

Strøm, A. 1948. "Examination into the Diet of Norwegian Families during the Years 1942–1945." *Acta Medica Scandinavica* 131 (supplement 214):1–47.

Webster, C. 1982. "Hungry or Healthy Thirties?" *History Workshop* 13:110–129.

Wold, K. G. 1938. *Vår Sosialpolitikk: Midler, Mål og Muligheter*. Oslo: Norges Venstrelag.

―――. 1941. *Kosthold og Levestandard: En Økonomisk Undersøkelse*. Oslo: Fabritius & Sønners Forlag.

Zebich, M. L. 1979. *The Politics of Nutrition: Issue Definition, Agenda-setting, and Policy Formulation in the United States*. Unpublished Dissertation. Albuquerque: University of New Mexico.

13

The Social Construction of Dietary Standards: The British Medical Association–Ministry of Health Advisory Committee on Nutrition Report of 1934

DAVID SMITH

Introduction

Across the political spectrum, nutrition was much debated in Britain during the "hungry thirties." For the left-wing strategists who attempted to build alliances of "progressive forces," the issue was sometimes almost as important as world peace and the rise of fascism. Harry Pollitt, Secretary of the Communist Party, commented in 1936:

> Experience has proved . . . [that] where struggles have developed against malnutrition which have brought in sections of the population like teachers, doctors, small shopkeepers, professional people . . . inevitably political discussion on other questions arises. Ultimately there comes . . . a deeper understanding of the class struggle and the aims of the working class movement. (Pollitt 1936:802)

But "malnutrition" was not as simple a campaigning issue as Pollitt might have wished. The definition, extent, causes of, and solutions to malnutrition were all highly contentious. One view that questioned the link between malnutrition and poverty suggested that the poor could feed themselves adequately if only they would adopt more economical shopping and food-preparation habits.[1] Pioneer nutrition scientist Wilbur O. Atwater developed a similar argument, which was employed in debates about nutrition-related social problems in late nineteenth-century America (Aronson 1982).

However, in Britain during the 1930s, there were additional levels of complication. One complicating factor, potentially to the advantage of the left-wing campaigners, arose from scientific advances that showed the importance of the more expensive foods such as milk as sources of essential vitamins and minerals. But complete scientific and medical consensus as to the practical importance of vitamins and minerals in human diets had not been achieved. In addition, allies of the Establishment who wished to resist claims that a large proportion of the poor were underfed and suffering from malnutrition could even claim that "state of nutrition" was a "clinical concept," with food constituting only one of many contributing factors. In 1928, for example, in a lecture on "The Foundations of National Health," George Newman, Chief Medical Officer of the Board of Education and the Ministry of Health, remarked that the "elements of nutrition for the body are six in number": food, warmth, fresh air and sunlight, cleanliness, exercise, and rest (Newman 1928:14).[2] Nevertheless, dietary standards were central to much of the malnutrition debate. Estimates of the levels of calorie and nutrient intakes that were essential for health were compared with the results of dietary surveys. In addition, dietary standards were converted into estimates of the minimum cost of an adequate diet, which were compared with actual or potential expenditure on food.[3] The question of how the dietary standards were arrived at is therefore an important aspect of the complete description of the construction of malnutrition as a social problem during the 1930s.

We might expect the analysis of the construction of the scientific resources such as dietary standards to involve the analysis of scientists' activities in the laboratory or in the field. Since the pioneering ethnographic studies of scientists at work (Knorr-Cetina 1981; Latour and Woolgar 1979), there has been a great deal of interest in these locations of scientific practice. But if the importance of the laboratory and the field is that they are sites of knowledge-generation, then there are other important sites of scientific practice to consider, such as, in the case of the construction of dietary standards, the committee room.

Aronson (1984) has discussed the implications of advances in science studies for the sociology of social problems, and has, in setting out a classification of scientific forms of claimsmaking, produced a schema that emphasizes processes internal to the scientific community in the production of scientific knowledge. She refers to the "work of scientists" as being concerned, primarily, with making "cognitive claims . . . concerning research findings directed towards a specialized research community for the purpose of transforming claims to be certified scientific knowledge" (Aronson 1984:8). But, she continues, scientists who are well-established and who are working largely in senior administrative positions also frequently engage in "interpretive claims-making directed towards non-specialist audiences." She defines one form of "interpretive claim" as the "social problem interpretive claim" that asserts "the existence of a social problem which a scientific specialty is uniquely equipped to solve." However, scientists who meet in committees to establish dietary standards may address themselves toward both the "research community" and nonspecialist audiences at the same time. The knowledge generated may be subsequently used, not only in policy-making, but also in future research. In other words, the distinction between "cognitive claims" and "interpretive claims" may not always be entirely appropriate; knowledge-construction and knowledge-deployment are not always easily separated.

This chapter will concentrate upon the construction of one particular set of dietary standards published in a 1934 Report issued as a result of two joint conferences of the Nutrition Committee of the British Medical Association (BMA) and the Advisory Committee on Nutrition of the Ministry of Health (ACN). This Report included the following table:

Sliding Scale of Calorie Requirements per Day[4]

Individuals	Calories Gross
Man: heavy work	3,400–4,000
Man: moderate work	3,000–3,400
Man: light work	2,600–3,000

The table included further figures for a woman engaged in active work, for a housewife, and for children of various ages. A section that discussed first-class (i.e., animal) protein intake concluded that "a diet to be reasonably adequate should always contain a proportion of animal origin; . . . this proportion should not be lower than one-third of the total protein consumed, and may perhaps with advantage be increased to one-half" (*British Medical Journal* 1934:901).

This chapter will explore the processes by which these statements about dietary standards were arrived at, and will take advantage of some unusually rich archival resources, including verbatim minutes of the Conferences in which the standards were negotiated. It will become apparent that the revision of the accepted dietary standards that these figures represented was not the result of the production of any new experimental or survey data. Instead, the new figures were the outcome of a process involving professional rivalry and public controversy, followed by the emergence of common interests in preventing the reoccurrence of that controversy.

The Advisory Committee on Nutrition of the Ministry of Health

The Advisory Committee on Nutrition (ACN) of the Ministry of Health, which first met in January 1931, was formed partly as a result of long-standing pressure from some scientists who argued that the health administration was neglecting the application of modern nutritional knowledge.[5] The Committee was chaired by a former Medical Officer of the Ministry, Major Greenwood, Professor of Epidemiology at the London School of Hygiene and Tropical Medicine. The other members included F. G. Hopkins, Professor of Biochemistry at Cambridge, and E. Mellanby, Professor of Pharmacology at Sheffield. Hopkins had shared a Nobel Prize for the discovery of vitamins, while Mellanby, Hopkins's student and colleague, had carried out important work on rickets as a vitamin deficiency disease. Another member, E. P. Cathcart, Regius Professor of Physiology at Glasgow, was highly skeptical about the practical importance of vitamins. This division of opinion was long-standing, and had been most clearly expressed in a controversy over the etiology of rickets during the late 1910s and early 1920s.[6] Cathcart's expertise was concerned with other aspects of nutrition: he had conducted a series of dietary surveys supported by the Medical Research Council (MRC), which aimed to provide estimates of calorie requirements from studies of the population's dietary habits (for example, Cathcart and Murray 1931, 1932). Cathcart was recognized internationally as an expert in this field and had chaired a League of Nations Conference concerned with the "Standardisation of Certain Methods Used in Making Dietary Studies" (League of Nations 1932). V. H. Mottram, who occupied the relatively humble position of Professor of Physiology at King's College of Household and Social Science in London, was also appointed to the ACN, and became responsible for drafting most of the documents produced.

The first two reports of the ACN aimed to assist local authority Medical Officers of Health in the performance of their duties. Recent changes to Poor Law regulations had given Medical Officers additional responsibilities in respect to the quality of institutional diets (Ministry of Health 1930). A Medical Officer, G. F. Buchan, was coopted on to the Committee. Mottram drafted both reports. *Diets in Poor Law Childrens' Homes*, based on visits to eight institutions, urged that the variety of the meals should be enhanced. Specimen menus, reduced to nutrients per child and recipes were included, but there was no discussion of dietary standards (Ministry of Health 1932a). In view of the number of requests for guidance that the Committee began to receive in connection with other problems, they decided to produce a more general memorandum that would allow Medical Officers to form their own views of diets. This led to *Criticism and Improvement of Diets*, which used the standards of 3,000 calories and 37 grams of animal protein per day for the average adult male (Ministry of Health 1932b). The requirements of mixed groups of men, women, and children were to be worked out from these figures by the application of a scale of "man values," which had been published by Cathcart. Women and children of various ages were calculated as fractions of men. The scale was based upon a study of food consumption within a small number of families, but Cathcart also observed that the figures amounted to a "combination" of the Atwater's scale and that of his fellow-American, Graham Lusk (Cathcart and Murray 1931:7). There is no evidence that the ACN experienced any difficulties in agreeing on these standards, and the report introduced the 3,000 calorie standard without explanation. Cathcart's dietary surveys had shown that the average supply of calories per "man" was about 3,000 calories, while the 37 grams of first-class protein was a rule-of-thumb representing 5% of 3,000 calories as protein. As will be seen, Mottram admitted, on more than one occasion, that he was unable to trace the origins of this method of calculation.

Despite the apparent consensus, Cathcart privately warned T. C. Carnwath, Senior Medical Officer who helped to administer the work of the ACN, that *Criticism and Improvement of Diets* could potentially be a source of trouble. Carnwath explained to Newman that Cathcart thought that the Report was "an admirable ideal . . . but [he] fears its economic implications. The diet recommended . . . is something much better than the average working man can afford, and he [Cathcart] is afraid that if it is embodied in an official document it may be seized upon by transitional beneficiaries and others as a yard stick to measure what their allowances should be."[7] While there was little immediate response of the kind that Cathcart foresaw, the eventual public contradiction of the standards by a Committee of the BMA did lead to a very difficult situation.

After the initial burst of activity by the ACN, the Committee's work scaled down, partly due to the financial crisis of the Autumn of 1931, and partly because of the difficulties of reaching unanimity on the issues under discussion. The Committee did not meet formally between February 1932 and July 1933, but during this period it dealt with several matters by post. One of these episodes illustrates the division of opinion among the members of the ACN, and the response of some members of the medical profession toward the centralized provision of nutritional advice. This concerned a memorandum on the practical importance of

MRC nutrition research findings, prepared by Mottram. The memorandum did not meet with unanimous approval, as Cathcart could not agree that the evidence that rickets and dental disease would be reduced by increasing the consumption of vitamin D and calcium was describable as "cogent." Carnwath commented to Newman:

> .From the conversations I have had with him [Cathcart], I believe his objections are fundamental rather than specific. He simply does not believe that the cure for our national ills is to be found in . . . daily spoonfuls of cod liver oil and his cautious mind is offended by the extravagant . . . claims that are made by his fellow workers . . . . When he comes to the bedrock of everyday experience he finds large numbers of families in poor circumstances . . . arriving at vigorous mental and physical maturity on a diet that by most standards of modern research appears to be deficient.[8]

However, Cathcart's dissent did not prevent the preparation of a Ministry of Health Circular that was sent to the Clerks of Town Councils (Ministry of Health 1932c). This advised that nutritional anemia in infants could be reduced by the administration of iron ammonium citrate, that foods rich in vitamin D and calcium mitigate or prevent rickets and dental disease, and that milk is of "paramount importance" for growing children. But the way that this advice was communicated did not please some Medical Officers of Health, and aggravated existing tensions with the Ministry. A meeting of the Public Health Committee of the BMA asked G. C. Anderson, the BMA's Medical Secretary, to complain to Sir Arthur Robinson, the Permanent Secretary at the Ministry of Health. Anderson declared that his Committee "felt that to address advice of this kind to a lay body, trusting that the Medical Officer of Health would adopt it, might result in the giving of instructions by the lay committee of a Council to its Medical Officer regarding the course of treatment in certain cases . . . information of a medical nature should be communicated directly to medical men."[9] The sentiments manifested by this letter are symptomatic of a general tension between the organized medical profession and the government over professional autonomy. Since it was founded in 1832, the Association had engaged in many campaigns, of varying scale, that aimed to protect the profession against the encroachment of state control, or exploitation by the local or central authorities. On many occasions these campaigns sought to address the problems of practitioners such as the Medical Officers of Health who were engaged in the least prestigious forms of employment. The BMA's involvement in nutrition during the 1930s, and the clash with the ACN, may be seen, partly as a result of perceptions that the activities of the Ministry of Health threatened the status of the medical profession as expert advisers in dietary matters, but also partly as a public relations exercise: this activity displayed the social engagement and responsibility of the medical profession to the general public.

Public Debate

While the members of the ACN, the Ministry Officials, and the representatives of the BMA conducted these exchanges, malnutrition was becoming a matter for public debate. One such debate took place in early 1933 in *Week-End Review*, a journal that had been associated with the technocratic "think tank," Political and Economic Planning. The *Review* published a series of letters that was stimulated by a correspondent who referred to an inquest into a death of a mother of seven, who had allegedly died from "pneumonia aggravated by voluntary starvation" because of inadequate unemployment benefits (Meynell 1933). After several weeks of discussion, *Week-End Review* (1933a) appointed a committee of experts to prepare a report on the minimum cost of an adequate diet. Mottram was among the members of the "Hungry England" Committee, and its report was based upon the physiological standards that had been used in the ACN's *Criticism and Improvement of Diets* (*Week-End Review* 1933c). An editorial accompanying the report concluded that since several of the destitute families mentioned in the correspondence now appeared to have been receiving insufficient financial support for an adequate diet, the next step "is evidently to have the implications and validity of the Report discussed by those concerned" (*Week-End Review* 1933b).

The "Hungry England" Report was soon under consideration in the Ministry of Health. Carnwath advised Newman that he thought the report largely the responsibility of Mottram, that it seemed "admirable," and that it was "an attempt to express in practical form . . . the principles of the Ministry's memorandum."[10] The ACN was asked for its opinion. Cathcart suggested that perhaps the calorie standard may need revising downwards,[11] because the majority of the members of League of Nation Committee that he had chaired thought that "the historic 3,000 Calories" was probably too high "even for a man doing a good day's work" (League of Nations 1932:478). Cathcart pointed out that the Hungry England Committee was concerned not with working men, but with the unemployed. However, when the Advisory Committee on Nutrition discussed these matters in July 1933, the historic 3,000 Calories" survived, and they agreed that the calculations carried out by the Hungry England Committee were physiologically sound.[12]

The Nutrition Committee of the British Medical Association

Prior to the formation of the "Hungry England Committee," a letter in *Week-End Review* from an anonymous BMA member pointed out that the BMA regularly appointed advisory committees, and asked "Could it not now be persuaded to appoint a committee . . . to tell us exactly how much a family needs to keep it in good health?" (BMA Member 1933). *The Review* agreed to approach the BMA about the matter (*Week-End Review* 1933b) and subsequently the BMA's Science Committee considered a proposal to appoint a special committee to investigate and report upon "the minimum dietary necessary to maintain the individual in a state of proper nutrition." A supporting document argued that "in view of the economic position . . . and the interest recently exhibited in the problems of nutrition . . . it would appear that the time is ripe for the medical profession to make an authoritative statement of what a proper diet should be."[13] The Science Committee suggested that the proposed "authoritative statement" would be of value to those responsible for "feeding certain sections of the population and to the authorities providing financial aid for this purpose." They also argued that by issuing a statement on minimum diets the BMA would be "associating itself with a health problem of immense public interest and importance, an action not without propaganda value."

The BMA Council subsequently appointed a Committee to "determine the minimum weekly expenditure on foodstuffs which must be incurred by families of varying size if health and working capacity are to be maintained." Two members of the ACN were appointed to the new Committee: Mottram and Buchan, and the other members included G. C. M. M'Gonigle, Medical Officer of Health for Stockton-on-Tees, G. P. Crowden, Lecturer in Industrial Physiology at the London School of Hygiene and Tropical Medicine, and S. J. Cowell, Professor of Dietetics at St. Thomas's Hospital.[14] The BMA Nutrition Committee met for the first time at the end of April, but the first substantive discussion of methodology took place at the second meeting, 3 weeks later. Mottram presented an analysis of the data from a number of dietary surveys (mainly those carried out under Cathcart). He found that the un-weighted mean calorie intake was 3,004, but observed that several objections could be taken to using this as a standard. First, he noted that while this figure might be the normal intake, it was not necessarily the optimal one, and second, it was lower than what would be instinctively taken, because many of the data were collected from poor and unemployed families. He referred to an allowance of 10% to take account of "loss in cooking etc." and pointed out that the rations for troops at home stations amounted to 3,535 calories, while the territorial army received 4,251 calories during training. He concluded that the calorie requirement should be set at 3,000 for sedentary males, and 3,400 for those in work. For the first-class protein requirement, Mottram suggested 5% of total calories, and calculated this at 37 grams for an intake of 3,000 calories. However, Mottram admitted: "I have not been able to discover the source of this estimate, though my impression is that it is American in origin (Graham Lusk?)."[15] M'Gonigle supplied several papers for the meeting, including one that noted that army rations provided 62.7 grams of first-class protein, and 90.5 grams during active operations.[16] Crowden presented a memorandum that drew attention to the fact that Cathcart's scale of "man values" was based upon an analysis of the food intake of members of only five families, and argued that it was desirable for much more data to be collected.[17] But despite all the doubts that Mottram, M'Gonigle, and Crowden cast upon the established standards, the meeting decided to use the 3,000 calories and 37 grams standards, and the Cathcart scale of "man values."[18]

At the next Committee meeting, held three weeks later, Crowden again questioned the paucity of the existing "man values," and argued that a worker should be employed to collect new data. It was pointed out that the BMA Council did not desire a "lengthy or exhaustive inquiry" but the Committee agreed to support an application for a Leverhulme Fellowship for a project to be conducted under Crowden. They appointed a Drafting Sub-Committee, consisting of Crowden, M'Gonigle, and Mottram.[19]

The report was drawn-up almost entirely by M'Gonigle, and contrary to the previous decisions of the Nutrition Committee, the draft that he sent to Mottram and Cowell in September 1933 employed the standards of 3,400 calories and 50 grams of animal protein. Mottram and Cowell appear to have approved the Report "with only very minor modifications," even in advance of a meeting of the Drafting Sub-Committee,[20] but the Drafting Sub-Committee met twice to refine the document further, before it was placed before the main Committee. The minutes of the latter meeting record that the report was approved after "considerable discussion and some emendation," and that they decided to recommend to the BMA's Council that it should be published at once.[21]

The report, as published, gave three objections to the 3,000 calorie standard, which were identical to those in Mottram's memorandum discussed at the second meeting of the Committee. It stated that it was doubtful whether "3,000 calories in the food as purchased are sufficient to maintain 'working capacity'," but that 3,400 would be "reasonably safe" allowing for "wastage in preparation and digestion" (British Medical Association 1933:2).

But since the second meeting of the Nutrition Committee, when Mottram admitted that he could not remember where "five percent of total energy" had come from, it seems that an alternative rationale for the 37 grams of first-class protein had been discovered. However, while this rationale was alluded to, it was not made explicit: "The minimum requisite daily quantity of first-class protein has been assessed at 37 grams per day. It appears that this figure was calculated upon the protein of milk, which has a high biological value, and there is some doubt as to the adequacy of this quantity when supplied by other animal proteins" (British Medical Association 1933:4). The Committee, it was explained, settled on 50 grams because this was about half-way between the 37 and 62.7, the ration for the peace-time army.

The ACN–BMA Controversy

The publicity for the BMA Report was well-planned. The British Broadcasting Corporation was provided with a draft several weeks in advance, and on the day of the launch it was the subject of a special broadcast.[22] On the same day the press used the report to criticize government policies. The popular left-wing *Daily Herald* included a front-page article using the headlines "B. M. A. Exposes Inadequacy of Unemployment Pay" and "Food Leaves only 6/8 1/2d for Everything Else," and for subheadings "Challenge to Ministry" and "Malnutrition." In bold print the article declared: "The Ministry of Health's figure is 3,000 calories. The members of the British Medical Association committee of investigation say bluntly that this is not enough" (Special Correspondent 1933). Later in the week further headlines and articles appeared in the *Daily Herald* and other newspapers, the major points being the parsimonious nature of the ACN standards, and the assertion that the minimum diet as laid down by the BMA was too expensive for poor families to afford. M'Gonigle was delighted with this treatment of the Report.[23] The BMA's Assistant Medical Secretary remarked "The Nutrition Report really has 'gone' extremely well," and regularly sent sales figures to M'Gonigle.[24]

By the beginning of December the Labour Party had prepared speakers' notes on the issue. Figures were supplied to show that "The amount left after purchasing the minimum foodstuffs laid down by the BMA would not pay the rent alone in many thousands of unemployed households. The only possible conclusion . . . is that in order to pay the rent and purchase the bare necessities, the housewife must economise on food."[25] Spokesmen for the Ministry of Health rebutted the Labour Party's arguments with references to the Chief Medical Officer's *Annual Reports*, which claimed that the nutritional status of children, as assessed by clinical inspection, had not deteriorated with increasing unemployment. Mr. Geoffrey Shakespeare, Parliamentary Secretary of the Ministry of Health, was able to correctly point out at a meeting during the evening of the day that the BMA Report was released: "There is not one single word in the BMA Report about the Ministry of Health's conclusion on unemployment and national health . . . nor are any of its conclusions questioned or doubted."[26] But when a Labour Member of Parliament submitted a parliamentary question that asked whether, in view of the BMA Report, the Government would "consider the necessity of making provision for more adequate allowances for unemployed persons and their dependents" (Tinker 1933) the House of Commons was told that the report was being looked at by the ACN (Hudson 1933).

But it seems that the Minister of Health, Sir Hilton Young, and his officials had no intention of asking the ACN to consider the financial implications of the BMA Report. Young remarked at a meeting with his Chief Officials that they needed to decide "how to make the best of a bad job. It was obviously impossible to overtake the harm done by the BMA report but something might be done to mitigate its . . . effects . . . the important thing now was to impress on the Advisory Committee that they must justify their 3,000 calorie standard which has been controverted . . . . Would the Advisory Committee be willing to make a simple statement that the BMA report was wrong?"[27] Buchan was at pains to emphasize that he had protested the abandonment of the accepted standards, and apologized to Newman for the embarrassment that the BMA Report had caused.[28] He subsequently resigned from the BMA Committee.[29] But Mottram thought that there was little to be concerned about: "There is so little discrepancy between the . . . estimates that I think no-one need worry about it. We [the ACN] wrote that the 3,000 calorie standard was not very generous and made no allowance for wastage."[30] However, the ACN, at a meeting that Mottram was unable to attend, obliged the Ministry by agreeing to a statement that was quoted in a Circular issued in early January 1934: "no evidence known to the Advisory Committee, and no argument stated in the BMA Committee's Report, justify the increase of 3,000 Calories to 3,400 Calories or of 37 grammes of first class protein to 50 grammes" (Ministry of Health 1934). But the Circular only fueled the controversy. The Director of the Conservative and Unionist Central Office wrote to Young to inform him that Circular was "causing a great deal of difficulty in the industrial areas"[31] and Mr. Shakespeare requested advice on how to tackle hecklers at a number of politically important meetings . . . in his constituency."[32]

Mottram wrote to *The Times* to point out that he should not have been included as a signatory of the ACN statement on the BMA Report and that he disagreed with the statement (Mottram 1934). The BMA issued a statement that defended their position, and *The Times* quoted Anderson pointing out that the terms of reference of the BMA Committee was to "specify a minimum standard, not a mere existence level, but for the maintenance of health and working capacity" (*The Times* 1934a). Greenwood responded with a letter that was sarcastic toward Anderson and bitter toward Mottram. He also complained that "The 'expert' committee . . . [meaning the BMA Committee] conceived itself competent . . . to overrule the judgment of physiologists whose life work has been in the field of nutrition and metabolism" (Greenwood 1934). The issue was rapidly becoming one focusing on the scientific credentials of the two Committees, and the controversy in *The Times* resulted in a new spate of sensational articles and headlines in other newspapers. *The Daily Herald*'s front page headlines were "Medical Storm over Ministry Food Minimum," "B.M.A. Retorts that Cooking Loss has been Overlooked," and "Attempt to Foster Underfeeding." After quoting Anderson's view that 3,400 calories and 50 grams of first-class protein were "absolutely essential" the article continued, "The Ministry of Health's circular . . . recommending a much lower standard, is regarded as a deliberate attempt to encourage the under-feeding of unemployed women and their families" (Political Correspondent 1934). Lord Dawson, President of the Royal College of Physicians, suggested a possible way of resolving the controversy in *The Times*. Dawson thought that the two Committees ought to meet in a "joint session" (Dawson of Penn 1934), an idea that was backed by an editorial under the heading "A Wise Proposal" (*The Times* 1934b). Robinson commented to Young: "Politically . . . I suppose there is a good deal to be said for it"[33] but warned that the ACN, consisting of the "most eminent medical scientists," might not be prepared to meet the BMA Committee, "a mixed lot of people of very varying status."[34] Greenwood suggested that the joint meeting could be confined to those ACN members with "special knowledge of physiology" (Hopkins, Cathcart, and Mellanby) and three members of the BMA Committee, and that the discussion could be confined to "purely physiological" questions. When Robinson invited the BMA's participation, he stated to Anderson that the Minister had instructed him to communicate about "one major point"—the 3,400 calories and 50 grams of first-class protein.[35]

When the BMA Committee met in mid-January 1934 to consider the proposed Joint Conference, the Ministry of Health's Circular and the correspondence in *The Times*, 9,000 copies of the report had already been sold. The Committee resolved to "reiterate unanimously the views expressed in the report on the necessary calories and grams of first class protein," but agreed to participate in the Conference, provided Anderson could be associated with the secretariat, and the BMA Committee would receive the report of the Conference at the same time as the

Minister. Mottram, Cowell, and Crowden were appointed as the BMA's representatives.[36]

Young sent a very flattering letter to Hopkins, Mellanby, and Cathcart, but while Hopkins and Mellanby readily agreed to attend the Joint Conference, and struck a conciliatory note in their replies, Cathcart responded, "As I am fully convinced the BMA cannot justify their conclusions . . . it seems to me the real difficulty will be to find a formula which will allow the BMA to retract and at the same time to 'save face'."[37]

Carnwath spared no effort in trying to smooth the way for a satisfactory outcome, frequently writing to and meeting with members of both sides. Of the BMA side, Carnwath reported that he did not "anticipate much difficulty" with Cowell, but he remarked to Newman that Crowden was "stubborn" and "rather stupid."[38]

However, Crowden was soon taking the initiative in the formulation of a possible compromise. He sent Anderson a copy of a "sliding scale" of calorie requirements according to occupation and habits that he had found in an American journal. He had already shown the scale to Mellanby and Carnwath and remarked "I sincerely hope it will form a basis on which agreement can be come to and on which a really practical and workable proposition can be put forward to the authorities."[39] Crowden included the idea of a "sliding scale" in a "Note on Calorie and Protein Requirements" that he sent to Anderson and to H. E. Magee, a Medical Officer of the Ministry who was acting as secretary to the conferences.

The officials regarded Cathcart's role as crucial, but as the conference drew closer there seemed to be no sign of Cathcart softening his line. He told Carnwath: "believing as I do that the evidence against the 3,400 is as complete as that against 3,200, if any attempt is made to reach an agreement on this basis . . . there will be a minority report . . . . Why should we argue with idiots who are placing mere assumptions . . . against what has been accepted as sound scientific fact . . . the present set of intuitions . . . are based . . . on nothing but loose thinking and sloshy sentiment."[40] A few days later he asked: "how is the withdrawal of this silly 3,400 Calories for the unemployed to be achieved? It must not be allowed to stand. Indeed it cannot be left or you [the Ministry] will always be coming up against it in the future. The BMA must be put in their proper place . . . Mottram and Cowell better prepare to do the noble hero stunt and go to their scientific (such as it is) deaths."[41]

The First ACN–BMA Joint Conference

The first Conference was held in early February 1934. Hopkins, who was elected Chairman, introduced the discussion by immediately alluding to the possibility of compromise. He stated that there was a need for "some sort of demonstration that the differences between the committees are not such as have been assumed."[42] According to Hopkins the task was to decide "what sort of statement . . . we can draw up, what line it should take, what character it should have, and to endeavour to reassure the public and straighten matters out."

Hopkins stressed that the ACN's standards had not been given as dogmatic figures, and said that he understood that the BMA Committee had used 3,400 to allow for wastage. But Crowden, speaking first for the BMA, did not take up the question of wastage, and instead explained that the BMA Committee was considering "a man actually engaged in muscular work or engaged in work on allotments or engaged in physical training to keep him fit."

Cathcart, speaking next, stated that he was especially aggrieved that the BMA Committee had described 3,000 calories as a "bare subsistence level" and pointed out that "all the people of international reputation in this field have said for a doctor 2,700 calories is ample." Crowden repeated the point that the BMA Committee was considering "a man of good physique keeping fit" and said that he thought such a man would be unable to maintain body weight on 3,000 calories. He also asserted "There is 10 percent loss by absorption," a point that Cathcart doubted, but Crowden continued: "There is very little data about the digestibility of food. I think our feeling was that, having regard to the scarcity of data, we must err on the generous side."

Already, it seemed, the conference was moving into territory in which even Cathcart, the international expert, was unable to give definitive answers. Hopkins repeated an earlier question about what evidence there was for the 3,400 calorie standard, and Cowell then took up the issue of wastage: "there was no new evidence . . . . We considered that we were getting data from . . . Professor Cathcart's investigations and so on, and making allowances for wastage." At this point Cathcart introduced some new figures, recently published by the American Department of Agriculture, which described 2,930 calories as a "liberal diet." Responding to this, Crowden again emphasized that the BMA Committee was considering a man working on an allotment, but Cathcart argued, on the basis of estimates of the total gross supply of calories available in the country, that 3,400 calories could not possibly represent the calorie consumption of the population at large. He then asserted: "I think that you can place very little stress on calories as a whole. I took figures for thirty-six . . . unemployed families and the figures ranged all over the place." He developed this theme later: "If you had said in your Report . . . that it was up to the Public Health Authorities to see that necessitous children got a square meal . . . it would have covered the whole thing, rather than put down a flat rate, because to put down a flat rate for anything is futile." Crowden replied "We are all agreed to that," and Cathcart continued: "To put down 3,000 Calories is equally futile. I do not think I would say that one figure is better than another. Anyone who puts down a flat rate is asking for trouble." Crowden concurred: "a standard is a dangerous thing because it is bound to be excessive for some and too little for others" and asked "Would you define men in categories, active and moderately active?" Cathcart thought that this would be the approach to adopt, and in this way a basis for an agreement on the question of calorie requirements began to emerge.

Mellanby then picked up on the issue of protein requirements and said that he approved of the increase in the first-class protein standard, if it was to allow for extra milk consumption. Cathcart asked where the 37 grams standard came from, which initiated the following exchange:

> *Crowden:* I think the figure comes from 5 percent of total calories in first class protein . . . .
>
> *Cathcart:* Who said so?
>
> *Crowden:* It is an American statement. I cannot trace where it comes from.
>
> *Chairman:* I have seen it.
>
> *Mellanby:* Is it Sherman?
>
> *Chairman:* No, it is not Sherman.
>
> *Cathcart:* As a matter of fact there has been no experiment on the relation of first class protein to any other protein.

Mottram was not present at this point in the meeting, but when he arrived, he confirmed the basis for the calculation, and that he did not remember its origins.

Later Cathcart explained why he had agreed to the 37 grams standard in the ACN Report: "I did not object at the time . . . because I have always worked it out in my own diets that if you get one third protein as first class protein you are quite safe, but if you want to improve the diet, raise it from one third." Like Mellanby, Cathcart stated that he was inclined to support the increase in the first-class protein requirement. Soon after this point in the discussion Hopkins revealed and read the paper that Crowden had prepared, and that opened as follows:

> It must be clearly recognized that owing to individual differences in physique, personal habits, likes and dislikes, and the variation in the degree of muscular effort involved in different occupations it is not only impossible to define but also there does not, in fact exist any standard food requirement which could be rigidly applied to all men alike . . . a workable solution of the problem of physiologically desirable dietary standards . . .

would be provided by a sliding scale . . . based on individual physique, occupation and habits.[43]

Cathcart stated that subject to some minor amendments, he would agree to the document.

The discussion then ranged over many areas, but eventually Hopkins said that it was becoming clear that "there will be no difficulty in our agreeing on a little give and take" and suggested that a sliding scale of calorie requirements could be formulated that would "more or less cover up our differences." The meeting adjourned with a feeling that an agreement was in sight, and they decided to meet again later in the month.

The officials were pleased. Robinson advised Young "I think we can safely let this run on now to the stage of an agreed report on the basis outlined in Dr. Crowden's paper."[44] Confident that a satisfactory solution was in sight, the Officials were relatively inactive during the period between the two conferences. Cathcart prepared a memorandum, which was circulated to the members of the Joint Conference, and which began as follows: "Dietetics is not and cannot be an exact science dealing as it does with unknown metabolic phenomena in the living organism. If, as is generally admitted, our ignorance about the qualitative aspect is profound that concerning the true inwardness of the caloric aspect of the problem is perhaps even deeper. The faith placed by many in calories almost amounts to fetish worship."[45] Cathcart again quoted the new lower American calorie requirement figures and included a sliding scale of calorie requirements, for men engaged in light, moderate, active, and heavy work.

Anderson urged the BMA physiologists not to weaken. He emphasized to Crowden that "it would be difficult, if not impossible, for the Nutrition Committee to accept anything less than the position you have set out in your draft"[46] and told Mottram that if the BMA representatives "fail to convince the Ministry's representatives on the wastage point and on the question of the man we had in mind" then Crowden's memorandum should be "our last word."[47]

The Second ACN–BMA Joint Conference

Hopkins introduced the second conference with a few paragraphs that he had drafted on the train. He pointed out that the "purposes and intentions" of the BMA and the ACN Reports differed, and went on to explain why the calorie figures had varied. He then showed that there was little difference between the BMA diets for children, and those in the ACN's *Diets in Poor Law Childrens' Homes*. With these paragraphs he hoped to dispel the belief of the press and the public "that there was a wide divergence between the two Committees, that one wanted to starve the poor and the other wanted to do them well."[48] Cathcart stated, "The only thing is to avoid discussion in the Press" and Hopkins agreed "that should be the chief guiding motive."

A substantial part of the debate that followed concerned the details of a scale that incorporated features of the statements by Cathcart and Crowden. The following exchange is a typical example of the way the calorie categories and figures were negotiated. Cathcart's scale gave 2,700–2,800 as the requirement for a "man engaged in light work." Crowden wanted to revise the figures upwards:

Dr. Crowden:	Would you agree to make it 2,700 to 3,000 because we find many people engaged in light occupations are now participating in physical exercises . . . . The money question is of no significance in regard to this really. [Meaning that the extra calories, in the form of bread or potatoes, could be bought very cheaply.]
Chairman:	The only question in my mind was to remember the history of all those articles.
Secretary:	Dr. Crowden has asked the question, would the other people be agreeable to 2,700 to 3,000 calories instead of 2,700 to 2,800 calories for light work?
Chairman:	I will agree to that.
Professor Cowell:	Is it not better to have the heavy range from 3,400 to 4,000 and then it is a continuous scale.
Professor Mellanby:	Would you like to see 2,500 to 3,000?
Professor Cathcart:	2,600, to include old age.
Secretary:	For the over 65?
Professor Cathcart:	Light, 2,600.
Professor Mellanby:	That makes 400 different in each case.
Chairman:	What are the figures now?
Secretary:	Man in heavy work 3,400 to 4,000, man in moderate work 3,000 to 3,400, man doing light work, inactive man, and man over 65 2,600 to 3,000.
Dr. Crowden:	Do not mention "inactive" and "over 65," but just call it light.

The discussion on the figures for first class protein proceeded along similar lines. Mellanby suggested that the protein question could be handled in the same way as the calories, that a range could be given:

Professor Mellanby:	We should say that we consider there are wide variations required in these first class proteins, varying from 37.5 up to 50 . . . .

Professor Cathcart:	I would rather put it in fractions and say one-third to two-fifths of the proteins to be in first class form.
Secretary:	It is saying the same thing.
Dr. Crowden:	I do not know about that . . . .
Professor Cathcart:	I do not think an adult would be harmed in the slightest by one-third . . . .
Professor Mottram:	. . . whereas I am willing to accept 37 to 50 I do not feel I can accept two-fifths, because one-third of one hundred is 33 1/3 and two-fifths of hundred is 40 and I want 50.
Professor Mellanby:	37 to 50 seems to be about right.
Professor Cathcart:	I do not like the 37.
Professor Mellanby:	We mentioned 37 and they mentioned 50.
Professor Cathcart:	Nobody can justify the 37. I think it is ridiculous that we should give a hard and fast figure.
Professor Mellanby:	Your one-third is just as ridiculous, except that it is a round figure.
Doctor Crowden:	I suggest that we agree on 37 to 50 . . . .
Professor Cathcart:	The Vegetarian gets along with nothing.
Professor Mellanby:	He drinks milk
Professor Cathcart:	Not many of them do.
Chairman:	Is it agreed that it should be actual figures or fractions.
Doctor Crowden:	. . . I prefer the figures.
Professor Mellanby:	I propose that the figures be given . . . .
Professor Cathcart:	I feel so uncertain about the whole thing.
Professor Mellanby:	Your suggestion is just as ridiculous.
Professor Cathcart:	I am quite prepared to admit that, but it looks less ridiculous.
Professor Mellanby:	Really it is more so.

When Cathcart asked if there was any evidence for the 37 grams, Mottram introduced the alternative method of calculation that was alluded to in the BMA Report: "Take the output of nitrogen, minimum output 3 grammes, calculating that as protein 18.75 and doubling that, assuming . . . milk proteins . . . [have] a biological factor of 50, that means that the intake has to be 37.5." Cathcart was initially very impressed by this, but quickly went on to reemphasize his view that the source of the protein did not really matter.

As the time approached for the conference to break for lunch, it became apparent that little further progress could be achieved in committee, and so they agreed that the details of both the sliding scale, and the formulation regarding protein requirements, could be left to Crowden and Cathcart to decide, with the assistance of Magee and Anderson.

The "Nutrition Agreement"

Crowden prepared a draft of what he called the "nutrition agreement,"[49] and during the weeks that followed adjustments were made to the text in response to comments made by other members of the Joint Conferences. Anderson took a hard line over some seemingly minor matters of wording, as may be seen in the following quotation from a letter to Magee. With reference to a passage in the report explaining the limits of applicability of the 3,000 calorie standard, Anderson remarked:

> I am prepared to agree to the document as it stands provided one word is altered, but the alteration I suggest I consider is one upon which, as representing the Association, I must insist. I refer to the last sentence on page 5. In place of the words "It might not be applicable" I suggest the words "it would not be generally applicable" so that the sentence would read: "This figure can safely be employed for calculation of mass requirements, but, of course, it would not be generally applicable to individuals or single families for the reasons indicated."[50]

After a series of similar exchanges, Magee finally sent the report to Anderson in early May,[51] and to Carnwath[52] who passed it on to Newman: "I hasten to pass this to you . . . especially in view of the fact that Dr. Magee has already 'liberated' a copy to Dr. Anderson."[53] Newman passed the report to Robinson, whom he advised, "You will observe the BMA have got it and anything may happen."[54] Robinson advised the Minister that publication was the only possible course because "we cannot suppress the report altogether." However he warned: "Judging from what happened before I . . . suppose that the ordinary press line . . . will be that the BMA have won since the table . . . shows an ascent to 4,000 Calories."[55] Certainly some members of the BMA's Committee saw the report as a victory. M'Gonigle remarked to Anderson that one part amounted to "a throwing over of the Advisory Committee" and was "a triumph for the BMA."[56] Anderson agreed: "the Report is a score for us."[57]

The report was published and sent to local authorities[58] and was also published in the *British Medical Journal*. However, despite Newman's fears, it received very little attention in the press. *The Times* included an article under the heading "Divergent Views Reconciled" that quoted extensively from the report and an editorial that amounted to a summary (*The Times* 1934c, 1934d). *The Daily Herald* ignored the report entirely.[59]

Summary and Conclusions

Using Aronson's terminology, the establishment of expert committees such as the Ministry of Health's Advisory Committee on Nutrition may be regarded as expressions of the partial success of interpretive claims. Such committees may become the arenas in which interpretive claims are pursued. However, when the proceedings of expert committees are characterized by conflict between the experts, the aims of the claims-makers may be frustrated. For the government, the creation of expert committees in which conflict is endemic may form part of a "damage-limitation" strategy. If a committee can reach few conclusions, there is less possibility that the government will find itself under pressure to implement challenging and costly recommendations, although there is a risk that committees in this situation may become vulnerable to challenges from alternative sources of expertise. From the government's point of view "damage limitation" was certainly one role of the Advisory Committee on Nutrition.

As nutrition and malnutrition were increasingly debated in the public arena during 1933, the Advisory Committee was initially uninvolved. The British Medical Association, in contrast, perceived an opportunity to intervene and to display the social engagement and importance of the medical profession. The BMA Nutrition Committee included some people who might be regarded as "scientific/medical statespeople" of the kind that, in Aronson's view, usually engaged in interpretive claims-smaking, but also some more junior figures, for example, Crowden, for whom the activity of interpretive claimsmaking formed part of a process of career development.[60]

When the BMA Committee contradicted the basic scientific data that the Advisory Committee had previously endorsed, causing great public political embarrassment for the Ministry, the expertise and integrity of the members of the Advisory Committee were called into question. Cathcart, who had made his reputation in the area of nutrition in which the BMA Committee had controverted existing opinion, felt especially aggrieved. However, the main members of the Advisory Committee, including Cath-cart, were eventually persuaded that it was in their interests to meet with the other side in an attempt to find a resolution to the dispute. For the Ministry, the Joint Conferences, like the Advisory Committee on Nutrition, constituted a damage-limitation exercise, but in this case it was a reduction of conflict between the experts that was required to alleviate the pressure on the government. During the conferences, it soon emerged just how little real substance there was in the data that were at the center of the dispute. Cathcart was unable to maintain his indignation. It would appear to be the desire to avoid further political controversy that prevailed, and the final formulation allowed both sides to emerge with their reputations as nutrition experts intact. The new "Sliding Scale of Calorie Requirements," and the formulation regarding first class protein requirements in the Report of the Joint Conferences, may be seen largely as a modification of some generally accepted data as a result of a series of clashes, and realignments of professional, personal, and political interests. The modifications protected the public image and credibility of the parties involved.

Medical and scientific knowledge was clearly central to the social construction of nutrition as a social problem in Britain during the 1930s, but in this chapter it has been possible to give an account of only a very limited aspect of the whole process. However, it has been possible to use some unusually rich archival sources, and to reveal the great extent to which the dietary standards set out in the Report of the Joint Conferences were the products of personal, professional, and political struggles. Such struggles are normally played out largely in private meetings, the records of which do not often become available to researchers. When such material is available, there are rarely verbatim reports of meetings, which there were in this case. This chapter therefore serves to emphasize the point that in the analysis of the social construction of any nutrition-related social issue, underlying the data deployed by the actors involved, there are likely to be important medical and scientific interests, which are rarely explicitly displayed, but which should be considered, whenever possible, if a comprehensive analysis is to be achieved.

Acknowledgment

During the preparation of this chapter, Dr. Smith has been in receipt of financial support from the Wellcome Trust to whom he wishes to record his gratitude.

Notes

Abbreviations for archival sources used in notes: PRO = Public Records Office, Kew, London; WI CMAC = Contemporary Medical Archives Centre, Wellcome Institute, London.

1. For a discussion of the recurrent debates about the causes of nutritional problems of the poor in Britain during the twentieth century see Smith and Nicolson (1993).

2. Sometimes Newman mentioned even more factors as contributing to "nutrition." In 1915, for example, he listed a total of 22 causes of "defective nutrition" (Board of Education 1915:67). Webster (1982) and Mayhew (1988) have discussed the various ways in which the health administration presented an optimistic interpretation of health statistics, and often consciously attempted to suppress the findings of and to silence critics who claimed that malnutrition was associated with poverty and unemployment during the 1930s.

3. The latter approach was used most effectively in the report *Food Health and Income* published in 1936 by John Boyd Orr, Director of the Rowett Research Institute in Aberdeen (Orr 1936).

4. The report was published by the Ministry of Health, but was also printed in the *British Medical Journal*. See *British Medical Journal* (1934:901).

5. See, for example, Mellanby (1927). Brief discussions of the Advisory Committee may be found in Mayhew (1988), op. cit. note 1, and Petty (1989).

6. For typical comments about vitamins see Cathcart (1931). For an account and analysis of the rickets controversy see Smith and Nicolson (1989).

7. Carnwath to Newman 12/1/31. PRO MH 56/51.

8. Carnwath to Newman and Beckett 4/18/32. PRO MH 56/46.

9. Anderson to Robinson 12/22/32. WI CMAC BMA F12.

10. Carnwath to Newman 4/4/33. PRO MH 56/40.

11. Cathcart to Hudson 7/24/33. PRO MH 56/46.

12. Minutes of Advisory Committee Meeting of 7/28/33. PRO MH 56/46.

13. "Supplementary Agenda" BMA Science Committee Minutes 3/10/33. WI CMAC BMA G44.

14. Council Minutes 1932–33, 203. WI CMAC BMA.

15. V. H. Mottram "Basic Calorie and Protein intake" (memorandum discussed at BMA Nutrition Committee Meeting 5/18/33). WI CMAC BMA G44.

16. G. C. M. M'Gonigle "Analysis of Diet in H. M. Forces (Army)" (memorandum discussed at BMA Nutrition Committee Meeting 5/18/33). WI CMAC BMA G44.

17. G. P. Crowden "Memorandum on the Minimum Cost of a Physiologically adequate diet" (discussed at BMA Nutrition Committee Meeting 5/1833). WI CMAC BMA G44.

18. Minutes of the BMA Nutrition Committee Meeting 5/1833. WI CMAC BMA G44.

19. Minutes of the BMA Nutrition Committee Meeting 6/8/33. WI CMAC BMA G44.

20. M'Gonigle to Hill 9/10/33. WI CMAC BMA G50.

21. Minutes of the BMA Nutrition Committee Meeting 10/20/33. WI CMAC BMA G44.

22. Hill to Seipmann 11/9/33, Seipmann to Hill 11/15/33, Hill to Seipmann, 11/16/33. WI CMAC BMA G47.

23. M'Gonigle to Hill 11/27/33. WI CMAC BMA G50.

24. The report had sold 3,200 copies by 11/29/33, 5,000 by 12/4/33, and 7,330 by 12/12/33. Hill to M'Gonigle 11/29/33, 12/4/33, 12/12/33. WI CMAC BMA G50.

25. Labour Party Notes for Speakers on the BMA Report 12/1/33. PRO MH 56/55.

26. Press statement 11/24/33. PRO MH 56/55.

27. Minutes of meeting called by the Minister of Health, Sir Hilton Young, attended by Robinson, Newman, Carnwath, and Hamill, 12/11/33. PRO MH 56/43.

28. Buchan to Newman 11/30/33. PRO MH 56/55.

29. Minutes of the BMA Nutrition Committee Meeting 1/18/34. WI CMAC BMA G44.

30. Memorandum on the BMA Report by Mottram, circulated 12/13/33. PRO MH 56/55.

31. H. Robert Topping, General Director of the Conservative and Unionist Central Office to Young 1/12/35. PRO MH 56/56.

32. KMG to 1. Sir Arthur Robinson, 2. CMO. PRO MH 56/55.

33. Robinson to Young 1/11/34. PRO MH 56/56.

34. Minute of meeting of Young, Robinson and Greenwood, 1/11/31. PRO MH 56/56.

35. Robinson to Anderson 1/17/34. WI CMAC BMA G45.

36. Minutes of the BMA Nutrition Committee 1/18/34. WI CMAC BMA G44.

37. Cathcart to Young 1/15/34. PRO MH 56/56.
38. Carnwath to Newman and Robinson 1/26/34. PRO MH 56/47.
39. Crowden to Anderson 2/3/34. WI CMAC BMA G48.
40. Cathcart to Carnwath 1/20/34. PRO MH 56/56.
41. Cathcart to Carnwath 1/30/34. PRO MH 56/47.
42. This, and the quotations until the next footnote, are all taken from the verbatim report of the "Meeting between Nutrition Advisory Committee and British Medical Association Committee" taken by Treasury Reporters 2/6/34. PRO MH 56/56 and WI CMAC BMA G45.
43. G. P. Crowden "Notes on Calorie and Protein Requirements" paper prepared for the Meeting between the Nutrition Advisory Committee and British Medical Association Committee 2/6/34. PRO MH 56/56.
44. Robinson to Young 2/8/34. PRO MH 56/56.
45. Memorandum by Cathcart 2/14/34. PRO MH 56/56.
46. Hill to Crowden 2/22/34. WI CMAC BMA G48.
47. Anderson to Mottram 2/26/34. WI CMAC BMA G50.
48. This, and the quotations until the next footnote, are all taken from the verbatim report of the "Meeting between the Nutrition Committee and British Medical Association" 2/27/34. PRO MH 56/56 and WI CMAC BMA G45.
49. Crowden to Magee 3/15/34. PRO MH 56/56.
50. Anderson to Magee 4/13/34. Anderson had already made representations to Magee about the wording of this passage: Anderson to Magee 3/27/34. WI CMAC BMA G45. The version finally agreed was "This figure can safely be employed for calculation of mass requirements, but in the case of individuals or single families due regard should be paid to the sliding scale" (*British Medical Journal* 1934:901).
51. Magee to Anderson 5/3/34. PRO MH 56/56.
52. Magee told Carnwath that he had sent the Report to Anderson and that members of the conference had taken it for granted that it would be published. Magee to Carnwath 5/3/34. PRO MH 56/56.
53. Carnwath to Newman 5/3/34. PRO MH 56/56.
54. Newman to Robinson 5/3/34. PRO MH 56/56.
55. Robinson to Minister 5/7/34. PRO MH 56/56.
56. M'Gonigle to Anderson 5/9/34. WI CMAC BMA G50.
57. Anderson to M'Gonigle 5/11/34. WI CMAC BMA G50.
58. The report was sent, with a Circular, to County Councils and Sanitary Authorities in England and Wales.
59. Partly as a result of the public controversy of November 1933–January 1934, the days of the ACN, as original constituted, were numbered. For the next episode in the life of the Advisory Committee on Nutrition see Smith (1987).
60. Aronson's own work on Atwater's early career supports the view that interpretive claimsmaking is not confined to upper echelons of science. See Aronson (1982).

References

Aronson, N. 1982. "Nutrition as a Social Problem: A Case Study of Entrepreneurial Strategy in Science." *Social Problems* 29:475–487.
_____. 1984. "Science as a Claims-making Activity: Implications for Social Prob-

lems Research." Pp. 1–30 in *Studies in the Sociology of Social Problems,* edited by J. W. Schneider and J. I. Kitsuse. Norwood, NJ: Ablex.

BMA Member. 1933. "Letter to the Editor." *Week-End Review* February 18:169.

Board of Education. 1915. *Annual Report of the Chief Medical Officer of the Board of Education for the Year 1914.* London: HMSO.

British Medical Association. 1933. "Report of Committee on Nutrition." *Supplement to the British Medical Journal* November 11.

British Medical Journal. 1934. "The Nutrition Question. An Agreed Report." *British Medical Journal* 1934 I:900–901.

Cathcart, E. P. 1931. "The Foundations of a National Diet." *Medical Officer* 45:131–134.

Cathcart, E. P., and A. M. T. Murray. 1931. "A Study in Nutrition: 154 St. Andrews Families." Medical Research Council Special Report Series 151. London: HMSO.

———. 1932. "Studies in Nutrition: An Enquiry into the Diets of Families in Cardiff and Reading." Medical Research Council Special Report Series 165. London: HMSO.

Dawson of Penn, L. 1934. "Diet and Health. Committees at Cross-Purposes. A Joint Session Proposed." (Letter to the Editor.) *The Times* January 11:13e.

Greenwood, M. 1934. "Diet and Health. Needs of an Average Man. The Minister and His Advisers." (Letter to the Editor.) *The Times* January 8:13e.

Hudson, R. S. 1933. Parliamentary Reply on "Sustenance." *Parliamentary Debates* 283 (1933–34), c1031.

Knorr-Cetina, K. 1981. *The Manufacture of Knowledge: An Essay on the Constructivist and Contextual Nature of Science.* Oxford: Pergamon.

Latour, B. 1987. *Science in Action.* Milton Keynes: Open University Press

Latour, B., and Woolgar, S. 1979. *Laboratory Life The Social Construction of Scientific Facts.* Beverly Hills, CA: Sage.

League of Nations. 1932. "Standardisation of Certain Methods Used in Making Dietary Studies." *Quarterly Bulletin of the Health Organization of the League of Nations* I:3.

Mayhew, M. 1988. "The 1930s Nutrition Controversy." *Journal of Contemporary History* 23:445–464.

Mellanby, E. 1927. "Duties of the State in Relation to the Nation's Food Supply." *British Medical Journal* II:633n636.

Meynell, V. 1933. "Letter to the Editor." *Week-End Review* February 4:117.

Ministry of Health. 1930. *Statutory Rules and Orders 1930 No 185 Poor Law England: The Public Assistance Order 1930: To Come into Operation on the 1st April 1930.* London: HMSO.

———. 1932a. *Advisory Committee on Nutrition Report to the Minister of Health on Diets in Poor Law Childrens' Homes, 30th Nov. 1931.* London: HMSO.

———. 1932b. *Advisory Committee on Nutrition Report to the Minister of Health on the Criticism and Improvement of Diets 5th Dec. 1931.* London: HMSO.

———. 1932c. *Certain Recommendations of the Advisory Committee on Nutrition: To County and County Borough Councils, and Other Maternity and Child Welfare Authorities, Oct. 27, 1932 (Circular 1290).* London: HMSO.

————. 1934. *Nutrition. To County Councils and Sanitary Authorities in England and Wales, Jan 4, 1934 (Circular 1370).* London: HMSO.

Mottram, V. H. 1934. "The Committee on Nutrition." (Letter to the Editor.) *The Times* January 6:6c.

Newman, G. 1928. *The Foundations of National Health.* (The Sir Charles Hastings Lecture.) London: HMSO.

Orr, J. B. 1936. *Food, Health and Income: A Report on a Survey of Adequacy of Diet in Relation to Income.* London: Macmillan.

Petty, C. 1989. "Primary Research and Public Health: The Prioritization of Nutrition Research in Inter-war Britain." Pp. 83–108 in *Historical Perspectives on the Role of the MRC,* edited by J. Austoker and L. Bryder. Oxford: Oxford University Press.

Pollitt, H. 1936. "Building the People's Front." *The Left Review* 2:797–803.

Political Correspondent. 1934. "Medical Storm over Ministry Food Minimum. B. M. A. Retorts that Cooking Loss Has Been Overlooked. Attempt to Foster Underfeeding." *Daily Herald* January 6:1c.

Smith, D. F. 1987. *Nutrition in Britain in the Twentieth Century.* Unpublished Ph.D. thesis, Edinburgh University.

Smith, D. F., and M. Nicolson. 1989. "The 'Glasgow School' of Paton, Findlay and Cathcart: Conservative Thought in Chemical Physiology, Nutrition and Public Health." *Social Studies in Science* 19:195–238.

————. 1993. "Health and Ignorance—Past and Present." Pp. 221–244 in *Locating Health: Sociological and Historical Explorations.* London: British Sociological Association and Avebury.

Special Correspondent. 1933. "B. M. A. Exposes Inadequacy of Unemployment Pay. Food Leaves only 6/8 1/2 for Everything Else. Standard Lower Than That for Convicts." *Daily Herald* November 24:1a.

The Times. 1934a. "Diet and Health. Reply to Ministry's Circular. A Defence of the B. M. A. Committee." January 6:7a.

————. 1934b. "A Wise Proposal." (Editorial) January 11:11d.

————. 1934c. "Minimum Diet for a Man. Divergent Views Reconciled. A Sliding Scale." May 16:18d.

————. 1934d. "Standards of Nutrition." (Editorial) May 16:17d.

Tinker, R. H. 1933. Parliamentary Question on "Sustenance." *Parliamentary Debates* (Commons) 283 (1933–34), c1030.

Webster, C. 1982. "Healthy or Hungry Thirties." *History Workshop Journal* 110–129.

Week-End Review. 1933a. "Editorial." March 11:264.

————. 1933b. "Hungry England Inquiry: Report of a Committee." April 1:357.

————. 1933c. "Minimum Cost of an Adequate Dietary." April 1:358–360.

14

Making an Issue of Food Safety: The Media, Pressure Groups, and the Public Sphere

DAVID MILLER and JACQUIE REILLY

Media coverage of health issues or public concern about those issues does not mirror the incidence of disease or the severity of the health problem (calculated in terms of human misery or death). While widely recognized, the reasons for this remain poorly explained. For some commentators, this relates to inadequacies in human perception, sometimes allied with "irresponsible" or "sensational" reporting by the mass media. Such explanations oversimplify and misrepresent the complex social processes that combine in the production of news media accounts and public perceptions of social problems. Most obviously, such approaches assume that expert assessments are based on straightforwardly objective evidence. They also tend to identify disparate social events as part of more general phenomena by pointing to surface similarities such as gaps between "expert" assessments of social problems and public or media assessments. Such analyses tend, therefore, to be devoid of historical perspective and to neglect the social processes involved in the definition of social problems.

Ironically, this latter problem is also one result of adopting a strict constructionist approach to social problems since historical factors and social processes are held to be unknowable because they are socially constructed. Here the focus is not on the "objective facts" of a health problem as defined by experts, but on the claims made by both experts, interest groups, and lay people on the definition of social problems. The tendency is to eschew references to underlying realities since all knowledge is held to be socially constructed and therefore interest laden.

In the foregoing paragraphs we have already implicitly made references to material conditions. This is not because we are engaging in what Woolgar and Pawluch have called "ontological gerrymandering" (Woolgar and Pawluch 1985a), that is, talking of social constructions while assuming (implicitly or explicitly) an underlying reality against which they may be judged. Rather, we will be arguing that the construction of food safety does not rely simply on the claimsmaking activities of government, industry, and pressure groups, but is founded on the intimate interaction of material conditions and struggles for definitional advantage. We contend that the definition of social problems around food could not take place without the actually existing systems of production surrounding both food and the media (Fine and Leopold 1993; Fine and Wright 1991). We make no apologies for asserting our view on this as better than those that emphasize only symbolic factors or alternatively those emphasizing only material or economic factors. We do not regard this assertion as an exercise in epistemological imperialism, but as an attempt to get as close as possible to understanding the world. Such attempts will always be flawed, but this does not mean that there are no criteria for separating fact from fiction and truth from lies, or for preferring some accounts over others.

This chapter focuses on the high profile food "scares"[1] that received extensive publicity in the British media in the late 1980s. We will try to outline some of the key factors that provided the context for the major crisis of public confidence in food that occurred as a result. We also examine the strategies of industry, government, and interest groups in their attempts to manage the media coverage of food issues. Finally we outline the ways in which some food safety issues can decline in media importance while others remain in the public eye.

Changes in Government Policy

In the post-World War II period, food safety rarely received extensive coverage in the British media. The most notable major public issue prior to the *Salmonella* in eggs crisis of 1988 was a 1964 outbreak of typhoid in an Aberdeen hospital associated with canned corned beef (Franklin 1994; North and Gorman 1990). Sir Michael Franklin, Permanent Secretary at the Ministry of Agriculture Fisheries and Food (MAFF) until 1987, is an important witness here:

One of my earliest political lessons—that the time Ministers need to devote to a subject is not in proportion to its intrinsic importance nor to the extent to which they can really do anything about it but to the volume of public concern—came from the typhoid outbreak in Aberdeen in the early 60s, which was traced to corned beef from South America. But by and large, this aspect of the Ministry's work trundled along without too much publicity until the late 1980s. (Franklin 1994:5)

A key reason why MAFF policy on food "trundled along" in this way is that food policy was seen straightforwardly as a means to encourage the production of more food. The Ministry of Food was disbanded with the end of rationing in 1955. In the official account, it was amalgamated with the Ministry of Agriculture. But civil servants in the Ministry of Food were concerned at the proposed merger: "Such a Ministry would be subjected to heavy pressure from the National Farmers Union at Ministerial level [and] it would rapidly degenerate into the kind of department that the Ministry of Agriculture is today, i.e. primarily looking after the farmers' interests" (MAFF 127/269, cited in Smith 1991:238). According to Sir Michael Franklin, this is precisely what happened: "Much as we pretended to our new colleagues that it was a true merger of the Ministries of Food and Agriculture, in fact it was a take-over" (Franklin 1994:4). Policy analysts agree that the farmers' influence in the Ministry of Agriculture was immense (Mills 1991, 1992; Smith 1989, 1991). This meant that health concerns were not of great importance. As Sir Michael Franklin has acknowledged:

food policy, if it existed at all was very much the junior partner in the MAFF. This was so from the outset. For the rest of my official career (and I retired in 1987), agriculture policy was in the driving seat . . . . Even the efforts to protect the consumer were carried out with more than half an eye on the interests of the food manufacturers. (Franklin 1994:4–5)

Policy was "developed in the absence of much in the way of effective intervention from elsewhere in government, in particular from the treasury and the cabinet" (Grant 1989:139). But the political influence of the agricultural lobby has declined over the past 20 years or so partly reflecting the decline in importance of agriculture in economic terms.

More important for our present purposes is the steadily widening split between health and agriculture policy within government. For much of the postwar period agriculture and health policy had the same goal: to make sure that everyone had enough to eat. With the end of food scarcity, the major problems of food policy related to overproduction and growing concerns about public health. Scientific arguments about the role of diet in coronary heart disease have led the Department of Health (DoH) and the Ministry of Agriculture to develop increasingly different sets of priorities. However, such concerns developed slowly and have had a low priority. This has been attributed, in part, to the predominance of curative rather than preventive medicine in health policy making (Mills 1992). The DoH's Nutrition Unit is, according to its director, Martin Wiseman (1990:397), a "small group of professionals" with few resources, compared with the major divisions of the DoH, which deal with the National Health Service. Other factors that have prevented the DoH from taking a stronger policy line on diet and nutrition have included the professed ideology of successive Conservative governments since 1979, which have preferred to place responsibility for health on the public or the "consumers," together with the influence of the Ministry of Agriculture as advocate for the food industry. The government's Chief Medical Officer, Sir Donald Acheson, has acknowledged such factors: "It is a . . . difficult matter for it [government] to propose that the consumption of pleasurable by perhaps harmful [food] factors should be reduced, particularly when the employment and prosperity of a large part of the nation depend on the production of these substances" (Acheson 1986:137).

Such difficulties have resulted in the government suppression or censorship of the reports of government appointed expert committees, which concluded that there was a strong relationship between dietary fats and coronary heart disease (Cannon 1987; Farrant and Russell 1986). Nevertheless, there has been an increasing sense in which the policy directions of MAFF and the DoH have diverged. This is important because of the reliance of the media on "credible," "authoritative," and "expert" sources. Thus, an announcement by the DoH of a serious public health problem is likely to be taken seriously by most of the mainstream media. Similarly, "disagreement," "conflict," "conspiracy," and "cover-up" are important components of newsworthiness, especially if the conflict is between "authoritative" sources, such as government departments. Both of these factors were especially important in the *Salmonella* and (in a different way) bovine spongiform encephalopathy (BSE) crises in Britain, as we shall see.

Trends in the Food Industry

Within the food industry there has been an increasing globalization of markets and a shift from the rhythms of agriculture to the needs of industry. This has led to an increasing "entanglement of the food and chemical industries" (Mennell et al. 1992:71), with a consequent proliferation of pesticides, additives, and methods of preservation and the rise of "fast-foods." Such technological advances have brought with them new hazards. So, while the causes of the increase in *Salmonella* and *Listeria* and the emergence of BSE have all been contested, it is common ground to all sides of such arguments that food safety worries have emerged as a result of recent changes in the production of food.[2]

The uses to which technological change have been put has also been an important impetus for changes in food distribution and retailing. Supermarkets, in particular, have become more important, with a small number of large firms dominating the British retail market by the early 1990s (Henson 1992). This dominance has meant a shift in the balance of power within the food industry in the retailers' favor (Gardener and Sheppard 1989). Retailers have been able to exert pressure on food producers and processors over the safety of food production in the absence of changes in government policy (Smith 1993).

Pressure Groups and Public Culture

Parallel with the increasing divergence at the heart of government policy, there has also been a significant growth in the moral, ethical, and environmental aspects of food in public culture. There are a myriad of factors here, but we can note the increase in vegetarianism, the impact of animal rights activism, campaigning by aid agencies and others about famine, particularly the Band Aid phenomenon in 1984 and 1985, and the growth of environmentalism. In the latter two cases, at least, public awareness and concern have been underestimated by the media or have preceded major interest from the mass media (Anderson 1991; Philo 1993; Schoenfield et al. 1979).

Although some pressure groups, such as the Vegetarian Society, have a long history, a large number of food-related pressure groups have appeared much more recently.[3] One of the first was the Coronary Prevention Group (CPG). Formed in 1979 the CPG saw its role as one of public education and campaigning to change government policy. While the main coronary heart disease-related charity since the 1960s had been the British Heart Foundation, the founders of the Coronary Prevention Group felt that there was a need for a more campaigning body (Rayner 1992).

During the 1980s a plethora of other groups came into existence. The London Food Commission was set up in 1985 as an independent watchdog on food. Emphasizing the crucial role of material resources, the Commission secured funding from the Labour controlled Greater London Council. Other examples include the National Food Alliance in 1985 and the Public Health Alliance in 1987. There has also been a growth in animal welfare organizations such as Chicken's Lib and the Farm Animal Welfare Network. The food safety crises of 1989 also sparked the creation of other campaigning groups, most notably, Parents for Safe Food in 1989.

In another overlapping sphere, we can note the rise of the consumer movement in Britain since the 1970s. The Consumers Association (CA) (the counterpart of the United States' Consumers Union) was founded in 1957 and has grown beyond traditional concerns with product testing (Grose 1978). Its magazine *Which?* now has a regular section on food and health information and the CA now produces a separate health magazine, *Which? Way to Health* (National Forum for Coronary Heart Disease Prevention 1988:72). One key factor in the emergence of such pressure groups has been their relationships with the media. In contrast with some sections of the food industry, pressure groups have had to use the media to raise the profile of their campaigning demands.

Changes in Journalism

Growth in interest in food as "newsworthy" is a relatively recent development within the British media. Food writing in the 1920s consisted mainly of recipe columns like those, for example, of Agnes Jekyll in *The Times*. Writing during this period, "she could still assume that her readers were not actually doing the cooking themselves. Her instructions for Gigot de six heures begin 'instruct your cook to treat it thus'" (Crawford-Poole 1993:19). By the 1970s it seemed that not much had changed. The emphasis remained clearly on domestic cookery with national daily newspapers relegating food writing to the "ghetto of the womens page" (Crawford-Poole 1993:19).

Yet, it was on the Women's page that the politics of food began to be first taken seriously in the British press.[4] As in the United States, food came to be seen as increasingly "newsworthy" (Hanke 1989). One of the first regular columnists in the British press to raise the politics of food as an issue for cookery or gourmet writers was Colin Spencer. Following the publication of his book, *Gourmet Cooking for Vegetarians* in 1978, Spencer was given a column by the editor of the *Guardian* Women's page, Liz Forgan in 1980. As early as 1981 he was complaining about the shortcomings of his cookery writing colleagues:

> I find the cookery clan unnerving, not only because it appears to be an insular elite but because it pretends a total ignorance of the politics of food in the most comprehensive sense . . . . Here were nearly a hundred fairly intelligent beings discussing food and the various qualities of different recipes, for a couple of hours, without relating food to anything else. I felt tempted to stand on a chair and shout: Malnutrition, Third World Famine,

Exploitation of world food resources by the West. Obscene realities in this context, yet I suspect to the gathering merely irrelevant. (Spencer 1981:9)

It is striking that Spencer did not feel tempted to shout about factory farming, pesticides, additives, or food poisoning. It was only later that these became central concerns of critical food journalists. The creation of the Guild of Food Writers in 1984 was one indication of the widening conception of the place of food in the media. Other journalists' associations, such as the Medical Journalists Association, the Association of British Science Writers, and the Guild of Agricultural Journalists, have close, some would say overclose (Lycett 1988), relationships with industry, in the form of sponsorship. The Guild of Food Writers, by contrast, sees its function as campaigning against the influence of vested interests in food writing. In a founding statement, journalist Derek Cooper argued that

> The power that such a guild could exercise for the public good is limitless. This present year, with its spate of radio and TV programmes questioning the whole basis of our national diet and the way in which our food is produced and processed, demonstrates that such concern is no longer confined to medical and nutritional experts. Thanks to investigative journalism, millions of shoppers are beginning to demand healthier food. (Cooper 1985:17)

This campaigning agenda has filtered into television and radio. Most notable here is *The Food Programme* on Radio 4 that deals with food issues from production to consumption, and the BBC's *Food and Drink* program that, although it still retains a cookery demonstration format, has increasingly featured information on the politics of food and health. Yet programs like this are still the exception rather than the rule and media coverage is generally concentrated only when food becomes a politically sensitive issue. As food journalism has expanded, so too has the number of consumer correspondents on national newspapers. By the early 1990s all Broadsheet papers and most tabloids had appointed consumer correspondents. Environment correspondents are also a recent innovation in British newspapers, most being appointed in 1988 and 1989 (Anderson 1991).[5]

The declining importance of farming in British politics has also has its impact on journalism. At the end of the 1970s there were agriculture correspondents on all the broadsheet newspapers and on the mid-range tabloids. British press agency, the Press Association had up to three reporters covering the agriculture beat. By 1994 there were only two agriculture correspondents on national papers, the *Times* and the *Daily Telegraph*. The beat covered by these correspondents has also widened,

its focus having shifted away from agricultural policy and a close relationship with the National Farmers Union and MAFF to a more diverse
"countryside" brief incorporating conservation and other rural issues.[6]

The Process of a "Scare"

The factors outlined above were necessary but not sufficient to create
the crisis of confidence in the food supply that ensued in 1989 and 1990.
The growth of pressure groups campaigning around food and the increase in coverage of the politics of food in the media have mutually
reinforced each other. Indeed in some cases, there has been an overlap
between media and activist personnel. The Guild of Food Writers includes both journalists and activists, and can be seen as a pressure
group. Geoffrey Cannon was one of the first journalists to make coronary heart disease a media issue when he revealed the government
suppression of an official report on the front page of the *Sunday Times*
(Cannon 1983). Cannon went on to become a key activist and chair of the
National Food Alliance (Cannon 1987; Cannon and Walker 1985). This
example also highlights the interaction of changes in government policy
with the media. The appointment of an official committee was a symptom of changes in government policy. The suppression of its report and
the revelation of this by the *Sunday Times* put coronary heart disease at
the center of the public sphere, pressuring government to go further and
giving a boost to coronary heart disease campaigners. However, it was
not until the end of 1988 that food safety really hit the headlines in the
form of the *Salmonella* in eggs crisis.

Immediate Factors

The crisis was sparked by a statement by Junior Health Minister Edwina Currie. On December 3, 1988 she said that "we do warn people
now that most of the egg production in this country, sadly, is now
infected with salmonella" (ITN 1988). Yet, while these remarks were
neither unusual nor dramatic, a number of factors did help to give them
more impact.

First, she was speaking to television cameras, not writing in a medical
journal. Currie also enjoyed a certain amount of credibility as a government Minister, enhanced by a reputation for speaking her mind and
media friendly conduct. Earlier controversial statements had made her
well known to the public. One poll in September 1988 (before the eggs

controversy) found that 78% of people recognized the junior heath minister, five times more than her boss, Health Secretary Kenneth Clarke (*Daily Mirror*, September 3, 1988:2). Because of her notoriety and the public response to her statements, Currie became the only junior minister to have her own press officer (Currie 1989:19).

Second, by December 1988, there had already been a considerable amount of official and industry activity on *Salmonella*. By late 1988 government scientists were arguing in the *Lancet* that *Salmonella enteritidis* was

> a new and important public health problem. The consequence for the public is that all eggs, including intact clean eggs, should be regarded as possibly infected. Raw egg consumption may therefore be unsafe. Furthermore, temperatures within the yolk of soft boiled eggs have been shown experimentally not to reach bactericidal levels, and the outbreak data presented here suggest that scrambled eggs, hard boiled eggs, and scotch eggs may be sources of infection. (Coyle et al. 1988:1296)

Indeed, the director of the relevant division at the Public Health Laboratory Service[7] had already advocated as the "remaining option" a campaign "to increase public awareness of food poisoning hazards, particularly among those concerned with the handling and preparation of foods, especially poultry. This approach would necessitate intensive campaigns to provide relevant information and instruction" (Humphrey et al. 1988:182).

There had been a dramatic rise in recorded cases of *Salmonella enteritidis* strain. In 1981, *enteritidis* constituted 11% (1,087) of reported cases of *Salmonella* in humans in Britain. By 1988 it had risen to 56% (15,427) (Public Health Laboratory Service 1989). There has been no suggestion that these figures have been affected by changes in reporting procedures or other factors. The rise in *Salmonella enteritidis* poisoning was not challenged by the egg industry, and it was widely agreed that there was a real increase in *Salmonella enteritidis* poisoning. The question was, how had this occurred? As early as December 1987 government scientists at the Public Health Laboratory Service suspected eggs as a factor in the increase in *Salmonella* and a report appeared in the *Sunday Times* to that effect (Deer 1987). Following the publication of similar findings in the United States in early 1988 (St. Louis et al. 1988), the egg theory became more established. On the other hand, the egg industry maintained that there was insufficient evidence of vertical transmission (from chicken to egg) and attributed the dramatic rise in food poisoning to cross-contamination and poor kitchen hygiene (British Egg Industry Council 1989; North and Gorman 1990).

Following several official meetings throughout the first half of the year, DoH representatives tried to convince the egg industry to accept at least the theoretical possibility that eggs were implicated in the rise of *enteritidis* infections. By June 1988 the DoH considered three options: (1) to do nothing, which might look bad if the media got hold of the story, (2) to advise the National Health Service (NHS) only about raw eggs, which might also leak to the media, and (3) to issue public advice (North 1989).

By this time the DoH had prepared a defensive briefing to be used in the event of media inquiries. But nothing was done. It was not until the end of July that the second option was taken; a letter was sent to NHS caterers and dieticians and District Medical Officers and Nurse Advisors (Thomson 1988) but not to Environmental Health Officers. It was picked up 6 days later by only one national newspaper (*The Independent* August 4, 1988). Almost a month after this (August 26) the first press release was issued after further consultation with the egg industry. This warned only about the risks of raw eggs, especially for the "vulnerable" (Department of Health and Social Security 1988a). This time the information was issued to Environmental Health Officers, who were asked to publicize it. It seems that this process led to an increasing interest in the provincial media and to consequent pressure on the DoH press office for a ministerial statement. According to Edwina Currie (1989:58): "For weeks my office had been fending off demands for a comment or remark from me all over the country, from local radio and television stations which had picked up their local Environmental Health officers warnings. But I referred them to the Chief Medical officer's two statements."

The local interest was also filtering back to the national media, prompting the interest of specialist food and consumer programs. In late 1988 BBC TV's *Food and Drink* covered *Salmonella* on November 15, BBC Radio Four's *Food Programme* on November 18, and BBC consumer program *Watchdog* on November 21. As a result of the increased media interest the DHSS issued a further statement on November 21 aimed at reassuring the public about the risks of eating lightly cooked eggs. This was interpreted by the press as downgrading the gravity of the risk.[8] Yet it was plain that the text masked serious divisions between the DHSS and MAFF when the Chief Medical Officer went further than the press release and said in an interview that the elderly, the sick, and the pregnant should "in my personal opinion be advised to stick to hard-boiled eggs" (*Evening Standard*, November 23 1988). By this time, pressure groups such as the London Food Commission, critics such as Professor Richard Lacey, and the Institute of Environmental Health Officers were also supporting the conclusion that even lightly cooked eggs were potentially risky. Finally on December 2, the Plymouth Health Authority announced that it was banning fresh eggs from the kitchens of its 25 hospitals. The next evening, Edwina Currie's statement prompted the reaction that placed *Salmonella* in eggs at the center of the political arena.

The next section reviews some of the key factors that helped to shape the form, duration, intensity, and outcome of the various crises.

Divisions within Government

Divisions within government, preeminently between the DoH and the Ministry of Agriculture, were a key factor in both the *Listeria* and *Salmonella* crises. At the DoH there was pressure from scientists at the government's Public Health Laboratory Service. As Edwina Currie has put it: "The laboratories had been screaming at us for months" (1989:262). During the crisis:

> Officials speak of "hellish rows" between the Departments of Agriculture and Health. "It was Agriculture who behaved quite appallingly," said one [health] official who observed the row at close quarters. "It is the egg producers who are guilty of allowing salmonella to spread, but now they are to be baled out with millions of pounds. I thought the Tory party was no longer in the pocket of such interests." The most overt sign of this furious interdepartmental split came on Friday, with the publication of an ambiguously worded advertisement in the national press. The text, which the Government said was designed to "clarify" the issue, begged as many questions as it answered. (Lustig et al. 1988:15)

This account is broadly confirmed by our own interviewees. Very senior medical sources in the Department of Health have reported that MAFF put "intense pressure" on the Chief Medical Officer to say "forget about it, she was quite wrong, eggs are safe" (Interview with the authors, February 1994).[9] Instead the DoH issued a press statement on the Monday following Currie's remarks, hardening the advice: "Although the risk of harm to any healthy individual from consuming a single raw or partially cooked egg is small, it is advisable for vulnerable people such as the elderly, the sick, babies and pregnant women to consume only eggs which have been cooked until the white and yolk are solid" (Department of Health and Social Security 1988b:1).

In any "scare," relationships between government departments and the media are fundamental to the form and content of the coverage. The news media depend on government sources as a staple source of information supply. But this does not mean journalists always believe the government. The ability of a government department to successfully manage the media is related to (1) the extent to which the department is unified internally and with other official sources and (2) the ability to portray the department as united and purposive by a strategy involving a varying mix of publicity and secrecy.

Government Secrecy

The British approach to information management relies heavily on secrecy. Britain has no freedom of information legislation. A central criticism of government action in all three food safety crises discussed here was that they had failed to inform the public about the risks associated with eating particular foods. We have seen how interdepartmental and government industry divisions delayed public advice in the *Salmonella* affair. Similarly, from the start the MAFF approach on BSE was to say nothing to the public or the media. Sensitivities centered on the similarities between BSE and the sheep disease scrapie. If the new cattle disease was found to be an equivalent of scrapie, this raised the possibility that the poorly understood scrapie might have jumped the species barrier. If this was so, there was more reason to suppose that it could do so again, possibly even infecting humans. Colin Whitaker, the vet who noted the first cases of BSE in 1985, discovered that the brains of infected cattle had a spongy texture similar to those of sheep infected with scrapie. According to Whitaker: "The Ministry seemed to keep very quiet about it in the early stages . . . . They didn't seem to want publicity with the disease . . . . It did seem to me a little odd that we were asked to keep somewhat quiet" (BBC Radio Four 1989). By 1987 Whitaker was preparing to publish a scientific paper on BSE but the Ministry would not allow him to use the term "scrapie like disease" because "The word 'scrapie' was deemed to be emotive and I was asked not to use it" (BBC Radio Four 1989).

Secrecy is of course intimately bound up with public relations and the pursuit of definitional advantage. The publication of the report of the expert committee on the risks of BSE was apparently delayed by officials nervous about its contents. "Attempts are being made to persuade the authors to change the report's emphasis. Officials also want some of the findings omitted from the version to be published" (Ballantyne and Norton-Taylor 1989:1).

Government Public Relations

The press office of a government department performs several functions. It both releases and suppresses information. It controls and coordinates information from the department and polices the public image of the department. In a crisis situation one of the key functions of the press office is to project the department as a unified body. Tight control of information is one method of trying to ensure this. Early in the BSE crisis the Agriculture Minister John Gummer took a close personal interest in the presentation of the Ministry. This meant that Gummer became the preeminent spokesperson on BSE and that the Ministry's veterinary scientists were not at the forefront of the public relations effort. Equally, the Chief Medical Officer was not routinely called upon to defend the official position.[10] During the BSE crisis the press office of the Ministry of Agriculture was awarded no plaudits for its media relations. The most memorable public relations stunt involved the Minister of Agriculture force-feeding his 4-year-old daughter a beef burger in front of TV cameras to underline the message that beef was safe to eat (Caulkin 1990:25).[11] Aside from such high profile public relations events, journalists were given very little information and the press office acted as a barrier between the media and government vets and scientists. This had two results: first, it made it easier for journalists to write about government cover-ups and conspiracies and second, it created a news vacuum that journalists tried to fill by approaching other sources. These included alternative experts as well as professional associations such as the British Veterinary Association (BVA). If BVA officials were unable to answer detailed technical and scientific questions, they would try and find out from expert sources who were also BVA members and then ring the journalist back.[12] With BSE, the major expert sources were Ministry of Agriculture vets. In this way the stonewalling of the MAFF press office was bypassed and journalists got information from official scientific sources via the BVA. As one tabloid journalist confirmed, the BVA "became one of the best sources of getting a definitive statement, not MAFF."[13]

Food Industry Public Relations/Secrecy

The approach of the food production and processing industries has been to try and play down food poisoning stories. Media enquiries are often rebuffed, and facilities refused. Such an approach is not unusual in business public relations, especially in the face of a perceived crisis in public confidence (Tumber 1993; Downing 1986; Gandy 1982, 1992).

For example, Wendy Sweetster, deputy cookery editor of *Woman's Realm*, has commented that during the *Salmonella* controversy she "didn't find the egg people desperately helpful. They seemed to be so anxious to defend their product that they couldn't supply me with any useful or unbiased information" (Slade 1989:16). Prior to Edwina Currie's statement it seems to have worked quite effectively, at least until November 1988. A letter from the Chair of the British Egg Industry Council (BEIC) to the National Farmers Union, dated November 2, 1988, reveals the strategy of the industry:

> we do not want to create public debate as this will only result in further publicity linking salmonella and eggs. The BEIC will continue its "behind the scenes" work which has so far been successful in limiting publicity for the subject and in ensuring that the industry is kept informed of all developments. I would be grateful if you could convey the industry position to your members as quietly and confidentially as possible. (Coles 1988)

The progress of the rash of food safety "scares" in 1988 and 1989 seems to have further convinced certain elements of the food industry that silence is the best policy.[14]

Pressure Groups and Campaigning

One consequence of a reluctance on the part of business and government to talk to the media is the creation of a partial news vacuum. This can either go unfilled and contribute to the disappearance of a story, as desired in the current examples by both industry and the Ministry of Agriculture, or it can be filled by enterprising pressure groups or alternative experts. So we find, for example, government critic Professor Richard Lacey featured a total of 18 times in television news bulletins on *Salmonella*,[15] equaling the number of interviews with the DoH's Chief Medical Officer and more than any other scientist. On BSE, where the Ministry of Agriculture was giving out very little information, Lacey was the most quoted scientist in one sample of newspapers.[16]

Willing alternative experts can be used as "balance" for official statements, and scientists can be given media space precisely because they disagree with the official line. This brings us to the other factor in such an equation, the role of news values.

News Values

Newspaper demands for controversy, novelty, or exclusives can affect even those known for their support of the Conservative government. Thus a statement by Professor Richard Lacey that "people should not eat beef until half the herds in Britain, each of which had at least one infected cow, had been destroyed" (Palmer and Birrell, 1990) became attractive to the Conservative supporting *Sunday Times* partly because of its novelty:

Andrew Neil, editor of the *Sunday Times*, was a happy man, nine days ago. He had picked up a scoop . . . and nothing so pleases an editor as beating his news desk to a story. The result was displayed across the top of the front page in a report stating that the risks of humans catching "mad cow" disease were so great 6m cattle need to be slaughtered. (MacArthur 1990)

Secrecy and conspiracy became major criteria of "news value" in British food safety crises. "One of the major organising themes throughout the BSE coverage" was the "notion that the Government [was] guilty both of complacency and repression of information" (Hansen 1992:10). The perception of secrecy and cover up, in turn, made some journalists more interested in the story. As Derek Cooper (1989:9) wrote of his research for a Channel Four series: "We shall be doing a lot of scrutinising in *This Food Business*, [although] many doors still remain closed to investigation. The fact that they are closed and subject to official secrecy hasn't made things easy—but it's certainly made them interesting." Such assessments have also interested tabloid newspapers. *Today*, a mid-market tabloid became very interested in consumer and environmental stories.[17] According to News Editor Colin Myler, MAFF's "bald statements" about the danger of raw eggs caused people to be more concerned than they needed to be, and retailers had "to realise they can only be secretive to a degree or it becomes counter-productive and throws up more questions" (cited in Bidlake and Falconer 1988:1).

The Process of a "Scare"

While the *Salmonella* "scare" may have been originated with government divisions, food industry secrecy, and pressure group activities, an abrupt shift in the tactics of food industry public relations helped to maintain a high level of media interest. Following Edwina Currie's statement (that "most of the egg production in this country, sadly, is now infected with salmonella") the farming industry attempted to keep the media interest alive in order to force the government to disown Edwina Currie and compensate egg producers. Indeed media coverage of the crisis really took off only with the reactions to Currie's December 3 statement. It was not until Tuesday, December 6 that press coverage escalated dramatically (see Figure 14.1). According to Warren Newman, head of public relations at the National Farmers Union (NFU):

It was in our interest at the NFU to make it stay in the news as an issue because of the distress that was going to be happening down there on the farm . . . . What we had to do was refocus on the consequences of what she (Edwina Currie) said and for that reason we had nothing to lose. We

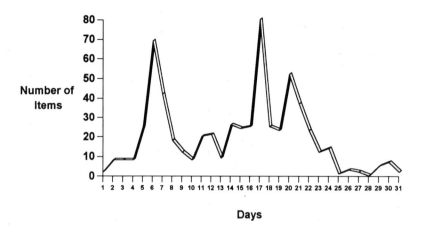

Days

Figure 14.1. British press coverage of *Salmonella*, December 1988.

were pressing for compensation, we had to make it embarrassing for the government. We had to force the government to introduce compensatory measures and we had to force the government to disown what Edwina had said. You could only do that by keeping it alive. (Interview with the authors, April 8 1993)

Ironically, the industry with the most to lose from the egg crisis played a part in keeping the "scare" alive. However, this public relations strategy was reasonably successful in forcing government action, if not in regaining public confidence. A £19 million compensation package was announced on December 19, three days after Edwina Currie had resigned.

Decline of a "Scare"

News values are also important in the process of deamplification. The rise and fall of the *Salmonella* "scare" occurred in a comparatively short period (see Figure 14.2). The story all but disappeared as Christmas approached. It resurfaced in January and February of 1989 when there was extensive coverage based around the proceedings of the Agricultural Select Committee, but it never again reached anything like the level of December 1988.

This was because first, "something was being done." The Agriculture Select Committee was investigating the affair (Commons Agriculture Committee 1989a, 1989b) and Currie's resignation had resolved the controversy at the level of political scandal. Second, and partly as a conse-

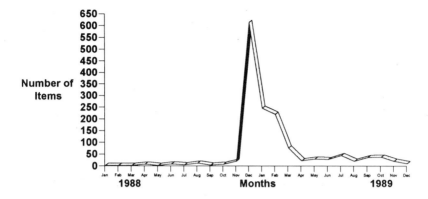

Figure 14.2. British press coverage of *Salmonella*, January 1988 to December 1989.

quence of the first factor, the news worthiness of government divisions and government and food industry secrecy had been displaced onto a concern with consumer practice. From being a problem of egg production, *Salmonella* became more centrally a problem of kitchen hygiene. This in itself made the story less interesting for journalists. According to Paul Crosbie, Consumer Editor of the *Daily Express*, an additional (economic) reason for the decline of the story was the fact that food consumers are also newspaper consumers:

> Producers are an easy target to attack. They're the people who should know better. Whereas it's very difficult to tell people who've got a jippy stomach one day that it was a problem with their cooking the previous day because in a way they don't want to read about it, and they're the ones who buy the paper. (Interview with the authors, February 1994)

By contrast the BSE crisis was never resolved in this way. While there was some conflict at the level of science over the behavior of the BSE agent, it was common ground that there was very little solid evidence either way about the safety of eating BSE-infected animal products. For the government this translated in public relations statements such as "British Beef is Safe." For critics of the government it meant there was a danger that beef was not safe. The decision about what to tell the public and what course of action to take thus related very strongly to questions of public confidence and perception. Although the government maintained that it was acting on the best available scientific advice, it is clear that its decisions were not based on bare evidence alone. Equally, the public uncertainty and continued news value of BSE has related not

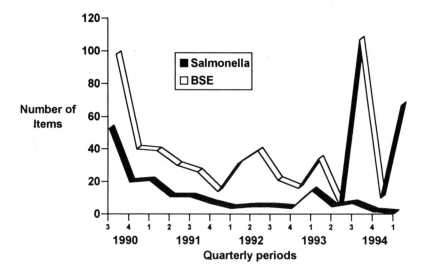

Figure 14.3. British press coverage of *Salmonella* compared with BSE, July 1990 to March 1994.

simply to contending claims but to the inability to judge the superiority of one set of claims over another.

Figure 14.3 compares the amount of press coverage devoted to BSE as compared with *Salmonella*. Although the peaks of coverage appear roughly comparable, it is the aftermath of the two issues where differences are manifest. The *Salmonella* story peaked comparatively quickly and then receded through 1989. Although there was a major interest in food safety and food poisoning throughout the year, *Salmonella* was often a passenger story invoked in the course of discussions of a new Food Safety Act, *Listeria*, the safety of microwave ovens, and irradiation. After 1989 the story more or less disappeared from the British press. At the same time the number of cases of *Salmonella enteritidis* had increased from 12,931 in 1989 to 16,151 in 1990 (Public Health Laboratory Service and State Veterinary Service 1993). Press coverage of BSE, on the other hand, developed more slowly than that of *Salmonella*, peaking in May and June 1990. The keen media interest in BSE evident in 1990 did decline partly because the story exhausted its news value. There were simply not enough unfolding events to maintain a critical mass of media interest. It is also true that there was a resolution of sorts on a political level. A number of European countries had banned British beef. A compromise solution was instituted that reinstated beef imports so long as they were certified to come from BSE free herds. Press coverage peaked on May 17, 1990 with a total of 63 items in the British press. However, the central issue of human transmission was not resolved by the European Community decision. Indeed, it can be argued that the certification of British beef exports to Europe made the official British position less credible.

Because the issue of human transmission was (and remains) unresolved, BSE still periodically reappears on the front pages of the press. It is the very uncertainty about BSE that makes it a continuing story, although its impact on human health is so far as is known inconsequential. This is, of course, quite different than the relationship between the media and *Salmonella enteritidis*. *Salmonella* has a much greater known impact on human health and the number of cases has continued to rise since 1988. The story of food safety as a public issue in Britain illustrates the crucial importance of definitional strategies in the construction of social problems and the centrality of the media to contests over social problems. Equally, it is our argument that the food safety "scares" arose at a particular juncture in history for particular historical and material reasons, which cannot be divorced from the strategies of the claimsmakers.

On Social Constructionism

Woolgar and Pawluch (1985a) are right to point to the inherent tension in the selective relativism of much work in the social constructionist tradition. However, such problems also affect their own writing. In their response to critics Woolgar and Pawluch claim that there are "differences" between the four responses to their arguments (Gusfield 1985; Hazelrigg 1985; Pfohl 1985; Schneider 1985). Such differences, they say, "lend support to our view that the constructivist approach subsumes a diversity of perspectives" (1985b:159). Presumably, if we follow their line of argument, the assertion that there are differences between the accounts is a social construction. And if this is the case it is difficult to see how their assertion can undermine or lend support to their position. Woolgar and Pawluch are actually engaged in their own "ontological gerrymander" in contravention of their plea for radical relativism. Woolgar and Pawluch (1985b:161) go on to berate their critics for accusing them of selectivity, saying that this is a "general response strategy." If Woolgar and Pawluch are "made out" to be wrong in their charge by the critics then contextual constructionism can "continue as before" (1985b:161). We have already seen that Woolgar and Pawluch have used a rhetorical device ("response strategy") to bolster their own argument. However, in both cases the real question is not "is this charge an example of a more general response strategy?" (since by their argument all arguments are rhetorical devices), but "is the charge true?"

When Woolgar and Pawluch (1985a) write that other academics are engaged in an ontological gerrymander, we are entitled to ask the criteria by which this statement is asserted to be true. If there are no criteria, then we might justifiably ask why we should pay attention to an argument that does not even claim to have any truth value. But if there are criteria, then the strict constructionist view collapses. One consequence of such an approach is that any statement is as good as any other in the claims it makes about the world. It certainly becomes impossible to favor some explanations or facts over others on the grounds of their truth value. It also makes it very difficult to analyze the use of lies, secrecy, and propaganda in the service of power. Indeed, as Woolgar and Pawluch acknowledge (1985b:162), the strict constructionist position "will not contribute . . . to our understanding of the world as we have traditionally conceived that pursuit." It is in this sense that Gusfield (1985:17) is correct to say that it is a sociological "dead-end." The retreat of the strict constructionist to a position of chronic disinterest in the world allows an escape into a self-referential universe of academic production that cannot be judged by reference to reality or indeed any criteria, but only by the exclusive club of agnostic cognoscenti.

The problem for social constructionism is how to reconcile the doctrine that all knowledge is socially constructed with the practicalities of making meaningful statements about the world. It seems to us, however, that the doctrine is wrong: not everything is socially constructed. Disagreements in this area have a long history in sociology, and are still the subject of substantial and mostly unproductive debate, particularly under the rubric of postmodernism. Here we are in sympathy with the formulation drawn up by Edward Thompson. Thompson distinguishes between experience I—lived experience and experience II—perceived experience. The first type of experience

> walks in without knocking at the door, and announces deaths, crises of subsistence, trench warfare, unemployment, inflation, genocide. People starve: their survivors think in new ways about the market. People are imprisoned: in prison they meditate in new ways about the law. (1981: 406; cf. Eldridge 1993; Gellner 1979; Thompson 1978)

We might add that the experience of food poisoning does not wait for the niceties of introduction through perceived experience. The lived experience of vomiting is one way in which it announces itself! The experience of food poisoning is one aspect of the experience each of us has with food. In addition we all experience material limitations on the food we can eat (whether they be in the lack of choice of food stuffs on sale, our inability to afford what we might like, or some form of allergy to particular foods, for example).

The way in which people react to the experience of food poisoning or the way in which they conceptualize it might vary, and this might be linked to particular social constructions about who is to blame for the poisoning. This might, in turn, shape eating habits and public views about the regulation of food safety in particular ways. Nevertheless, it would be foolish to deny that reality does pose limits for human actions.

Contextual Constructionism

One alternative to strict constructionism is what Joel Best (1989) calls "contextual constructionism." While our approach is closer to contextual rather than "strict" constructionism, we have a number of reservations about Best's outline of a research agenda on social problems. We think that spelling them out might help to clarify our position on the social constructionist debate.

Best argues that claimsmaking can be studied by adopting a three part research strategy: "This requires focusing on the claims themselves, the claims-makers, and the claims-making process" (1989:250). He goes on to highlight research that is outside the focus of social constructionism:

> It is important to avoid being distracted by the social conditions about which claims are being made. This does not necessarily mean that conditions cannot figure into the analysis . . . . Certainly conditions should never become the focal point. Strict constructionists are likely to ask how claims-makers perceive conditions, or how they describe these conditions. Contextual constructionists may also ask whether it is likely that claims-makers have misrepresented or inaccurately described the conditions, or how conditions may account for claims or the reaction to them. (Best 1989:251)

Claims are not free floating, they are generated out of particular social conditions. Best's account lacks enough emphasis on structure. The social and historical context and the political economy of particular claims are fundamental. Social problems explanations need to focus on a much wider horizon than simply on claimsmaking strategies. As Derné has recently put it, "partly because their main concern is an analysis of the processes that generate commonsense knowledge, social constructionists have often neglected the causal issues of greatest interest to sociologists" (Derné 1994:269). For us it is self-evident that the success or failure of social movements, governments, and industries in placing an issue on (or keeping it off) the public agenda is related not only to their claimsmaking (public relations and lobbying) strategies (Miller 1993; Schlesinger 1990), but to their cultural, financial, and institutional resources, as they interact with and help to constitute the balance of forces at any one time. It is, in our view, ludicrous to analyze claimsmaking outside of its social, material, and historical context. Whatever the claims to the contrary, much writing in the constructionist tradition neglects questions of causation and material determination.

The interaction of the material and the symbolic or definitional creates the social problem. Without real threats to real interests there would be no social problems. If problems are created by means simply of contending claims, it is impossible for us to explain why some claims are successful and why others fail, unless we are to attribute such outcomes to "better" or "worse" arguments or presentational skills. But even mentioning presentational skills should lead us to ask sociological questions about the social distribution and resource base of such skills, and the processes by which they are learned and incorporated into the strategies of claimsmakers. Some writers on social problems have attempted to do this.

Public Arenas

The "public arenas" model advanced by Hilgartner and Bosk is an attempt to "move beyond natural history models" (1988: 54) of social problems (e.g., Blumer 1971; Spector and Kitsuse 1973, 1977) and as such provides a more sophisticated account of the process by which contending problems compete for public attention.

The model stresses the "arenas" where social problems evolve. It proposes that issues compete for space on the public agenda, but that space is limited by the "carrying capacities" of public institutions. There are obviously more potential public issues vying to get on to public agendas than issues that actually become publicly important. Once an issue is defined as important it is subject to continuing pressure for attention: "Growth is constrained by the finite 'carrying capacities' of public arenas, by competition and by the need for sustained drama" (Hilgartner and Bosk 1988:53).

It seems to us that the chief difficulty with the public arenas model is that it tends not to focus on factors external to the arena. This causes problems in explaining both the generation and decline of social problems. For Hilgartner and Bosk "public arenas" include

> the executive and legislative branches of government, the courts, made for TV movies, the cinema, the news media (television news, magazines, newspapers, and radio), political campaign organizations, social action groups, direct mail solicitations, books dealing with social issues, the re-

search community, religious organisations, professional societies, and private foundations. (1988:58–59)

This seems to us a rather broad definition, which raises the question of what is not a public arena? Since almost everything is a public arena the airing of public issues is seen as being determined by factors internal to the arena. We might therefore characterize the model as "arena-centered" in that almost all fora are described as public arenas. There is little space for activity *outside* an arena, i.e., in private or in secret. Therefore there is little interest in assessing the part that such factors play in setting the agenda in a public arena. In fact Hilgartner and Bosk explicitly state that the model examines "the effect of [public] arenas on both the evolution of social problems and the actors who make claims about them" (1988:55). This is certainly one part of a research agenda, but it concentrates on arenas at the expense of considering the effect of the strategies of social groupings on the arenas and, therefore, on social problem definition.

The model is also too arena centered in explaining the decline of social problems. In relation to the public arena(s) provided by the mass media, we would not want to deny the importance of media factors (internal to the arena) in maintaining issues on the public agenda. News values, novelty, and the economic logic of media organizations clearly have an important impact on the emergence and coverage of public issues such as food safety or coronary heart disease, but it seems to us that the public arenas model approaches the discussion from an overly "media-centric" (Schlesinger 1990) perspective. In the *Salmonella* epidemic, our argument is that the key limiter was not a technical phenomena such as the exhaustion of the carrying capacity, but that interest declined because some arguments are apparently won or lost and others resolved. This is more than saying it was impossible to maintain interest because of a lack of drama and novelty. If enough news sources stop pushing an issue, then it will disappear. In the *Salmonella* crisis the food industry managed to shift media coverage toward blaming the consumer (the victim) and the government agreed to introduce food safety legislation thus (at least) giving the appearance of moving toward some of the campaigning demands of food pressure groups. In such circumstances the rationale for the story is removed or symbolically resolved; something is being done. As Hilgartner and Bosk emphasize, it does not matter whether the problem has actually been solved. According to official figures *Salmonella* poisoning in Britain in 1993 was much greater than it was in 1988 when the crisis emerged as a public issue (Public Health Laboratory Service and State Veterinary Service 1993). The public arena provided by the mass media is a key terrain on which arguments are won or lost. It should not be forgotten that while this arena is subject to all sorts of media priorities these are also bound up with the priorities of all sorts of social institutions. These institutions are the focus of the widely influential concept of "moral panic" that attempts to explain social problems.

Moral Panics

The term "moral panic" appears to have originated with criminologist Stan Cohen and his well known study *Folk Devils and Moral Panics* (1972). Cohen argues that inegalitarian social orders create problems for powerless and marginalized sections of society and then use their rebellion to reinforce the social order via the mechanism of a "moral panic," which he defined as follows:

> A condition, episode, person or group of persons emerges to become defined as a threat to societal values and interests: its nature is presented in a stylised and stereotypical fashion by the mass media; the moral barricades are manned by editors, bishops, politicians and other right-thinking people; socially accredited experts pronounce their diagnoses and solutions; ways of coping are evolved or (more often) resorted to. (Cohen 1972:9)

Panics function as a mechanism of control by the "control culture" in which the mass media act as a means of deviancy "amplification." Stuart Hall and his colleagues developed and "politicized" (Harris 1992) this analysis in their widely influential book *Policing the Crisis* (1978; cf. Hall 1988) in which they argue: "To put it crudely, the 'moral panic' appears to us to be one of the principal forms of ideological consciousness by means of which a 'silent majority' is won over to the support of increasingly coercive measures on the part of the state, and lends its legitimacy to a 'more than usual' exercise of control" (Hall et al. 1978:221).

The most widely noted problem with a deviancy amplification model is, as Cohen himself has noted, that it becomes difficult to explain how panics subside (1972:198; cf. Ditton 1979). Cohen's own answer is that panics subside when there is "a lack of interest" from the public and the mass media; this occurs "when it [is] felt that 'something is being done about it'" (1972:200).

Because the state (theoretically) creates and manages the moral panic as an instrument of control, there is no space for countervailing pressures to operate against the assumed might of the state. What is missing from the model, then, is a notion of active struggle at the level of the media. In the original study Cohen concludes:

> More moral panics will be generated and other, as yet nameless, folk devils will be created. This is not because such developments have an inexorable inner logic, but because our society, as present structured, will continue to generate problems for some of its members—like working class adolescents—and then condemn whatever solution these groups find. (1972:204)

Here again "society as present structured" is described as creating problems for marginalized groups, to which they only respond. This instrumental model assumes that the power to define social issues rests only with the "control culture" or the "structure" of society (cf. Miller 1993). However, we contend that the definition of social issues is drawn up in the struggle between different social groups and between humans who possess agency and the structures of society that they constitute and reconstitute by their actions (cf. Giddens 1984).

There is a further problem in using the concept of "moral panic," as some sociologists have recently done (Beardsworth 1990; Gofton 1990) to explain food safety crises. Food scares just don't fit the model. "Folk Devils" in Cohen's analysis are marginalized sections of society labeled "deviant" by the "control culture." In the case of the "scares" or "panics" over *Salmonella* or *Listeria* who are the folk devils? and who are the representatives of the "control culture"? Should we label the egg industry as a marginalized group for which society "as present structured" generates problems? Are we to label food pressure groups and consumers the "control culture"? A further issue is: to which side do we allocate the government in this analysis? According to policy analysts of differing persuasions and to the former Permanent Secretary at MAFF, Sir Michael Franklin, it is not the government, but the food industry that has been the most influential player in the policy arena in the entire postwar period (Franklin 1994; Mills 1991, 1992; Smith 1989, 1991).

However, it does not seem unreasonable to suppose that the state or industry (or sections of them) does on occasion launch public relations campaigns that result either in large scale media attention and widespread public concern or in a social issue being kept in (or returned to) the margins of the public sphere. In either case changes in legislation or official practice may result. However, it is possible, in principle (given official secrecy and the self-denying status of propaganda) to discover that this is the case.

The media are not simply the tools of one or other section of society, nor do they straightforwardly reflect the world. Nevertheless they are oriented toward the powerful and have their own sectional interests. The media can also on occasion act as an ally of relatively poorly resourced pressure groups, enabling the building of agendas that may result in new social problems taking their place at the center of the public sphere. The public arenas model and the concept of moral panic are similar in that they make insufficient distinction between the media and the social institutions with which they interact and on which they report. But the two concepts differ markedly in other respects. Hilgartner and Bosk (1988) emphasize public arenas, while moral panic relies on an all-embracing "control-culture" of which the media are assumed to be a part. We might go so far as to claim that there is a tendency in the work of Cohen (1972), and especially Hall (1988), that overemphasizes structure at the expense of agency and that Hilgartner and Bosk emphasize agency (claimsmaking) at the expense of structure.

In our view, Thompson's (1978) separation of lived from perceived experience, while crude, is an advance on the other formulations discussed here. It brings the relationship between power and truth into central focus and makes possible the empirical sociological investigation of public relations strategies and the analysis of lies and propaganda. Such an approach is ruled out by those theorists who are unable to separate truth from falsehood.

Concluding Comments

In this chapter we have analyzed the competition or struggle for definitions of food safety. We recognize that there is serious competition for definition in the public sphere but that it does not take place on a level playing field. Some participants (notably the state and big business) have immense material and cultural advantages. Yet, this does not make history a foregone conclusion. Social problems are not created from thin air. They are constructed by human beings but not in circumstances of their own choosing. There is a complex interaction between definitional struggle and material conditions, and the material world imposes clear limitations on the generation of claims. Definitional struggle is predicated on material relationships and results in changes in them, thus the importance of examining public relations, lobbying, and claimsmaking strategies and their material context and consequences. It ought to be a central task of social science to understand the relationship between the material and the symbolic. Instead, many social constructionists have abandoned this task, focusing instead on claimsmaking as a closed self-referential system.

Acknowledgments

The research for this chapter was funded by the (British) Economic and Social Research Council (ESRC) as part of their "Nation's Diet" research programme.

Our thanks to the ESRC for funding the research and to our colleagues John Eldridge and Sally Macintyre for help and advice.

Notes

1. We use the term "scare" in quotation marks throughout this chapter since to suggest that something is a scare generally means that there is no real substance to the problem. In other words the term "scare" is part of a definitional struggle that is itself the focus of this chapter.

2. On *Salmonella* the argument is either that vertical transmission has caused the infection of eggs, or that convenience foods are not being properly handled in the kitchen. *Listeria* has been associated with cook-chill methods of cooking and food production. The official scientific view of the cause of BSE is that cows, fed the scrapie-infected remains of sheep, developed a similar disease, or that organophosphate pesticides are to blame.

3. In general animal welfare and vegetarian organizations have a longer history than general food and health pressure groups. The Vegetarian Society was set up before 1950 and Compassion in World Farming was established in 1970 (Compassion in World Farming 1991).

4. "Hard news" is the staple of news pages and television bulletins. "Soft" news tends to be confined to feature pages. "Soft news" areas such as food have historically been seen as women's issues and, therefore, have been marginalized in news judgments.

5. By 1993, however, there were many fewer environment correspondents, as media interest fell off (Anderson and Gaber 1993).

6. Information from interviews with David Brown and Michael Hornsby, Agriculture Correspondents on the *Times* and *Daily Telegraph*, respectively, February 1994.

7. The government monitoring and surveillance center.

8. Only the *Daily Telegraph* and the *Daily Mirror* covered the press release, the *Telegraph* under the heading "Back to Work on an Egg" and the *Mirror* reporting "Cracking News," both on November 22, 1988.

9. It has been suggested that the DoH found it convenient to blame the rise in *Salmonella* poisoning on eggs, since there was a growing controversy about the links between "cook-chill" catering and food poisoning. If this emerged as a major issue, the DoH would find itself under pressure to allocate resources to upgrade the catering facilities in crown premises, particularly hospitals and prisons. As Oliver Gillie put it: "There is a conflict of interest inside the Department of Health. It sets food safety standards but also runs the largest catering organisation in Britain" (1989:3; see also North and Gorman 1990). Whether this was indeed a contributory factor or not, it is clear that there were serious divisions between the DHSS and MAFF.

10. The most interviewed person on British television news coverage of BSE between 1987 and 1991 was John Gummer, who appeared 49 times. The next most often interviewed were the president of the National Farmers Union, Sir Simon Gourlay (31 times) and the opposition (Labour Party) spokesperson (33 times). The Chief Vet was interviewed 15 times and the Chief Medical Officer only 4 times.

11. Caulkin (1990:25) writes:

First prize for the most counter-productive media image of 1990 must go to John

Gummer. The Agriculture Minister and his daughter cramming their mouths with what the nation instantly christened BSE-burgers turned over more stomachs than salmonella, listeria and lager and vindaloo combined. It was not just an isolated misjudgment but the latest in a line of systematic communications mismanagement which has allowed the issue of bovine spongiform encephalopathy, or mad cow disease to develop from a worrying problem to an international crisis.

12.   Interview with Frances Anthony, President, and Chrissie Nicholls, Head of Veterinary Services, British Veterinary Association, July 26, 1993.

13.   Interview with Paul Crosbie, Consumer Editor, *Daily Express*, February 1994.

14.   According to Derek Cooper (1989:8):

There is a strong feeling in the industry that whatever they say is not likely to improve their image. Salmonella, Listeria, botulism, additives, pesticides, hormones and antibiotics in the meat, nasties in the poultry feed, cruelty in the broiler sheds have not only upset tummies but, much more significantly, upset public perception of the way in which the food and farming industry is discharging its functions. What is really at stake is the credibility and integrity of the foodmakers, many of whom seem to feel a dignified silence is their wisest course of action.

15.   The sample here includes all British television news bulletins between December 1, 1988 and December 31, 1989.

16.   The sample here included the *Guardian*, the *Independent*, the *Daily Telegraph*, and *Today* for the period April 1988 to December 1991 (Hansen 1992:10). It should be noted, however, that the Minister for Agriculture, John Gummer, took personal charge of much of the public presentation of the BSE crisis. This resulted in government scientists and others supporting the official line, being interviewed less frequently. Gummer was quoted or referred to 750 times, Lacey was quoted 178 times, and the government's chief vet Keith Meldrum was referred to 72 times.

17.   There are also clear economic motives for such an approach. Katz (1994:B6) has revealed this as part of *Today* editor David Montgovery's approach: "At his first editorial conference Montgomery told senior staff the paper would be aimed at 'greedy people.' When environmental panic set in in the late eighties he refined his target audience to include 'green greedy people.' The timely cocktail of consumption and conservation helped to propel the paper's circulation to almost 600,000."

References

Acheson, D. 1986. "Food Policy, Nutrition and the Government." *Proceedings of the Nutrition Society* 45:131–138.

Anderson, A. 1991. "Source Strategies and the Communication of Environmental Affairs." *Media Culture and Society* 13(4):459–476.

Anderson, A., and I. Gaber. 1993. "The Yellowing of the Greens." *British Journalism Review* 4(2):49–53.

Ballantyne, A., and R. Norton-Taylor. 1989. "Meat Risks Report 'Held Back'." *The Guardian* 11 (February):1.

BBC Radio Four. 1989. *Face the Facts*. Broadcast on May 18.

Beardsworth, A. 1990. "Trans-Science and Moral Panics: Understanding Food Scares." *British Food Journal* 92(5):11–16.

Best, J. (ed.). 1989. *Images of Issues: Typifying Contemporary Social Problems.* Hawthorne, NY: Aldine de Gruyter.

Bidlake, S., and H. Falconer. 1988. "Angry Retailers Slam Food Poisoning Hype." *Supermarketing* 850 (December 2):1.

Blumer, H. 1971. "Social Problems as Collective Behavior." *Social Problems* 18:298–306.

British Egg Industry Council. 1989. *Salmonella in Eggs, First Report, Minutes of Evidence and Appendices.* Memorandum submitted to the Commons Agriculture Committee (February 28):54–55 .

Cannon, G. 1983. "Censored: A Diet for Life and Death." *Sunday Times* July 3:1.

——. 1987. *The Politics of Food.* London: Century.

Cannon, G., and C. Walker. 1985. *The Food Scandal.* London: Century.

Caulkin, S. 1990. "Mad Cows and a Pig's Ear." *The Guardian* July 16:25.

Cohen, S. 1972. *Folk Devils and Moral Panics.* London: McKibbon and Kee.

Coles, J. 1988. Letter to Representative of the National Farmers Union, November 2.

Commons Agriculture Committee. 1989a. *Salmonella in Eggs, Minutes of Evidence and Appendices.* London: HMSO.

——. 1989b. *Salmonella in Eggs, First report, Minutes of Evidence and Appendices.* London: HMSO.

Compassion in World Farming. 1991. *Compassion in World Farming* FS4874, November.

Cooper, D. 1985. "A New Voice." *The Listener* November 7:17.

——. 1989. "Conspiracy of Silence." *The Listener* July 27: 8–9.

Coyle, E. F., S R. Palmer, C. D. Ribeiro, H. I. Jones, A. J. Howard, and L. Ward. 1988. "Salmonella Enteritidis Phage Type 4 Infection: Association with Hens' Eggs." *The Lancet* December 3:1295–1296.

Crawford-Poole, S. 1993. "Consuming Passions." *The Guild of Foodwriters News* 9(Spring):19.

Currie, E. 1989. *Life Lines: Politics and Health 1986–1988.* London: Sidgwick & Jackson.

Daily Mirror. 1988. "Edwina's Face Fits." September 3:2.

Deer, B. 1987. "Eggs Blamed for Increase in Food Bugs." *Sunday Times* November 8:1.

Department of Health and Social Security. 1988a. "Salmonella and Raw Eggs." DHSS Press release, August 26.

——. 1988b. "Chief Medical Officer Repeats Advice on Raw Egg Consumption." DHSS Press release, December 5.

Derné, S. 1994. "Cultural Conceptions of Human Motivation and Their Significance for Culture Theory." Pp. 267–287 in *The Sociology of Culture*, edited by D. Crane. Oxford: Blackwell.

Ditton, J. 1979. *Controlology: Beyond the New Criminology.* London: Macmillan.

Downing, J. 1986. "Government Secrecy and the Media in the United States and

Britain." Pp. 153–170 in *Communicating Politics: Mass Communications and the Political Process*, edited by Peter Golding et al. Leicester: Leicester University Press.

Eldridge, J. 1993. "Whose Illusion? Whose Reality? Some Problems of Theory and Method in Mass Media Research." Pp. 331–350 in *Getting the Message: News, Truth and Power*, edited by Glasgow University Media Group. London: Routledge.

Farrant, W., and J. Russell. 1986. *The Politics of Health Information*. London: Bedford Way Papers, Institute of Education.

Fine, B., and E. Leopold. 1993. *The World of Consumption*. London: Routledge.

Fine, B., and J. Wright. 1991. "Digesting the Food and Information Systems." *Discussion Paper in Economics*. Birkbeck College, University of London.

Franklin, Sir M. 1994. "Food Policy Formation in the UK/EC." Pp. 3–8 in *The Politics of Food, Proceedings of an Inter-disciplinary Seminar*, edited by S. Henson and S. Gregory. Department of Agricultural Economics and Management, Reading University.

Gandy, O. H 1982. *Beyond Agenda Setting: Information Subsidies and Public Policy*. Norwood, NJ: Ablex.

———. 1992. "Public Relations and Public policy: The Structuration of Dominance in the Information Age." Pp. 131–163 in *Rhetorical and Critical Approaches to Public Relations* edited by E. Totn and R. Heath. Hillsdale, NJ: Lawrence Erlbaum.

Gardner, C., and J. Sheppard. 1989. *Consuming Passion: The Rise of Retail Culture*. London: Unwin Hyman.

Gellner, E. 1979. *Spectacles and Predicaments*. Cambridge: Cambridge University Press.

Giddens, A. 1984. *The Constitution of Society*. Cambridge: Polity.

Gillie, O. 1988. "Raw Eggs Banned on Hospital Menus." *Independent* August 4:2.

———. 1989. "How Health Officials Went to Work on Eggs." *Independent* February 15:3.

Gofton, L. 1990. "Food Fears and Time Famines: Some Social Aspects of Choosing and Using Food." *British Nutrition Foundation Nutrition Bulletin* 15(1):78–95.

Grant, W. 1989. *Pressure Groups, Politics and Democracy in Britain*. Hemel Hempstead: Philip Allan.

Grose, D. 1978. "Consumers' Association and *Which*." In *Marketing and the Consumer Movement*, edited by J. Mitchell. Maidenhead: McGraw-Hill .

Gruner, P. 1988. "Soft-boiled Eggs Are Dangerous Say Experts." *Evening Standard* November 23:5.

Gusfield, J. R 1985. "Theories and Hobgoblins." *SSSP Newsletter* 17:16–18.

Hall, S. 1988. *The Hard Road to Renewal: Thatcherism and the Crisis of the Left*. London: Verso.

Hall, S., C. Critcher, T. Jefferson, J. Clarke, and B. Roberts. 1978. *Policing the Crisis: Mugging, the State and Law and Order*. London: Macmillan.

Hanke, R. 1989. "Mass Media and Lifestyle Differentiation: An Analysis of the Public Discourse about Food." *Communication* 11: 221–238.

Hansen, A. 1992. "Newspaper Science: The Press Presentation of Science and Scientists." Paper presented at the Annual Meeting of the Association for Science Education, Sheffield, U. K.

Harris, D. 1992. *From Class Struggle to the Politics of Pleasure: The Effects of Gramscianisation on Cultural Studies.* London: Routledge.

Hazelrigg, L. E. 1985. "Were It Not for Words." *Social Problems* 32:234–237.

Henson, S. 1992. "From High Street to Hypermarket: Food Retailing in the 1990's." Pp. 95–115 in *Your Food: Whose Choice,* edited by National Consumer Council. London: HMSO.

Hilgartner, S., and C. Bosk. 1988. "The Rise and Fall of Social Problems: A Public Arenas Model." *American Journal of Sociology* 94(1):53–78.

Humphrey, T. J., G. C. Mead, and B. Rowe. 1988. "Poultry Meat as a Source of Human Salmonellosis in England and Wales." *Epidemiology and Infection* 100:175–184.

ITN. 1988. *Evening News* 1700 December 3.

Katz, I. 1994. "'Monty the Merciless." *The Guardian* Media Page, March 14:B6–B7.

Lustig, R., V. Smart, A. Ferriman, and J. Connolly. 1988. "When the Chickens Came Home to Roost." *The Observer* December 18.

Lycett, A. 1988. "Award for Integrity." *The Times* June 29.

MacArthur, B. 1990. "Front-runner in the Media Herd Sparks a Stampede of Newsmen." *Sunday Times* May 20:56.

Mennell, S., A. Murcott, and A. Van Otteroo. 1992. *The Sociology of Food: Eating, Diet and Culture.* London: Sage.

Miller, D. 1993. "Official Sources and Primary Definition: The Case of Northern Ireland." *Media, Culture and Society* 15 (3):385–406.

Miller, D., and J. Reilly. 1994. *Food 'Scares' in the Media.* Glasgow: Glasgow University Media Group.

Mills, M. 1991. "Food and Health Policy in Britain." Department of Government Papers, 76. Colchester: Department of Government, University of Essex.

———. 1992. *The Politics of Dietary Change.* Aldershot: Dartmouth Publishing Company Ltd.

National Forum for Coronary Heart Disease Prevention. 1988. *Coronary Heart Disease Prevention: Action in the UK 1984–1987.* Health Education Authority.

North, R. 1989. "Memorandum Submitted by Richard North." Pp. 252–326 in *First Report: Salmonella in Eggs, Volume 2, Minutes of Evidence and Appendices,* Commons Agriculture Committee, February 28. London: HMSO.

North, R., and T. Gorman. 1990. *Chickengate: An Independent Analysis of the Salmonella in Eggs Scare.* London: Institute for Economic Affairs.

Palmer, R., and I. Birrell. 1990. "Leading Food Scientist Calls for Slaughter of 6m Cows." *Sunday Times* May 13:A1.

Pfohl, S. 1985. "Toward a Sociological Deconstruction of Social Problems: A Response to Woolgar and Pawluch." *Social Problems* 32:228–232.

Philo, G.. 1993. "From Buerk to Band Aid: The Media and the 1984 Ethiopian Famine." Pp. 104–126 in *Getting The Message: News, Truth and Power,* edited by Glasgow University Media Group. London: Routledge.

Public Health Laboratory Service. 1989. "Salmonella and Eggs." Pp. 14–36 in *Salmonella in Eggs, First Report, Minutes of Evidence and Appendices*. Memorandum submitted by the Public Health Laboratory Service, in Commons Agriculture Committee.

Public Health Laboratory Service and State Veterinary Service. 1993. *PHLS-SVS Update on Salmonella infection* January 10.

Rayner, M. 1992. *The History of the Coronary Prevention Group*, Coronary Prevention Group, Unpublished manuscript.

Schlesinger, P. 1990. "Rethinking the Sociology of Journalism: Source Strategies and the Limits of Media-Centrism." In *Public Communication: The New Imperatives*, edited by M. Ferguson. London: Sage

Schneider, J. W. 1985. "Defining the Definitional Perspective on Social Problems." *Social Problems* 32:232–234.

Schoenfield, A. C., R. F. Meier, and R. J. Griffin. 1979. "Constructing a Social Problem: The Press and the Environment." *Social Problems* 27(1):38–61.

Slade, J. 1989. "A Hard Act to Swallow." *PR Week* February 3:15–16.

Smith, M. J. 1989. "Changing Agendas and Policy Communities: Agricultural Issues in the 1930's and the 1980's." *Public Administration* 67:149–165.

———. 1991. "From Policy Community to Issue Network: Salmonella in Eggs and the New Politics of Food." *Public Administration* 69:235–255.

———. 1993. *Pressure, Power and Policy*. London: Harvester-Wheatsheaf.

Spector, M., and J. I. Kitsuse. 1973. "Social Problems: A Reformulation." *Social Problems* 21:145–159.

———. 1977. *Constructing Social Problems*. Menlo Park, CA: Cummings.

Spencer, C. 1981. "Too Much Bourgeois Relish Spoils the Cookery Books." *Guardian* August 31:9.

St. Louis, M.E., D. L. Morse, and M. E. Potter. 1988. "The Emergence of Grade A Shell Eggs as a Major Source of Salmonella Enteritidis Infections." *Journal of the American Medical Association* 259: 2103–2107.

Thompson, E. P. 1978. *The Poverty of Theory*. London: Merlin Press.

———. 1981. "The Politics of Theory." Pp. 396–408 in *People's History and Socialist Theory*, edited by S. Raphael. London: Routledge and Kegan Paul.

Thomson, D. G. 1988. "'Raw Shell Eggs' Letter Issued to Catering Managers, Dieticians, District Medical Officers and Nurse Advisors." *Department of Health*, EL(88)P/136, July 29.

Tumber, H. 1993. "'Selling Scandal': Business and the Media." *Media, Culture and Society* 15:345–361.

Wiseman, M. J. 1990. "Government: Where Does Nutrition Policy Come From?" *Proceedings of the Nutrition Society* 49:397–401.

Woolgar, S., and D. Pawluch. 1985a. "Ontological Gerrymandering: The Anatomy of Social Problems Explanation." 32(3):214–227.

———. 1985b. "How Shall We Move Beyond Constructivism?" *Social Problems* 33(2):159–62.

Biographical Sketches of the Contributors

Clifton Anderson is Extension Editor at the University of Idaho College of Agriculture, where he has served since 1972. He is the author of chapters on biotechnology in two World Future Society conference volumes—*The Future: Opportunity Not Destiny* (1989) and *The Years Ahead: Perils, Problems, and Promises* (1993).

Alan Beardsworth graduated in 1969 from the University of Manchester with a degree in Sociology and Social Anthropology, and was awarded a Ph.D. in Sociology by the University of Loughborough in 1979. He is currently a lecturer in the Department of Social Sciences at the University of Loughborough. His research interests include the cultural and ideological context of contemporary vegetarianism, diet and poverty, food-related concerns and anxieties, and the dynamics of food scares. He has held grants for nutrition-related sociological research from such organizations as the Nuffield Foundation, the Joseph Rowntree Foundation, and the Leverhulme Trust.

Thomas A. Hirschl is an Associate Professor in the Department of Rural Sociology at Cornell University. His expertise is in social stratification, demography, and community organization. Dr. Hirschl's primary research interest is in the area of economy and society, and his 1986 Ph.D. dissertation in sociology from the University of Wisconsin analyzed the effect of Social Security transfers on the nonmetropolitan United States. His subsequent research has focused on the social problems and behaviors associated with poverty in the United States, including papers published on homelessness, welfare recipiency, and structural unemployment.

Thomas J. Hoban is an Associate Professor in the Department of Sociology and Anthropology at North Carolina State University. Much of his work focuses on how people accept new ideas and respond to change. He has completed several major national studies about consumer attitudes about biotechnology and provides advice on the social aspects of biotechnology to government, industry, and nonprofit organizations. Dr. Hoban received his Ph.D. in Rural Sociology from Iowa State University. He also has Master's degrees in Agricultural Journalism and Water Resource Management from the University of Wisconsin.

Unni Kjærnes has an M.Sc. in nutrition. She has been a research fellow at the University of Oslo, and is now a researcher at the National Institute for Consumer Research, Norway. Her main topics of research are nutrition policy and consumer policy. She is co-editor of *Regulating Markets–Regulating People: On Food and Nutrition Policy* (1993).

Donna Maurer is a doctoral candidate in the Department of Sociology at Southern Illinois University–Carbondale. Her research centers on the cultural aspects of the vegetarian movement, microlevel processes of dietary change, and food consumption and sharing as forms of communication.

Wm. Alex McIntosh is a Professor of Sociology in the Departments of Sociology and Rural Sociology and is a member of the Nutrition Faculty at Texas A & M University. His primary area of interest is in the sociology of food and nutrition, publishing this work in journals such as *Rural Sociology, Food and Foodways, Social Science Quarterly, Appetite, Medical Care, Review of Religious Research, Journal of the American Dietetic Association, Journal of Nutrition, Journal of Aging and Health,* and *Social Indicators Research*. He continues to investigate the impact of social support, stressful life events, and health and nutritional status among the elderly, and has recently completed data collection for a pilot study that investigates the effects of household structure and interpersonal relationships on adolescent obesity and lipid status. McIntosh is also completing *Sociologies of Food and Nutrition*.

David Miller is Lecturer in the Department of Film and Media Studies at Stirling University, Scotland and a member of the Glasgow University Media Group. He has written widely on the media politics of the Northern Ireland conflict. His books include *Don't Mention the War: Northern Ireland, Propaganda and the Media* (1994) and *Dying of Ignorance: AIDS, the Media and Public Belief* (1995). He and Jacquie Reilly are currently collaborating on *The Social Production of Risk: Food, Public Culture and the Mass Media*.

Janet Poppendieck teaches Sociology at Hunter College, City University of New York and is Director of the Hunter College Center for the Study of Family Policy. Her published works include *Breadlines Knee Deep in Wheat: Food Assistance in the Great Depression* (1986) as well as articles in journals of sociology, nutrition, social work, and philosophy. She is currently at work on a study of the emergency food system entitled *Reinventing Charity: Emergency Food and American Culture*. A long time antihunger activist, Dr. Poppendieck is chair of the Board of Directors of the Community Food Resource Center in New York City.

Mark R. Rank is an Associate Professor in the George Warren Brown School of Social Work at Washington University, St. Louis. He received his Ph.D. in sociology from the University of Wisconsin and has done extensive research in the areas of welfare, poverty, and families. Dr. Rank's scholarly work has been published in a number of the premier academic journals in sociology, demography, economics, and social welfare. In addition, his most recent books include *Living on the Edge: The Realities of Welfare in America* (1994) and *Diversity and Change in Families: Patterns, Prospects, and Policies* (1995).

Jacquie Reilly is Researcher in the Department of Sociology at Glasgow University, Scotland and a member of the Glasgow University Media Group. She is currently working on the relationship between expert media constructions of risk and on culture and national identity among women in Northern Ireland. She and David Miller are completing *The Social Production of Risk: Food, Public Culture and the Mass Media*.

David Smith is a graduate of Reading, London, and Edinburgh Universities, and Moray House College, Edinburgh, where he studied physiology and biochemistry of farm animals, human nutrition, sociology and history of science, and education. His Ph.D. thesis was on the history of nutrition science in Britain during the twentieth century (1987). Dr. Smith was a Wellcome Trust Research Fellow at the University of Glasgow from 1991 to 1994, and he is now Wellcome Lecturer in the History of Medicine at the Centre for Cultural History of the University of Aberdeen. His current project is entitled "Nutritional Sciences and Nutritional Politics 1918–1950." He is chair of the Society for the Social History of Medicine.

Jeffery Sobal is an Associate Professor in the Division of Nutritional Sciences at Cornell University. His doctoral training is in medical sociology, and he currently teaches undergraduate and graduate courses that apply social science perspectives to food, eating, and nutrition. His areas of research include the examination of the social epidemiology of body weight, stigmatization of obesity, vitamin/mineral consumption as a health behavior, and processes of food choice.

Kim D. Travers is Assistant Professor of Human Ecology at Mount Saint Vincent University, Halifax, Nova Scotia, Canada. She teaches in the areas of community nutrition and nutrition education and her research interests are in the area of the social organization of nutrition and health inequities. She holds a Ph.D. in Adult Education/Educational Sociology from Dalhousie University in Halifax. Her B.Sc. (Home Economics) and MA (Home Economics Education) are both from Mount Saint Vincent University. She has also completed a dietetic internship and is a registered professional dietitian (PDt).

Karen Way is a Ph.D. candidate in Sociology at American University in Washington, D.C. Her previous work on eating disorders includes *Anorexia Nervosa and Recovery: A Hunger for Meaning* (1993), based on interview research with 21 women recovering from anorexia nervosa. She is currently writing her dissertation on the effects of fame and celebrity on interpersonal relationships.

Index